Cutting-Edge Research on Physical Fitness Profile in Soccer Players

Cutting-Edge Research on Physical Fitness Profile in Soccer Players

Guest Editor

Ioannis Michailidis

MDPI

Basel • Beijing • Wuhan • Barcelona • Belgrade • Novi Sad • Cluj • Manchester

Guest Editor
Ioannis Michailidis
Department of Physical
Education and Sport Science
Aristotle University of
Thessaloniki
Thessaloniki
Greece

Editorial Office
MDPI AG
Grosspeteranlage 5
4052 Basel, Switzerland

This is a reprint of the Special Issue, published open access by the journal *Sports* (ISSN 2075-4663), freely accessible at: https://www.mdpi.com/journal/sports/special_issues/G45FPQ89DZ.

For citation purposes, cite each article independently as indicated on the article page online and as indicated below:

Lastname, A.A.; Lastname, B.B. Article Title. *Journal Name* **Year**, *Volume Number*, Page Range.

ISBN 978-3-7258-5903-0 (Hbk)
ISBN 978-3-7258-5904-7 (PDF)
https://doi.org/10.3390/books978-3-7258-5904-7

Contents

sports

MDPI

Editorial

Cutting-Edge Research on Physical Fitness Profile in Soccer Players

Yiannis Michailidis

Laboratory of Evaluation of Human Biological Performance, Department of Physical Education and Sports Sciences, Aristotle University of Thessaloniki, 54124 Thessaloniki, Greece; ioannimd@phed.auth.gr; Tel.: +30-231-099-2248

Soccer is one of the most popular sports in the world, with millions of athletes engaged in it. The sport evolves over time, and players continuously develop their physical, technical, and tactical skills in order to meet its increasing demands. Technological advances have enabled a detailed investigation of the physical fitness profile required for high performance, as well as the quantification of many factors related to training load.

However, despite these advances, in several areas of the game, the scientific literature remains limited or findings are inconclusive. Much of the research focuses on isolated performance indicators without examining their interactions, either with one another or in relation to competitive conditions. Furthermore, most studies involve elite male soccer players, with women, youth, and amateur athletes being underrepresented. In addition, there is still considerable scope for research into training protocols aimed at improving/maximizing performance, preventing injuries, and supporting return-to-play following injury.

This Special Issue of *Sports*, entitled *Cutting-Edge Research on Physical Fitness Profile in Soccer Players*, addresses some of these gaps by compiling scientific contributions on modern soccer. Specifically, the 15 articles included examine physical capacities, performance monitoring strategies, match analysis, recovery, and injury prevention frameworks. These studies also involve male and female players of different ages and competitive levels. Both experimental and review articles are included.

Within the Special Issue, several articles focus on tracking external load using GPS technology, both during matches and training sessions. Such studies aim to clarify the demands of different playing positions and inform the structuring of more effective training microcycles. Other studies investigate specific intervention programs and the role of feedback in performance and learning. Furthermore, bibliometric and review papers address topics such as decision-making, injury-prevention markers, and return-to-play criteria. Additional contributions examine the effects of contextual factors (e.g., temperature) on performance and explore the relationships between running performance and physical capacities. Taken together, this Special Issue offers a multidimensional and updated perspective on how profiling the physical fitness of soccer players can support evidence-based practice in the sport.

Looking ahead, long-term monitoring across different levels of play and both sexes is needed to clarify position-specific demands. Moreover, further research should focus on the use of artificial intelligence for more efficient training design, as well as on big data analytics for predicting performance and injury risk. A key goal of future studies must be the integration of findings into applied practice.

Conflicts of Interest: The author declare no conflict of interest.

sports

MDPI

Article

Associations Between Isokinetic Torque and External Load Metrics During Youth Soccer Matches

Yiannis Michailidis

Laboratory of Evaluation of Human Biological Performance, Department of Physical Education and Sports Sciences, Aristotle University of Thessaloniki, 57001 Thessaloniki, Greece; ioannimd@phed.auth.gr; Tel.: +30-231-099-2248

Abstract: Physical fitness, especially strength, is key for football performance and injury prevention, but its role in match running remains unclear. This study examined correlations between knee flexor and extensor isokinetic torque (60°/s, 180°/s, 300°/s) and running performance in 20 U17 players (age 16 ± 0.5 years, height 1.78 ± 0.05 m, weight 71 ± 7.1 kg) across 16 matches, with GPS tracking (Apex, STATSports, Newry, Northern Ireland). Results varied by position. Central defenders showed a negative correlation between non-dominant knee flexor torque at 300°/s and high-speed running distance (r = −0.975, p = 0.025). Side defenders displayed positive correlations between dominant knee flexor torque at 300°/s and both total distance and moderate running (r = 0.885–0.976, $p < 0.05$), but negative correlations with maximum speed (r < −0.89, $p < 0.05$). Central midfielders had several negative associations between dominant knee flexor torque at 300°/s and accelerations or decelerations (r < −0.88, $p < 0.05$). Side midfielders and forwards showed positive correlations between torque at higher speeds (180°/s, 300°/s) and sprint distance (r ≥ 0.85, $p < 0.05$). Overall, associations differed by position, velocity, and performance variable, reflecting tactical demands and the limits of single-joint testing. However, in SMFs, high positive correlations were observed, highlighting the importance of strength and its necessity in the training process.

Keywords: correlation; strength; football; GPS; running performance; association

1. Introduction

Football is a highly popular sport involving millions of athletes of various levels and ages [1,2]. Player performance depends on various factors such as technique, tactics, physical condition, etc., [3], which are developed over a long-term training process.

In modern football, physical fitness is particularly important for players to cope with the increasing pace of matches, as the frequency of high- and maximum-intensity actions—as well as player duels—has increased [4]. Physical fitness in football is not one-dimensional; a modern footballer must have highly developed aerobic capacity (endurance) as well as anaerobic capacity (strength, speed, power) [5].

One of the physical abilities of particular importance for football performance is strength, specifically the form known as power (explosive strength) [6,7]. Most high-intensity actions during a match—such as jumps, accelerations, decelerations, sprints, and duels—require the application of high levels of force in a short amount of time (high power). Power is a key attribute for all modern footballers, as it is directly related to the effectiveness of both their defensive and offensive actions [8].

Strength also influences a player's running economy. Running economy is defined as the oxygen or energy required to cover a certain distance or to maintain a specific submaxi-

https://doi.org/10.3390/sports13090311

mal running speed [9]. Recent studies have observed that strength training can improve running economy [10–13], particularly influencing running time trial performance [14,15]. Therefore, a similar improvement in footballers could enhance their running performance during matches, as they cover approximately 10–12 km per game, 2–3 km of which are at high speeds.

In recent decades, technological advances (global positioning systems) have enabled monitoring of the external load of footballers during matches [16,17]. From the GPS variables, the analysis included the distances covered by the players in zone 14.4–19.79 km/h, zone 19.8–25.19 km/h, zone $\geq$ 25.2 km/h), and the total distance covered. Also included were accelerations with an intensity between 2 and 3 m/s^2, above 3 m/s^2, as well as decelerations with an intensity between -3 and -2 m/s^2 and below -3 m/s^2. In addition, the player's maximum speed and match pace were used.

As mentioned above, several variables measured using GPS may be influenced by a player's strength level (e.g., maximum speed, accelerations, decelerations, distance covered at high intensity, etc.). Biomechanically, greater isokinetic strength in knee flexors and extensors enhances the ability to generate rapid, forceful contractions necessary for accelerations, decelerations, and changes in direction [18]. Stronger muscles improve joint stability and reduce injury risk, allowing players to maintain performance during demanding actions [19]. Physiologically, increased muscle strength contributes to improved neuromuscular efficiency and power output, which supports better sprinting speed and endurance by delaying fatigue onset during repeated high-intensity efforts [20,21]. Moreover, enhanced strength facilitates more effective energy transfer and reduces metabolic cost during running, thereby positively influencing total distance covered and high-speed running variables [22]. However, a review of the literature reveals a significant research gap, as only few studies [23–25] have investigated the relationship between strength parameters and running performance. Most studies focus on examining the relationship between strength and other physical abilities assessed via laboratory or field tests [26,27].

The difference in methodology between these studies is particularly important: in one case, correlations are sought between specific physical abilities (e.g., power and speed), which are easier to observe—especially when based on the same physiological mechanism (e.g., stretch-shortening cycle—jump ability and sprinting); in the other case, correlations are sought with indicators of match running performance, i.e., metrics used to evaluate football performance. Observing such relationships could enhance training effectiveness, as strength elements with a direct impact on in-game running performance would be specifically targeted.

Therefore, the aim of the present study was to investigate the relationship between the isokinetic torque of the knee flexors and extensors of young footballers and external load indicators during official matches. Based on the study objectives, we hypothesize that isokinetic torque of the knee flexor and extensor muscles will be positively correlated with key match running performance metrics, including maximum speed, high-speed running distance, and the number of accelerations and decelerations. Furthermore, we expect these correlations to vary according to playing position and angular velocity of assessment, with stronger associations anticipated at higher testing velocities and in positions that demand greater sprinting and change-of-direction activities, such as side defenders, side midfielders and forwards.

2. Materials and Methods

2.1. Participants

To conduct the study, 26 players from the under-17 team of a football academy were invited. Of these, only 20 footballers participated in the study (age 16.0 $\pm$ 0.5 years, training age 11.1 ± 1.3 years, height 180 ± 10 cm, weight 71.0 ± 7.1 kg, body fat percentage 11.6 ± 1.3), all of whom met the inclusion criteria, which were: (a) absence of injuries in the past month, (b) no use of medication, (c) participation in all pre-match tests (anthropometrics, isokinetic torque at three speeds: 60°/s, 180°/s, 300°/s), and (d) participation in at least 85 min of the match. The team competed in the national championship of its country and participated in 4 training sessions and 1 official match per week. The players were categorized based on their playing position as central defenders (CD, n = 4, 20%), side defenders (SD, n = 5, 25%), central midfielders (CM, n = 5, 25%), side midfielders-forwards (SMF, n = 6, 30%). Informed consent was obtained from all subjects and their parents involved in the study. The local institutional review board approved the study (approval number 217/2024) in accordance with the Helsinki Declaration.

2.2. Procedure

The footballers were already familiar with the tests, as these were part of the routine assessments conducted during their previous years of ergometric evaluations. The study was conducted over the course of the first 16 matches of the competitive season. All tests were conducted in the morning, between 9:00 and 12:00 AM, to control circadian variations in performance, within a laboratory setting maintaining stable temperature (~22 °C) and humidity (~40%) conditions. At the end of the preseason, the players visited the laboratory, where anthropometric measurements were taken first. This was followed by a 10 min warm-up (7 min of cycling and 3 min of stretching), after which the isokinetic torque assessment was carried out. During the procedure, participants were allowed to drink water ad libitumto ensure proper hydration during testing. Subsequently, once the competitive season began, the players' external load during the first 16 matches was recorded using GPS technology. Dominant and non-dominant legs were determined based on player self-report, with the dominant leg defined as the preferred limb for ball control and manipulation during match play.

2.3. Anthropometric Measurements

The players' body height was measured using a stadiometer with 0.1 cm precision (Seca 220e, Hamburg, Germany). Body weight and body fat percentage were measured using a dual-frequency body composition analyzer (TANITA DC-360, Tanita Corporation, Tokyo, Japan), based on the principles of bioelectrical impedance.

2.4. Isokinetic Strength Testing

Muscular strength of the hamstrings and quadriceps were evaluated under isokinetic conditions using a Cybex II dynamometer (Lumex Inc., Ronkonkoma, NY, USA). At each test velocity, the highest torque output was recorded, with corrections applied to exclude the effects of limb mass and equipment resistance. Participants were seated in a modifiable chair attached to the device, with stabilizing straps placed across the torso, hips, and thighs to restrict extraneous movements. The test leg was set at 90 degrees of knee flexion (where 0 degrees denotes full extension), ensuring proper alignment between the knee joint axis and the lever arm's axis at the distal lateral femoral condyle. Lever arm length and resistance pad position were adjusted individually, with the pad placed just above the medial malleolus. The opposite leg remained passive, unsupported.

Movements were executed in a fixed pattern: extension began from 90° flexion, while flexion started from full extension. Participants were instructed to exert maximal effort, moving their leg through the complete range of motion as quickly and forcefully as possible while maintaining crossed arms. Three trials were performed at each test speed, and the peak torque value was captured for analysis. Recovery between repetitions was set at 30 s, with one-minute intervals between velocity changes. Verbal cues were provided throughout to encourage full voluntary effort. Measurements were taken at speeds of 60°, 180°, and 300° per second which are reported to represent different strength qualities [28,29]. Specifically, testing at 60°/s reflects maximal strength, at 180°/s reflects muscular endurance, and at 300°/s reflects power. The purpose of selecting these three different velocities was to provide a comprehensive profile of strength capacity in young footballers and to examine the relevance of each strength quality to match-running performance variables. Peak isokinetic torque was considered the highest force output during the complete motion range for both muscle groups [28]. To assess muscle balance, the conventional hamstring-to-quadriceps (H:Q) ratio was determined by dividing the maximal concentric torque of the hamstrings (flexion) by that of the quadriceps (extension) at each velocity. All measurements were performed by the same person.

2.5. Global Positioning System Variables

To record the external load during the matches, the global navigation satellite system 10 Hz Apex (STATSports, Newry, Northern Ireland) was used. Previous studies have reported that the above GPS system is valid and reliable for measuring the external load of football players [30,31]. The device was placed in a special vest between the player's shoulder blades and was activated at the beginning of each half and deactivated at the end of each half. After the matches, the transmitters were placed in a special company docking station to transfer the data from the devices to the computer, from which the data were exported in CSV format. Each player always used the same GPS unit. The distances covered by players were categorized into three speed zones to capture different intensities of running performance during the match.

Zone 1 (14.4–19.79 km/h): This zone represents moderate-intensity running and is often associated with sustained efforts during the game, such as jogging or controlled running. Distances covered in this zone provide insights into the player's ability to maintain movement over prolonged periods without reaching maximal effort, reflecting aerobic endurance components.

Zone 2 (19.8–25.19 km/h): This zone corresponds to high-speed running (HSR), encompassing efforts that require substantial anaerobic capacity and neuromuscular power. Running at these speeds typically involves crucial phases such as offensive and defensive transitions, where players need to accelerate rapidly and cover ground effectively [32].

Zone 3 ($\geq$25.2 km/h): This zone captures sprinting efforts, representing maximal or near-maximal running speeds. Sprint distance is critical in football for decisive actions like breakaways, counters, and defensive recoveries. Due to the intermittent and high-intensity nature of these efforts, sprinting distance is highly sensitive to fatigue and training status, making it an important variable for assessing player readiness and physical condition [33].

Total Distance (TD): The total distance covered during the match sums all running intensities and provides a comprehensive measure of overall workload. TD is a fundamental variable frequently used to gauge player activity levels and has a low coefficient of variation between matches, enhancing its utility for monitoring and comparison purposes [34].

Accelerations between 2 and 3 m/s^2 and above 3 m/s^2: Accelerations reflect the ability of a player to rapidly increase running speed. The inclusion of two intensity categories allows differentiation between moderate- and high-intensity accelerative efforts. These actions are mechanically demanding and involve explosive muscle contractions, contributing significantly to match performance. Previous research indicates that acceleration counts correlate well with neuromuscular strength and power measures, supporting their relevance in performance analysis [33].

Decelerations between -3 and -2 m/s^2 and below -3 m/s^2: Decelerations represent the capacity to reduce speed rapidly, a critical component for change-of-direction and tactical positioning. Like accelerations, decelerations were categorized into moderate and high intensities to better characterize the physical demands placed on players. Previous research indicates correlations between strength and deceleration ability [35].

Maximum running speed attained during the match serves as an indicator of a player's top-end velocity capacity. It is a critical determinant of match-defining moments such as successful sprints and defensive recoveries. Maximum speed measurements are reliable and have been shown to correlate with strength and power metrics, making this variable valuable for evaluating player explosive capabilities [36].

Match pace was evaluated through variables such as total distance per minute (TD/min) and high-speed running distance above 19.8 km/h. These metrics provide insights into the intensity of activity relative to playing time and overall workload efficiency. Match pace is useful for standardizing comparisons between players with different playing durations.

2.6. Statistical Analysis

To assess the normal distribution of the data, the Shapiro–Wilk test was conducted, revealing that parametric statistical tests could be applied. Pearson correlation test was applied to examine potential correlations between the isokinetic strength indexes with GPS running performance indexes during matches. The strength of the correlation was determined based on the value of r: $r \leq 0.1$, trivial; $0.1 < r \leq 0.3$, small; $0.3 < r \leq 0.5$, medium; $0.5 < r \leq 0.7$, large; $0.7 < r \leq 0.9$, very large; and $r > 0.9$, almost perfect. Correlation heatmaps were performed using JASP version 0.19.3.0 for Windows (ASP Team: Amsterdam, The Netherlands) [37]. Statistical significance was set at $p < 0.05$. All analyses were performed using SPSS version 28.0 (SPSS, Inc., Chicago, IL, USA).

3. Results

From the correlation analysis of all players combined, negative associations were observed for the knee flexors of the dominant limb at 60° and 180° ($r = -0.495$, $p < 0.05$ and $r = -0.494$, $p < 0.05$, respectively) and for the non-dominant limb at 180° and 300° with HSR/min ($r = -0.645$, $p < 0.01$ and $r = -0.507$, $p < 0.05$, respectively). Negative correlations were also found between the flexors of the dominant and non-dominant limb at 180° and 300° with the number of high-intensity decelerations ($r = -0.481$, $p < 0.05$ and $r = -0.511$, $p < 0.05$; $r = -0.480$, $p < 0.05$ and $r = -0.629$, $p < 0.01$, respectively). All correlations are presented in Figure 1.

In central defenders (CD), a strong negative correlation was observed between the distance covered in zone 2 and the knee flexors of the non-dominant limb at 300°/s. No other significant associations were detected. All results of the statistical analysis are presented in Figure 2.

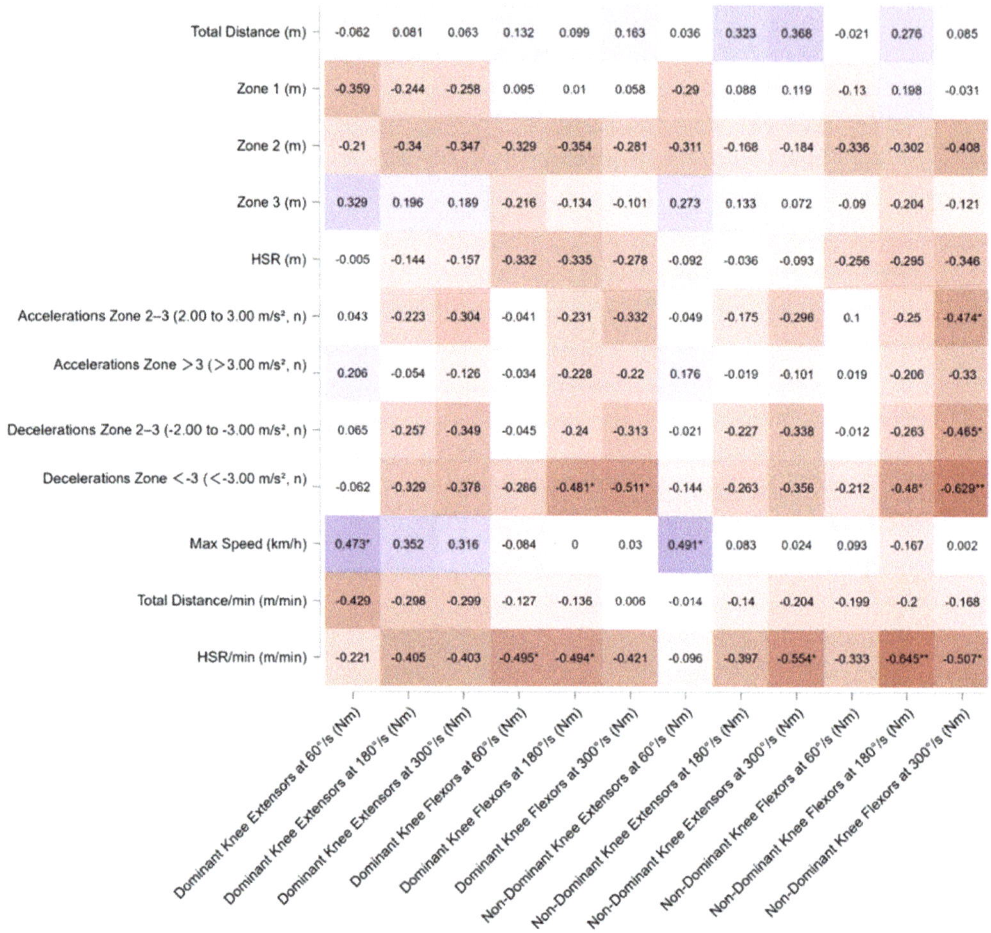

Figure 1. Pearson's correlation matrix of isokinetic variables of dominant and non-dominant extensors and flexors leg muscles across different angular velocities (60°/s, 180°/s, 300°/s) with match running variables for all players. The heatmap displays Pearson's correlation coefficients (*r*) between isokinetic variables of dominant and non-dominant extensors and flexors leg muscles across different angular velocities (60°/s, 180°/s, 300°/s) with match running variables for all players. Significant correlations are indicated with * $p < 0.05$, ** $p < 0.01$,. Warmer colors indicate negative correlations, while cooler colors represent positive correlations. Note: Significant relationships were observed between knee flexor strength and deceleration metrics, particularly for decelerations greater than -3.00 m/s^2 (r = -0.48 to -0.63, $p < 0.01$). Dominant knee extensor strength at 60°/s correlated positively with maximum speed (r = 0.47, $p < 0.05$). Additionally, negative correlations were identified between knee flexor strength at higher angular velocities and relative high-speed running per minute (r = -0.49 to -0.65, $p < 0.01$).

In side defenders (SD), strong positive correlations were observed between the flexors of the dominant limb at 300°/s and both TD and distance covered in zone 1 (representing tactical positioning running) (r = 0.885, $p = 0.046$ and r = 0.976, $p = 0.004$, respectively). Moreover, a strong negative correlation was observed between the flexors of both limbs at 300°/s and maximum speed (r < -0.89, $p < 0.05$). A summary of these findings is presented in Figure 3.

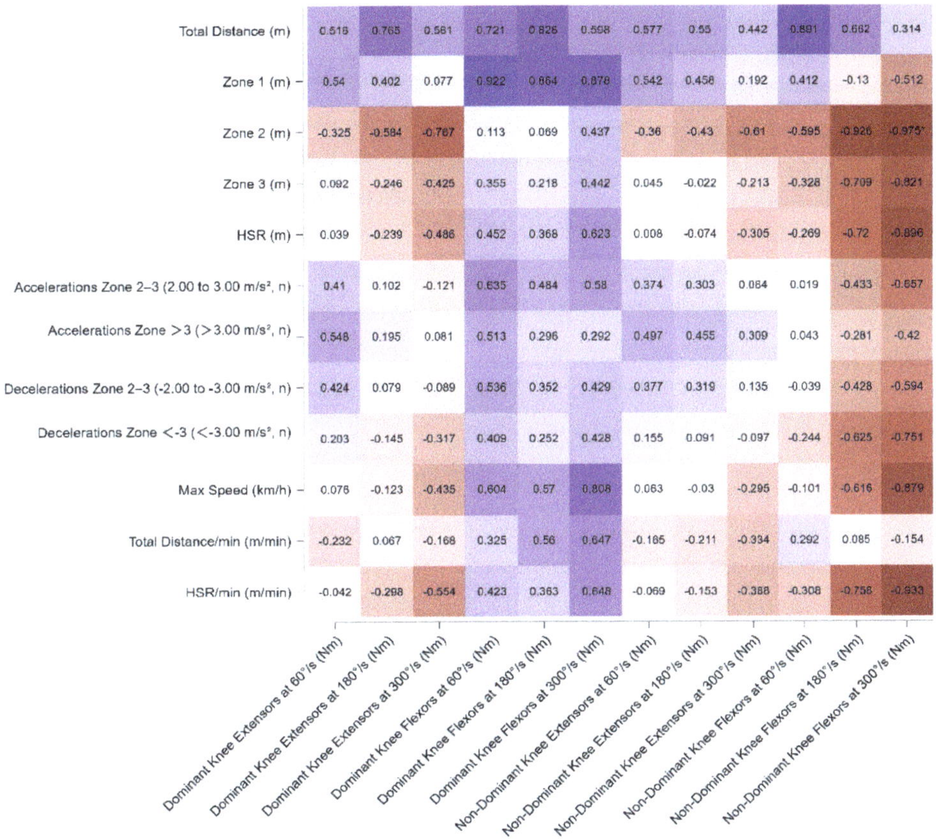

Figure 2. Pearson's correlation matrix of isokinetic variables of dominant and non-dominant extensors and flexors leg muscles across different angular velocities (60°/s, 180°/s, 300°/s) with match running variables for central defenders. The heatmap displays Pearson's correlation coefficients (*r*) between isokinetic variables of dominant and non-dominant extensors and flexors leg muscles across different angular velocities (60°/s, 180°/s, 300°/s) with match running variables for central defenders. Significant correlations are indicated with * $p < 0.05$. Warmer colors indicate negative correlations, while cooler colors represent positive correlations. Note: For CD, significant relationships were observed between GPS-derived external load indicators and isokinetic strength parameters. Strong positive correlations were found between total distance, Zone 1, HSR, and accelerations with dominant and non-dominant knee extension peak torque at 180°/s and 300°/s (r = 0.51–0.92, $p < 0.01$). Max speed also correlated strongly with dominant and non-dominant knee extensors at 180°/s (r = 0.57–0.81, $p < 0.01$). Conversely, Zone 2 running and HSR demonstrated strong negative correlations with knee flexor strength, particularly in non-dominant assessments at 180°/s and 300°/s (r = −0.59 to −0.98, $p < 0.01$).

In central midfielders (CM), strong negative correlations were found between the extensors of both the dominant and non-dominant limbs at 300°/s and HSR (r = −0.890, $p = 0.043$ and r = −0.923, $p = 0.025$, respectively). Furthermore, the knee flexors of the dominant limb at 300°/s were negatively correlated with all categories of accelerations and decelerations as well as with maximum speed (r < −0.88, $p < 0.05$). A summary of these results is presented in Figure 4.

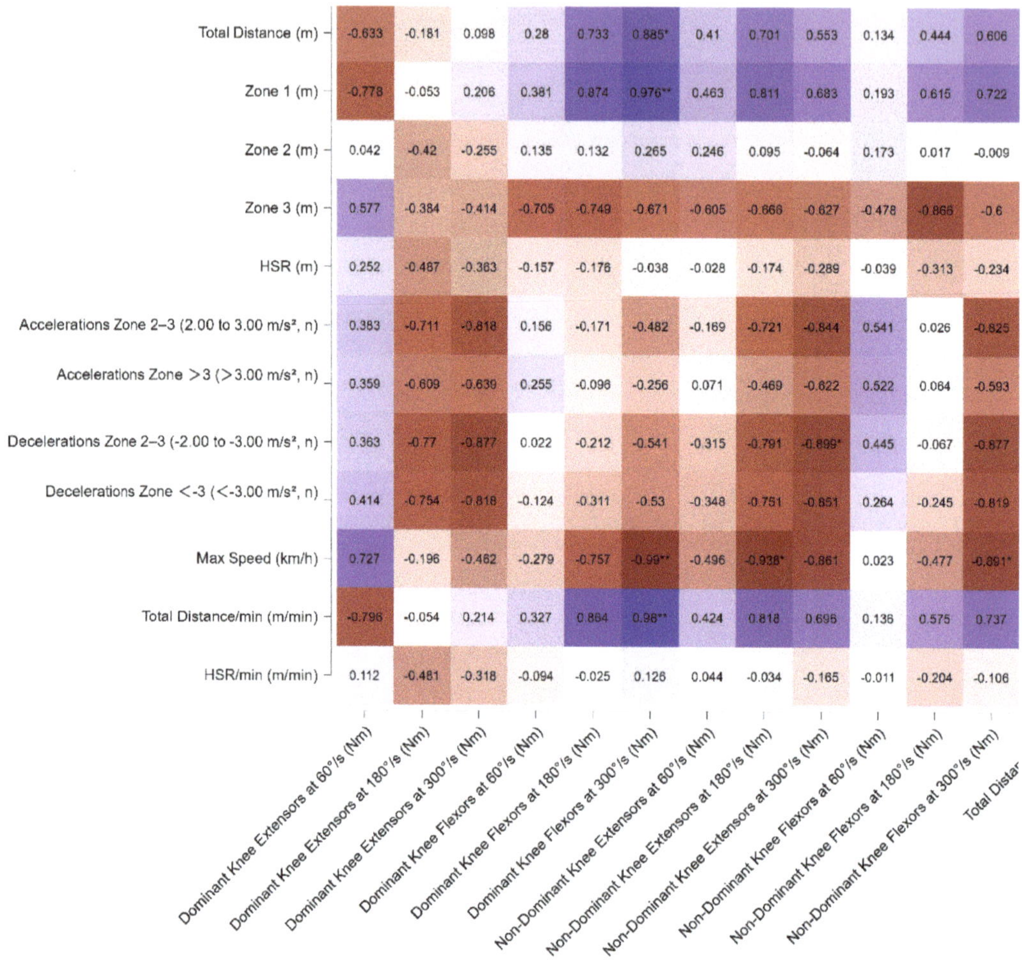

Figure 3. Pearson's correlation matrix of isokinetic variables of dominant and non-dominant extensors and flexors leg muscles across different angular velocities (60°/s, 180°/s, 300°/s) with match running variables for side defenders. The heatmap displays Pearson's correlation coefficients (r) between isokinetic variables of dominant and non-dominant extensors and flexors leg muscles across different angular velocities (60°/s, 180°/s, 300°/s) with match running variables for side defenders. Significant correlations are indicated with * $p < 0.05$, ** $p < 0.01$. Warmer colors indicate negative correlations, while cooler colors represent positive correlations. Note: For SD—Significant relationships were observed between GPS-derived external load indicators and isokinetic strength parameters. Strong positive correlations were found between total distance, total distance per minute, maximal speed, and both dominant and non-dominant knee extension torque at 180°/s and 300°/s (r = 0.73–0.99, $p < 0.01$). Zone 1 activity also correlated very strongly with knee extensor strength (r = 0.87–0.98, $p < 0.01$). In contrast, strong negative correlations were observed between accelerations (2–3 m/s^2 and >3 m/s^2) and decelerations (−2 to −3 m/s^2 and <−3 m/s^2) with dominant and non-dominant knee flexor strength at higher angular velocities (r = −0.59 to −0.90, $p < 0.01$).

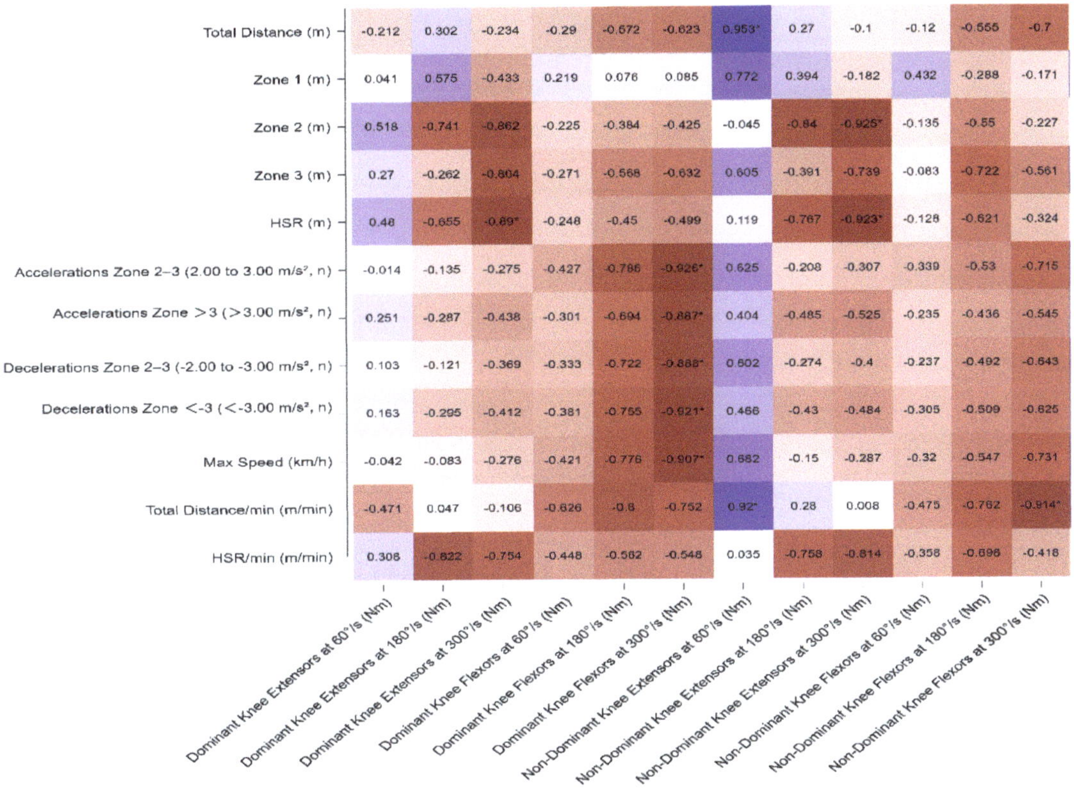

Figure 4. Pearson's correlation matrix of isokinetic variables of dominant and non-dominant extensors and flexors leg muscles across different angular velocities (60°/s, 180°/s, 300°/s) with match running variables for central midfielders. The heatmap displays Pearson's correlation coefficients (r) between isokinetic variables of dominant and non-dominant extensors and flexors leg muscles across different angular velocities (60°/s, 180°/s, 300°/s) with match running variables for central midfielders. Significant correlations are indicated with * $p < 0.05$. Warmer colors indicate negative correlations, while cooler colors represent positive correlations. Note: For CM—Significant relationships were observed between GPS-derived external load indicators and isokinetic strength parameters. Total distance and total distance/min showed very strong positive correlations with dominant knee extensors at 60°/s (r = 0.953 and r = 0.920, $p < 0.01$). HSR/min demonstrated strong negative associations with dominant knee extensors at 180°/s (r = −0.822, $p < 0.01$) and non-dominant knee extensors at 180°/s (r = −0.758, $p < 0.01$). Additionally, accelerations > 3 m/s^2 and decelerations < −3 m/s^2 were strongly negatively correlated with dominant knee flexors at 300°/s (r = −0.887 and r = −0.881, $p < 0.01$).

In side midfielders (SMF), positive correlations were observed between the extensors of both limbs at 180° and 300°/s and sprint distance (r > 0.84, $p < 0.05$). In addition, strong positive correlations were found between the flexors and extensors of the dominant limb at 60°/s and maximum speed (r = 0.869, p = 0.025 and r = 0.832, p = 0.040, respectively) (Figure 5).

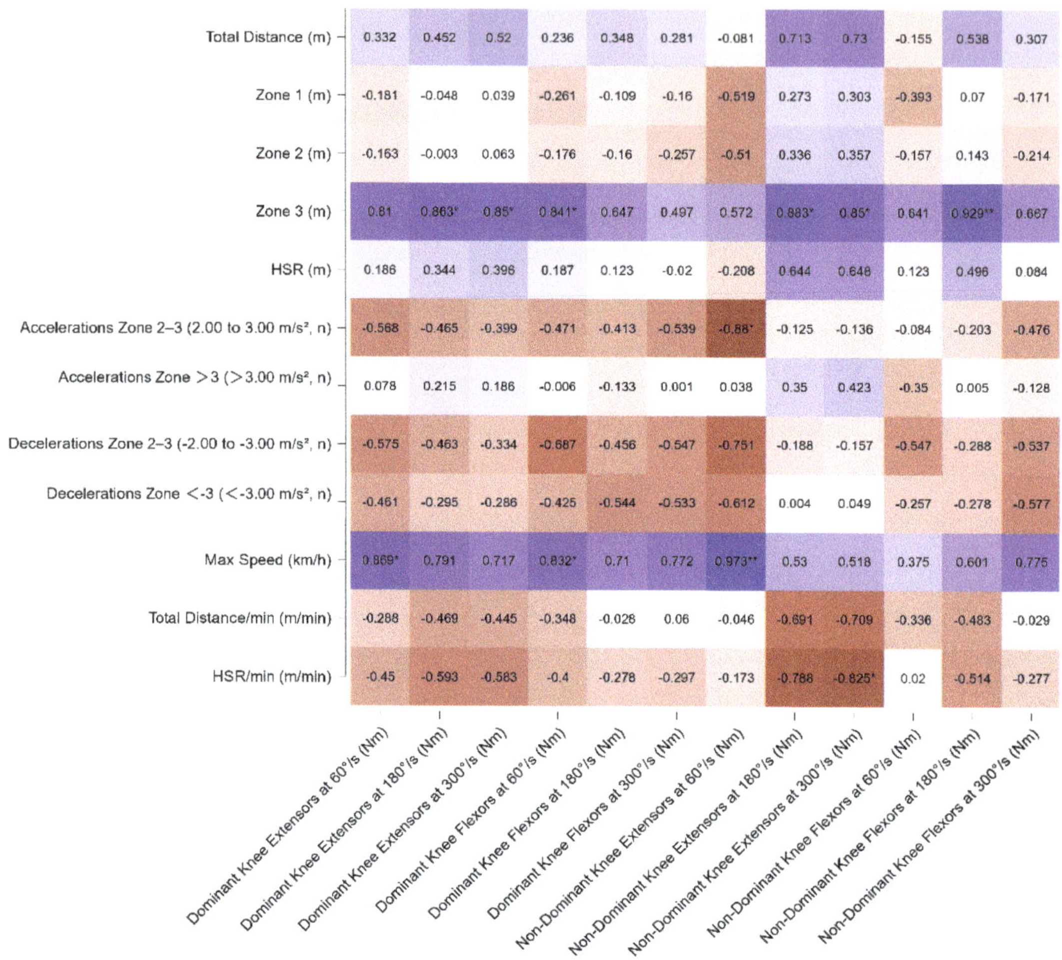

Figure 5. Pearson's correlation matrix of isokinetic variables of dominant and non-dominant extensors and flexors leg muscles across different angular velocities (60°/s, 180°/s, 300°/s) with match running variables for side midfielders and forwards. The heatmap displays Pearson's correlation coefficients (*r*) between isokinetic variables of dominant and non-dominant extensors and flexors leg muscles across different angular velocities (60°/s, 180°/s, 300°/s) with match running variables for side midfielders and forwards. Significant correlations are indicated with * $p < 0.05$, ** $p < 0.01$. Warmer colors indicate negative correlations, while cooler colors represent positive correlations. Note: For F and SM—Significant relationships were observed between GPS-derived external load indicators and isokinetic strength parameters. Strong positive correlations were found between Zone 3 activity and both dominant and non-dominant knee extension torque at 180°/s and 300°/s (r = 0.81–0.93, $p < 0.01$). Maximal speed correlated strongly with knee extensors at 60°/s, 180°/s, and 300°/s in both limbs (r = 0.77–0.97, $p < 0.01$). Additionally, negative correlations were observed between accelerations (2–3 m/s^2) and decelerations (−2 to −3 m/s^2; <−3 m/s^2) with knee flexor strength, particularly in non-dominant assessments at higher angular velocities (r = −0.47 to −0.82, $p < 0.01$). Table 1 presents a consolidated overview of all strong correlations identified in this study.

Table 1. Major correlations between lower-limb isokinetic torque at different angular velocities and running load parameters.

Position	GPS Variable	Strength Variable	r	p	95% CI		ES	SE ES
					Lower	Upper		
CD	Zone 2 (m)	Non-Dominant Knee Flexors at 300°/s (Nm)	−0.975	0.025 *	−1.000	−0.228	−2.192	1.000
CM	Total Distance (m)	Non-Dominant Knee Extensors at 300°/s (Nm)	0.953	0.012 *	0.442	0.997	1.861	0.707
CM	Zone 2 (m)	Non-Dominant Knee Flexors at 60°/s (Nm)	−0.925	0.024 *	−0.995	−0.231	−1.621	0.707
CM	HSR (m)	Dominant Knee Extensors at 300°/s (Nm)	−0.890	0.043 *	−0.993	−0.038	−1.424	0.707
CM	HSR (m)	Non-Dominant Knee Extensors at 300°/s (Nm)	−0.923	0.025 *	−0.995	−0.222	−1.612	0.707
CM	Accelerations Zone 2–3 (n)	Dominant Knee Flexors at 300°/s (Nm)	−0.926	0.024 *	−0.995	−0.239	−1.629	0.707
CM	Accelerations Zone >3 (n)	Dominant Knee Flexors at 300°/s (Nm)	−0.887	0.045 *	−0.993	−0.023	−1.409	0.707
CM	Decelerations Zone 2–3 (n)	Dominant Knee Flexors at 300°/s (Nm)	−0.888	0.044 *	−0.993	−0.028	−1.414	0.707
CM	Decelerations Zone >3 (n)	Dominant Knee Flexors at 300°/s (Nm)	−0.921	0.026 *	−0.995	−0.206	−1.595	0.707
CM	Max Speed (km/h)	Dominant Knee Flexors at 300°/s (Nm)	−0.907	0.034 *	−0.994	−0.124	−1.510	0.707
CM	Total Distance/min (m/min)	Non-Dominant Knee Extensors at 60°/s (Nm)	0.920	0.027 *	0.200	0.995	1.588	0.707
CM	Total Distance/min (m/min)	Non-Dominant Knee Flexors at 300°/s (Nm)	−0.914	0.030 *	−0.994	−0.166	−1.553	0.707
SMF	Zone 3 (m)	Dominant Knee Extensors at 180°/s (Nm)	0.863	0.027 *	0.170	0.985	1.304	0.577
SMF	Zone 3 (m)	Dominant Knee Extensors at 300°/s (Nm)	0.850	0.032 *	0.123	0.983	1.256	0.577
SMF	Zone 3 (m)	Dominant Knee Flexors at 60°/s (Nm)	0.841	0.036 *	0.091	0.982	1.223	0.577
SMF	Zone 3 (m)	Non-Dominant Knee Extensors at 180°/s (Nm)	0.883	0.020 *	0.251	0.987	1.388	0.577
SMF	Zone 3 (m)	Non-Dominant Knee Extensors at 300°/s (Nm)	0.850	0.032 *	0.126	0.983	1.258	0.577
SMF	Zone 3 (m)	Non-Dominant Knee Flexors at 180°/s (Nm)	0.929	0.007 **	0.476	0.992	1.650	0.577
SMF	Accelerations Zone 2–3 (n)	Non-Dominant Knee Extensors at 60°/s (Nm)	−0.880	0.021 *	−0.987	−0.239	−1.375	0.577
SMF	Max Speed (km/h)	Dominant Knee Extensors at 60°/s (Nm)	0.869	0.025 *	0.195	0.986	1.329	0.577
SMF	Max Speed (km/h)	Dominant Knee Flexors at 60°/s (Nm)	0.832	0.040 *	0.062	0.981	1.193	0.577
SMF	Max Speed (km/h)	Non-Dominant Knee Extensors at 60°/s (Nm)	0.973	0.001 ***	0.769	0.997	2.149	0.577
SMF	HSR/min (m/min)	Non-Dominant Knee Extensors at 300°/s (Nm)	−0.825	0.043 *	−0.980	−0.041	−1.173	0.577
SD	Total Distance (m)	Dominant Knee Flexors at 300°/s (Nm)	0.885	0.046 *	0.013	0.992	1.399	0.707
SD	Zone 1 (m)	Dominant Knee Flexors at 300°/s (Nm)	0.976	0.004 **	0.676	0.998	2.208	0.707
SD	Decelerations Zone 2–3 (n)	Non-Dominant Knee Extensors at 300°/s (Nm)	−0.899	0.038 *	−0.993	−0.082	−1.468	0.707
SD	Max Speed (km/h)	Dominant Knee Flexors at 300°/s (Nm)	−0.990	0.001 ***	−0.999	−0.847	−2.632	0.707
SD	Max Speed (km/h)	Non-Dominant Knee Extensors at 180°/s (Nm)	−0.938	0.018 *	−0.996	−0.325	−1.723	0.707
SD	Max Speed (km/h)	Non-Dominant Knee Flexors at 300°/s (Nm)	−0.891	0.042 *	−0.993	−0.041	−1.427	0.707
SD	Total Distance/min (m/min)	Dominant Knee Flexors at 300°/s (Nm)	0.980	0.003 **	0.719	0.999	2.292	0.707

CD, central defenders; SD, side defenders; CM, central midfielders; SMF, side midfielders and forwards; Zone 1 (14.4–19.79 km/h); Zone 2 (19.8–25.19 km/h); Zone 3 (≥25.2 km/h); HSR, high-speed running (>19.8 km/h); ES, effect size; SE ES, standard error effect size; Significant correlations are indicated with * $p < 0.05$, ** $p < 0.01$, *** $p < 0.001$.

4. Discussion

The aim of the present study was to investigate the existence of correlations between the isokinetic torque of the lower limbs in young football players and running performance indicators from official matches. The initial hypothesis of the study was partially confirmed, as correlations were found between isokinetic torque and variables such as sprinting, maximum speed, and high-speed running (HSR). However, these correlations did not follow a consistent pattern and appeared to vary depending on playing position, the angular velocity used for isokinetic evaluation, and the limb being tested.

Before discussing the results by playing position, it can be noted that there was no substantial effect of the dominant versus non-dominant limb, as the stronger correlations were evenly distributed between them. The type of correlations (positive vs. negative) was also similarly balanced. However, the angular velocity at which the majority of correlations were observed was 300°/s (19 out of 30). Finally, in SMF players predominantly positive correlations were found, whereas in CM players, negative correlations were more prevalent. This observation may be directly related to the functional role of each playing position, as will be discussed below.

Starting with central defenders (CDs), it was observed that higher isokinetic torque at 300°/s (power) was negatively correlated with high-speed running distance. This finding contradicts the initial hypothesis and may be better understood by considering the tactical role of this playing position. Previous research has shown that CDs cover the least distance in sprints and HSR [38], likely due to the increased defensive responsibilities and high player density in their zones. As previously noted, the literature on this topic is very limited. The most relevant study is that of Pedersen [23], conducted on female footballers, which found no significant correlation between strength (1RM) and match running performance indicators (max speed, accelerations, decelerations) in a friendly match. In that study, players were divided into central and wide roles. Additionally, studies that used jump tests to explore such correlations found no significant relationships [23,25,39]. In another study [40] investigating strength and speed demands in 4v4 and 8v8 small-sided games, a moderate correlation between power and accelerations was found. This is essentially the only study reporting such correlations; however, it should be noted that the smaller the game format (e.g., 4v4), the more frequent the duels and the higher the frequency of decelerations and accelerations—factors which could influence the results.

In side defenders (SDs), the observed correlations were limited to high angular velocities (180–300°/s), with positive correlations associated with TD, pace (TD/min) and distance in zone 1, while negative correlations were associated with high-intensity metrics (decelerations, max speed). Considering the fact that players in this position typically cover large distances, this observation might be explained by the impact of strength training on running economy [10–13]. It is possible that players with higher isokinetic strength perform better in medium-intensity running activities due to improved running economy. The negative correlations observed between isokinetic torque and high-intensity performance metrics (decelerations, and maximal speed) among side defenders may be explained by the influence of body composition and movement demands on match performance. Higher isokinetic torque values often reflect greater absolute muscle mass, which can increase total body mass and, in turn, reduce relative strength-to-weight ratios. For side defenders—whose tactical role requires frequent high-velocity sprints along the flanks, rapid changes in direction, and repeated accelerations over varying distances—excessive muscle mass may hinder movement efficiency and agility, thereby compromising their ability to perform these explosive actions effectively [41]. Moreover, the high-intensity running demands of this position are often more dependent on neuromuscular coordination, elastic strength, and reactive power than on maximal torque measured in isolated, controlled conditions [28]. As a result, players with greater absolute torque but lower relative power output may demonstrate reduced performance in GPS-derived high-intensity metrics.

For central midfielders (CMs), the positive correlations observed between isokinetic torque at 60°/s and pace TD/min) likely reflect the importance of maximal muscle strength at slower contraction speeds for sustaining prolonged, low-to-moderate-intensity efforts throughout a match. It has also been reported that strength training can improve running economy in well-trained runners, thereby affecting their performance [42]. Conversely, the negative correlations with high-speed running and torque measured at 300°/s suggest that maximal strength at very high contraction velocities may not directly translate to improved performance in explosive sprinting or high-velocity actions. High-speed running demands rapid force production and neuromuscular coordination that are not fully captured by isokinetic torque (single joint) at very high velocities. Furthermore, greater maximal strength at slow speeds may be linked with increased muscle mass, which could potentially impair acceleration and sprinting ability due to increased inertia [43]. This divergence underscores the complex relationship between strength characteristics at different contraction velocities and specific match-running demands. Also, it is important to consider the tactical role of this position. Specifically, these players are involved in all four phases of the game (defense, attack, offensive and defensive transitions), often covering long distances, typically at moderate intensities [16]. Additionally, they operate in areas with high player density and limited space, making it difficult to execute sprints. Their high-intensity efforts are mostly characterized by duels rather than frequent maximal sprints.

Finally, for side midfielders and forwards (SMFs), the study found exclusively positive correlations across all isokinetic testing velocities with high-intensity running performance variables and maximum speed achieved. This finding aligns with the positional demands placed on SMFs, who typically operate in wider and more advanced zones of the pitch where there is greater spatial freedom to execute frequent and intense sprints [44]. Unlike central midfielders (CMs), whose roles often require more frequent changes in direction and shorter bursts within congested areas, SMFs have more opportunities to utilize their maximal speed during offensive transitions and counterattacks [45]. Additionally, wide midfielders are tasked with rapid defensive recovery runs during transitions to disrupt opposition attacks, further emphasizing the need for high-speed and powerful running capacity [46]. The positive correlations suggest that players with higher isokinetic strength—reflecting greater muscle torque and power—are better equipped to perform repeated sprints and achieve elevated maximum speeds, critical for their tactical role. These findings are supported by previous research demonstrating that strength qualities, particularly eccentric and concentric muscle capabilities, underpin effective sprinting and high-velocity actions in football players [36,47].

As previously mentioned, studies investigating potential correlations between strength variables and running performance indicators during football matches are extremely limited, with most of them focusing on power indicators (e.g., jump performance) rather than maximal strength indicators (e.g., isokinetic torque, one-repetition maximum). In the present study, the results were inconclusive, as the correlations varied depending on playing position, limb (dominant vs. non-dominant), and the angular velocity used in isokinetic testing. Several factors may have contributed to the inconsistent pattern of correlations. For example, isokinetic strength assessments are generally conducted using isolated, single-joint movements—such as knee extension or flexion—at predetermined, fixed angular velocities. While such protocols provide precise and reliable measurements of maximal torque under standardized conditions, they do not fully capture the functional demands of match play. In competitive football, most high-intensity actions, including sprinting, jumping, tackling, and rapid changes in direction, involve complex, multi-joint movements that require the coordinated activation of several muscle groups. These movements are typically executed at much higher velocities and under variable, unpredictable conditions. Consequently, the biomechanical and neuromuscular demands encountered on the pitch differ markedly from those assessed in the controlled environment of isokinetic testing. Additionally, the study evaluated isokinetic torque, which may not represent the critical performance factor for high-intensity match activities. Relative strength might also be a more appropriate metric, as increased muscle mass can potentially hinder performance.

Finally, this is the first study to examine these correlations while also categorizing footballers into four distinct playing positions. This positional classification is particularly important, as the tactical role and physical demands associated with each position can vary considerably. Positional differences in movement patterns inevitably influence the physical performance variables recorded, which in turn affects the strength and nature of the correlations observed. By accounting for these tactical and positional variations, the present study provides a more nuanced understanding of the relationship between physical performance metrics and the demands of competitive football.

This study had several limitations. Firstly, the sample size was small, including players from only one team, which also limited the number of players per position. Additionally, data were collected during a single season, and the team employed only one tactical formation (1-4-3-3) throughout the study period. Isokinetic torque measurements were taken only at the beginning of the season and used in analyses alongside match data collected nearly 10 months later, without repeated assessments to account for changes over time. Furthermore, torque values were not normalized to body mass, which may affect the interpretation of strength relative to player size. The isokinetic assessment was limited to a few angular velocities, and multi-joint strength tests were not included. Future research should involve larger, more diverse samples from multiple teams, incorporate different tactical formations, normalize torque data to body mass, and include multi-joint strength assessments to better understand the relationship between strength and match running performance. All the above limitations restrict the generalizability of the study's results.

5. Conclusions

This study highlights that strength-performance relationships in youth soccer are both position-dependent and specific to the velocity of isokinetic assessment, yet overall, these correlations remain inconsistent. Positive associations between isokinetic strength and high-intensity running were observed in certain positions, such as SMFs, while other positions, like CM, showed negative correlations with accelerations and decelerations. Additionally, no clear links were found between strength and acceleration or deceleration metrics, suggesting that factors like rate of force development (RFD) may play a more pivotal role in these aspects of match performance.

Funding: This research received no external funding.

Institutional Review Board Statement: The Ethics Committee of the School of Physical Education and Sport Science at Thessaloniki hereby approved the study (11 December 2024, App. No. 217/2024).

Informed Consent Statement: Informed consent was obtained from the parents of all subjects involved in the study.

Data Availability Statement: The data presented in this study are available on request from the corresponding author (due to privacy).

Acknowledgments: The authors thank the players of the team who participated in the study.

Conflicts of Interest: The author declares no conflict of interest.

References

1. FIFA. Professional Football. 2021. Available online: https://publications.fifa.com/en/annual-report-2021/around-fifa/professional-football-2021/ (accessed on 1 January 2023).
2. FIFA. Advancing Football. Available online: https://inside.fifa.com/advancing-football (accessed on 18 June 2025).
3. Sarmento, H.; Anguera, M.T.; Pereira, A.; Araújo, D. Talent Identification and Development in Male Football: A Systematic Review. *Sports Med.* **2018**, *48*, 907–931. [CrossRef] [PubMed]
4. Barnes, C.; Archer, D.T.; Hogg, B.; Bush, M.; Bradley, P.S. The Evolution of Physical and Technical Performance Parameters in the English Premier League. *Int. J. Sports Med.* **2014**, *35*, 1095–1100. [CrossRef]
5. Hostrup, M.; Bangsbo, J. Performance Adaptations to Intensified Training in Top-Level Football. *Sports Med.* **2023**, *53*, 577–594. [CrossRef]
6. Ishida, A.; Travis, S.K.; Stone, M.H. Associations of Body Composition, Maximum Strength, Power Characteristics with Sprinting, Jumping, and Intermittent Endurance Performance in Male Intercollegiate Soccer Players. *J. Funct. Morphol. Kinesiol.* **2021**, *6*, 7. [CrossRef] [PubMed]
7. Wing, C.E.; Turner, A.N.; Bishop, C.J. Importance of Strength and Power on Key Performance Indicators in Elite Youth Soccer. *J. Strength Cond. Res.* **2020**, *34*, 2006–2014. [CrossRef]
8. Oliver, J.L.; Ramachandran, A.K.; Singh, U.; Ramirez-Campillo, R.; Lloyd, R.S. The Effects of Strength, Plyometric and Combined Training on Strength, Power and Speed Characteristics in High-Level, Highly Trained Male Youth Soccer Players: A Systematic Review and Meta-Analysis. *Sports Med.* **2024**, *54*, 623–643. [CrossRef]
9. Shaw, A.J.; Ingham, S.A.; Folland, J.P. The Valid Measurement of Running Economy in Runners. *Med. Sci. Sports Exerc.* **2014**, *46*, 1968–1973. [CrossRef]
10. Blagrove, R.C.; Howe, L.P.; Cushion, E.J.; Spence, A.; Howatson, G.; Pedlar, C.R.; Hayes, P.R. Effects of Strength Training on Postpubertal Adolescent Distance Runners. *Med. Sci. Sports Exerc.* **2018**, *50*, 1224–1232. [CrossRef]
11. Festa, L.; Tarperi, C.; Skroce, K.; Boccia, G.; Lippi, G.; La Torre, A.; Schena, F. Effects of Flywheel Strength Training on the Running Economy of Recreational Endurance Runners. *J. Strength Cond. Res.* **2019**, *33*, 684–690. [CrossRef]
12. Li, F.; Nassis, G.P.; Shi, Y.; Han, G.; Zhang, X.; Gao, B.; Ding, H. Concurrent Complex and Endurance Training for Recreational Marathon Runners: Effects on Neuromuscular and Running Performance. *Eur. J. Sport Sci.* **2021**, *21*, 1243–1253. [CrossRef] [PubMed]
13. Llanos-Lagos, C.; Ramirez-Campillo, R.; Moran, J.; de Saez Villarreal, E. The Effect of Strength Training Methods on Middle-Distance and Long-Distance Runners' Athletic Performance: A Systematic Review with Meta-Analysis. *Sports Med.* **2024**, *54*, 1801–1833. [CrossRef]
14. Eihara, Y.; Takao, K.; Sugiyama, T.; Maeo, S.; Terada, M.; Kanehisa, H.; Isaka, T. Heavy Resistance Training Versus Plyometric Training for Improving Running Economy and Running Time Trial Performance: A Systematic Review and Meta-Analysis. *Sports Med. Open* **2022**, *8*, 138. [CrossRef]
15. Hoogkamer, W.; Kram, R.; Arellano, C.J. How Biomechanical Improvements in Running Economy Could Break the 2-Hour Marathon Barrier. *Sports Med.* **2017**, *47*, 1739–1750. [CrossRef]
16. Michailidis, Y.; Stafylidis, A.; Vardakis, L.; Kyranoudis, A.E.; Mittas, V.; Leftheroudis, V.; Plakias, S.; Mandroukas, A.; Metaxas, T.I. The Running Performance of Elite Youth Football Players in Matches with a 1-4-3-3 Formation in Relation to Their Playing Position. *Appl. Sci.* **2025**, *15*, 3984. [CrossRef]
17. Modric, T.; Versic, S.; Sekulic, D.; Liposek, S. Analysis of the Association between Running Performance and Game Performance Indicators in Professional Soccer Players. *Int. J. Environ. Res. Public Health* **2019**, *16*, 4032. [CrossRef] [PubMed]
18. Ross, A.; Leveritt, M.; Riek, S. Neural influences on sprint running: Training adaptations and acute responses. *Sports Med.* **2015**, *38*, 839–855. [CrossRef]
19. Croisier, J.L.; Ganteaume, S.; Binet, J.; Genty, M.; Ferret, J.M. Strength imbalances and prevention of hamstring injury in professional soccer players: A prospective study. *Am. J. Sports Med.* **2008**, *36*, 1469–1475. [CrossRef] [PubMed]
20. Bishop, D.; Girard, O.; Mendez-Villanueva, A. Repeated-sprint ability—Part II: Recommendations for training. *Sports Med.* **2018**, *44*, 1027–1049. [CrossRef]
21. Meylan, C.; Cronin, J.; Oliver, J.; Hughes, M. The effect of maturation on adaptations to strength training and detraining in youth athletes. *J. Strength Cond. Res.* **2014**, *28*, 687–694. [CrossRef]
22. Impellizzeri, F.M.; Rampinini, E.; Marcora, S.M. Physiological assessment of aerobic training in soccer. *J. Sports Sci.* **2008**, *23*, 583–592. [CrossRef]
23. Pedersen, S.; Welde, B.; Sagelv, E.H.; Heitmann, K.A.; Randers, M.B.; Johansen, D.; Pettersen, S.A. Associations between Maximal Strength, Sprint, and Jump Height and Match Physical Performance in High-Level Female Football Players. *Scand. J. Med. Sci. Sports* **2022**, *32* (Suppl. S1), 54–61. [CrossRef] [PubMed]
24. Silva, J.R.; Magalhães, J.; Ascensão, A.; Seabra, A.F.; Rebelo, A.N. Training Status and Match Activity of Professional Soccer Players Throughout a Season. *J. Strength Cond. Res.* **2013**, *27*, 20–30. [CrossRef]

25. Michailidis, Y.; Vardakis, L.; Mikikis, D.; Mandroukas, A.; Metaxas, T. Match Running Performance of Elite Soccer Players and Correlations with Anthropometric and Power Indexes. *J. Sports Res.* **2019**, *6*, 44–51. [CrossRef]
26. Nuñez, J.; Suarez-Arrones, L.; de Hoyo, M.; Loturco, I. Strength Training in Professional Soccer: Effects on Short-Sprint and Jump Performance. *Int. J. Sports Med.* **2022**, *43*, 485–495. [CrossRef] [PubMed]
27. Yilmaz, H.H.; Seren, K.; Atasever, G. The Relationship between Isokinetic Strength and Anaerobic Performance in Elite Youth Football Players. *J. ROL Sport Sci.* **2023**, *4*, 457–468. [CrossRef]
28. Mandroukas, A.; Michailidis, Y.; Metaxas, T. Muscle Strength and Hamstrings to Quadriceps Ratio in Young Soccer Players: A Cross-Sectional Study. *J. Funct. Morphol. Kinesiol.* **2023**, *8*, 70. [CrossRef]
29. Kabacinski, J.; Szozda, P.M.; Mackala, K.; Murawa, M.; Rzepnicka, A.; Szewczyk, P.; Dworak, L.B. Relationship between isokinetic knee strength and speed, agility, and explosive power in elite soccer players. *Int. J. Environ. Res. Public Health* **2022**, *19*, 671. [CrossRef]
30. Beato, M.; Coratella, G.; Stiff, A.; Iacono, A.D. The validity and between-unit variability of GNSS units (STATSports Apex 10 and 18 Hz) for measuring distance and peak speed in team sports. *Front. Physiol.* **2018**, *9*, 1288. [CrossRef]
31. Beato, M.; Devereux, G.; Stiff, A. Validity and reliability of global positioning system units (STATSports Viper) for measuring distance and peak speed in sports. *J. Strength Cond. Res.* **2018**, *32*, 2831–2837. [CrossRef]
32. Di Salvo, V.; Baron, R.; Tschan, H.; Calderon Montero, F.J.; Bachl, N.; Pigozzi, F. Performance characteristics according to playing position in elite soccer. *Int. J. Sports Med.* **2007**, *28*, 222–227. [CrossRef]
33. Little, T.; Williams, A.G. Specificity of acceleration, maximum speed, and agility in professional soccer players. *J. Strength Cond. Res.* **2005**, *19*, 76–78. [CrossRef]
34. Doncaster, G.; Unnithan, V. Between-game variation of physical soccer performance measures in highly trained youth soccer players. *J. Strength Cond. Res.* **2019**, *33*, 1912–1920. [CrossRef]
35. Chen, Z.; Gu, Z.; Lyu, M.; Bishop, C.; Harper, D.J.; Ainsworth, B.; Dai, B.; Li, Y. Relationships between knee and ankle strength and horizontal deceleration performance at different sprint distances in multi-directional sports athletes. *Sports Biomech.* **2025**, 1–14. [CrossRef]
36. Wisløff, U.; Castagna, C.; Helgerud, J.; Jones, R.; Hoff, J. Strong correlation of maximal squat strength with sprint performance and vertical jump height in elite soccer players. *Br. J. Sports Med.* **2004**, *38*, 285–288. [CrossRef]
37. JASP Team. *JASP*, Version 0.19.3.0; Computer Software; JASP Team: Amsterdam, The Netherlands, 2025. Available online: https://jasp-stats.org (accessed on 20 June 2025).
38. Varley, M.C.; Gregson, W.; McMillan, K.; Bonanno, D.; Stafford, K.; Modonutti, M.; Di Salvo, V. Physical and Technical Performance of Elite Youth Soccer Players during International Tournaments: Influence of Playing Position and Team Success and Opponent Quality. *Sci. Med. Footb.* **2016**, *1*, 18–29. [CrossRef]
39. Savolainen, E.H.J.; Vänttinen, T.; Ihalainen, J.K.; Walker, S. Physical qualities and body composition predictors of running performance in national level women's official soccer matches. *Biol. Sport.* **2023**, *40*, 1187–1195. [CrossRef] [PubMed]
40. Rebelo, A.; Silva, P.; Rago, V.; Barreira, D.; Krustrup, P. Differences in Strength and Speed Demands between 4v4 and 8v8 Small-Sided Football Games. *J. Sports Sci.* **2016**, *34*, 2246–2254. [CrossRef]
41. Dharmajayanti, I.A.; Negara, A.A.; Artini, I.G. The correlation between the body mass index, speed, and agility among athletes: A literature review. *Kinesiol. Physiother. Compr.* **2023**, *2*, 81–86. [CrossRef]
42. Zanini, M.; Folland, J.P.; Wu, H.; Blagrove, R.C. Strength training improves running economy durability and fatigued high-intensity performance in well-trained male runners: A randomized control trial. *Med. Sci. Sports Exerc.* **2025**, *57*, 1546–1558. [CrossRef]
43. Ross, S.A.; Wakeling, J.M. Muscle shortening velocity depends on tissue inertia and level of activation during submaximal contractions. *Biol. Lett.* **2016**, *12*, 20151041. [CrossRef]
44. Bradley, P.S.; Di Mascio, M.; Peart, D.; Olsen, P.; Sheldon, B. High-intensity activity profiles of elite soccer players at different performance levels. *J. Strength Cond. Res.* **2013**, *27*, 2340–2350. [CrossRef]
45. Di Salvo, V.; Gregson, W.; Atkinson, G.; Tordoff, P.; Drust, B. Analysis of high intensity activity in Premier League soccer. *Int. J. Sports Med.* **2007**, *28*, 222–227. [CrossRef] [PubMed]
46. Dellal, A.; Chamari, K.; Wong, D.P.; Ahmaidi, S.; Keller, D.; Barros, R.; Carling, C. Comparison of physical and technical performance in European soccer match-play: FA Premier League and La Liga. *Eur. J. Sport Sci.* **2011**, *11*, 51–59. [CrossRef]
47. Hoff, J.; Helgerud, J. Endurance and strength training for soccer players: Physiological considerations. *Sports Med.* **2004**, *34*, 165–180. [CrossRef] [PubMed]

sports

MDPI

Article

Segmental External Load in Linear Running in Elite Futsal Players: A Multifactorial and Individual Variability Analysis Using Linear Mixed Models

Diego Hernán Villarejo-García †, Carlos Navarro-Martínez *,† and José Pino-Ortega †

Faculty of Sport Science, University of Murcia, 30100 Murcia, Spain; dvillarejo@um.es (D.H.V.-G.); josepinoortega@um.es (J.P.-O.)
* Correspondence: c.navarromartinez@um.es; Tel.: +34-685118928
† These authors contributed equally to this work.

Abstract: Limited evidence exists on how segmental external load is distributed during linear running and how it varies with speed, training intensity, and individual differences. This study examines the external load profile across six body segments in elite female futsal players during linear treadmill running, focusing on the effects of speed and training zone, as well as individual variability. Eight elite players, including six outfield players and two goalkeepers (mean age 23.9 ± 3.4 years, height 164.96 ± 4.22 cm, body mass 60.31 ± 4.56 kg), performed an incremental test and were measured using six WIMU PRO™ inertial sensors. The sensors recorded segmental PlayerLoad, speed, and training zones. Data were analyzed using Linear Mixed Models. The most important results show significant interactions between body location and speed and between body location and training zone ($p < 0.001$), with intraclass correlation coefficients (ICC) ranging from 0.437 to 0.515. These results indicate variability among players and specific and asymmetrical segmental load patterns. These findings offer practical insights for tailoring individualized training strategies that optimize performance and reduce segment specific overuse injuries.

Keywords: external load monitoring; female athletes; futsal; inertial measurement units; linear running; load distribution; segmental PlayerLoad; training load

1. Introduction

The monitoring of segmental external load in elite training is a key factor for achieving higher performance in athletes [1]. This individualization allows us to optimize athletic performance [2] and reduce the risk of injury [3]. In this way, external load [4] and, in particular, metrics such as PlayerLoad [5], which can be obtained using various inertial sensors, can provide valuable information regarding the mechanical demands placed on different body segments of high-performance athletes during their daily training. Specifically, one of the sports with the most intense physical demands is futsal. In this sport, players are exposed to very high heart rate intensities [6], frequent and numerous changes of direction [7], and intermittent effort throughout the match [8].

Physical preparation in female futsal players uses various training methodologies aimed at enhancing or replicating specific aspects of the game. Among the most common training methods are small-sided games (SSGs) [9], running drills involving changes of direction (COD) [10], and linear running [11]. Small-sided games (SSGs) are known for providing high contextual and cognitive specificity, although managing the training load in these activities tends to be more variable and challenging to measure [12]. Meanwhile, running drills with changes of direction (COD) are designed to replicate the multidirectional movement patterns typical of futsal, although they may lack the tactical complexity found in actual match play. Conversely, linear running, while less specific in terms of multidirectionality and the inherent intermittency of futsal, remains a prevalent training method due to its ease of prescription, precise speed control, and intensity monitoring.

In this regard, although running speed acts as a modulator of the total load imposed on the athlete, both in terms of internal load (e.g., heart rate) and external load (e.g., distance covered), a crucial question arises in the context of linear treadmill running: Does external load, measured segmentally, behave the same way across all body locations when speed varies? More importantly, is this segmental load profile consistent among all players, or does significant individual variability exist? In this respect, Gómez-Carmona et al. examined segmental external load profiles in young football players during an incremental treadmill test, providing an initial insight into how load is distributed across different body locations [13]. Their results show that PlayerLoad differs significantly between various body segments in response to linear running. However, the statistical analysis used in that study, based on Analysis of Variance (ANOVA), did not allow for modeling of the complex interactions between factors, nor the inherent variability of repeated measures within the same individual, which could limit the depth of interpretation of their findings. Therefore, there remains a gap in the detailed understanding of how speed and internal load (training zone) specifically modulate external load at the segmental level in elite female players, and how this manifests in inter-individual variability during linear running. Unlike previous studies, such as Gómez-Carmona et al. [13], which investigated external load in male futsal players and employed Analysis of Variance (ANOVA) to compare loads between different positions or game conditions without addressing individual variability or complex interactions between multiple factors, the present study utilizes Linear Mixed Models. This advanced statistical approach allows for a more robust analysis of multifactorial effects and individual differences, providing unprecedented insight into segmental load patterns. Furthe]. Understanding on elite female futsal players addresses a critical research gap, as this population experiences high physical demands and potential injury vulnerabilities, yet remains underrepresented in load monitoring research [14,15]. Understanding their specific load profiles is crucial for optimizing performance and injury prevention strategies tailored to their unique physiological and biomechanical characteristics.

Given that linear running is a widely used training method, addressing this knowledge gap is essential for optimizing the prescription of linear running training, enabling coaches to better understand the specific demands placed on each body segment and thereby contributing to performance enhancement and injury prevention. The application of a Linear Mixed Model (LMM) is key for this purpose, as it enables the analysis of complex interactions between factors and allows for modeling of the significant variability inherent in individual athlete data [16,17].

Accordingly, the present study aims to address this gap by investigating external load in elite female futsal players from a multifactorial and individual-centered perspective. Thus, the objectives of this work were as follows: (1) to characterize the differential influence of speed on segmental external load according to body location; (2) to determine specific patterns of external load by body location across different training intensity zones; and (3) to quantify the individual variability in external load attributable to differences between players. It was hypothesized that segmental external load (measured using the PlayerLoad index) would be influenced by speed and training zone and that these effects would vary substantially depending on body location, with considerable variability also expected among players. The results of this study offer valuable practical implications for coaches and strength and conditioning professionals, as they enable the individualization of linear running training, optimization of load management strategies, and contribute to the prevention of segment-specific injuries in elite female futsal players.

2. Materials and Methods

2.1. Participants

The study sample comprised 8 elite-level female futsal players (6 outfield players, 2 goalkeepers) (age: 29.9 ± 5.1 years; height: 164.96 ± 4.22 cm; body mass: 60.31 ± 4.56 kg) who participated in the Primera RFEF Futsal Femenina (Spanish first division) during the 2020/2021 season. The present study adopted an observational within-subject repeated measures design. All players were professional athletes with at least five years of experience in elite futsal and presented no musculoskeletal injuries or physical limitations that could have affected their performance during the study.

Following the Declaration of Helsinki guidelines, and to ensure participant confidentiality, all performance data were anonymized prior to analysis [18]. The study protocol was approved by the Ethics Committee of the University of Murcia (approval number: 3180/2020), which waived the requirement for written informed consent, as the research was deemed non-interventional, utilizing retrospective and anonymized routine performance data collected within a professional sports team setting. The study sample comprised 8 elite-level female futsal players... All players were actively participating in regular training with their professional team without current or recent (within 6 months) history of lower-limb or spinal injuries requiring medical intervention or preventing full participation.

2.2. Equipment

For external workload assessment during the incremental running treadmill test, six WIMU PRO™ inertial devices (Realtrack Systems, Almería, Spain) were utilized. These devices are equipped with triaxial accelerometers capable of detecting and measuring movement through a micro-electromechanical system. In the present research, the accelerometers' sampling frequency was set at 100 Hz. Data acquisition and initial processing were performed using the SPRO™ software (version 989). A motorized treadmill (HP Cosmos Pulsar 3P, HP Cosmos Sports & Medical GmbH, Nussdorf-Traunstein, Germany), with a minimum capacity of 20 km/h and electronic speed control, was also used for testing. To ensure proper sensor attachment, a back harness, elastic leg straps, and industrial-grade Velcro were employed.

2.3. Variables

2.3.1. Dependent Variable

PlayerLoad: PlayerLoad can be defined as a measurement that indicates the accumulated external load that an athlete—in this, case professional female futsal players—has to endure. This measurement is calculated based on acceleration data recorded in three directions (forward–backward, side-to-side, and up–down). The final value is obtained by summing all the high-speed changes in acceleration recorded across these three axes. This indicator was developed by Realtrack Systems (Almería, Spain), and is expressed in arbitrary units (a.u.). It is consolidated into a single value, resulting from the sum of the differences in acceleration between each moment across the three directions.

$$PlayerLoad = \sum \sqrt{\left((A_{\mathrm{xi}} - A_{\mathrm{xi-1}})^2 + (A_{\gamma \mathrm{i}} - A_{\gamma \mathrm{i-1}})^2 + (Az_{\mathrm{i}} - Az_{\mathrm{i-1}})^2 \right)}$$

In this formula, A_{xi}, A_{yi}, and A_{zi} denote the acceleration values on the X, Y, and Z axes at time point i, and n is the total number of samples. This parameter reflects the magnitude of instantaneous mechanical load fluctuations during movement, and has been widely used to monitor external workload in team sports [19,20].

2.3.2. Independent Variables

Speed: This is defined as the distance covered in a given period of time and is commonly expressed in kilometers per hour (km/h).

Training Zone: This is defined as the classification of exercise intensity based on the estimated percentage of an individual's maximal heart rate [21]. Five distinct training zones were defined for analysis: R0 (50–60% HRmax), R1 (60–70% HRmax), R2 (70–80% HRmax), R3 (80–90% HRmax), and R4 (>90% HRmax).

Location: This is defined as the anatomical placement of the inertial measurement units (IMUs) during the exercise, allowing for the recording of load data in different body regions (see Figure 1). Once the data were obtained using the SPRO™ software, they were processed in Microsoft Excel 365.

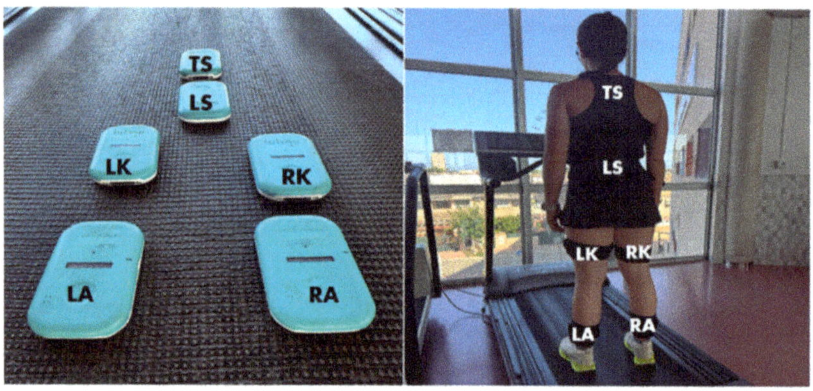

Figure 1. Anatomical placement of inertial measurement units (IMUs). Left ankle (LA), right ankle (RA), left knee (LK), right knee (RK), lumbar spine (LS), and thoracic spine (TS).

2.4. Statistical Analysis

The PlayerLoad variable was subjected to a natural logarithm transformation prior to the analysis. This transformation was performed primarily to address the positive skewness in the distribution of external load and to improve the normality and homoscedasticity of the model residuals [17]. To manage the high collinearity between speed and training zone, two separate Linear Mixed Model (LMM) analyses were employed. Both models included ID_jugadora as a random intercept to model individual variability among players. Additionally, Model 1 included speed as a random slope to account for individual variability in the response to speed. Model 1 investigated the effects of location, speed, and their two-way interaction (Location × Speed). Model 2 investigated the effects of location, training zones, and their two-way interaction (Location × Training Zone). Prior to LMM execution, statistical assumptions were verified for each model. The normality of the model's residuals was evaluated using the Kolmogorov–Smirnov test, complemented by visual inspection of Q-Q plots. For Model 1, the K-S test yielded $p < 0.001$; however, visual inspection of the Q-Q plot indicated a close approximation to normality, particularly in the central distribution, suggesting that the transformation substantially mitigated non-normality for practical inference, given the large sample size. For Model 2, the K-S test yielded $p = 0.093$; the Q-Q plot showed an excellent approximation to normality. The homoscedasticity of residuals and the linearity of the relationship between predictor variables and the response variable were visually inspected using scatter plots of the residuals versus predicted values, with no significant deviations observed in either model. Statistical significance for all fixed effects was set at $p < 0.05$. For a more complete interpretation of the practical magnitude of the effects, effect sizes were calculated using Partial Eta Squared (ηp^2). These values were interpreted, where 0.01 is considered a small effect, 0.06 a medium effect, and 0.14 a large effect [22]. For a detailed interpretation of significant interactions, conceptual simple effects analyses were performed based on parameter estimates and confidence intervals. All statistical analyses were carried out using Jamovi, version 2.6 [23], and its modules, along with supplementary computations in R Studio, version 4.5.0 [24], to derive the effect sizes (ηp^2).

2.5. Data Availability

The data used for statistical analysis and the results of this work are publicly available in the Research Data Repository (DIGITUM) under the following Digital Object Identifier (DOI): http://hdl.handle.net/10201/156980 (accessed on 1 July 2025).

2.6. Procedure

The research was conducted over three weeks, with one session per week. In the first week, participants were informed about the study's objectives and protocol. In the second week, they familiarized themselves with the treadmill test procedure and the experimental equipment (inertial sensors) by conducting a trial session. The incremental treadmill test was performed in the third week.

Prior to the placement of the inertial devices, they were manually calibrated according to the manufacturer's recommendations and synchronized. This process is fundamental for eliminating 3D accelerometer error sources (offset error, scaling error, non-orthogonal error, and random error). The devices were affixed to the following anatomical locations following a validated scheme: (i) upper back, on the interscapular line; (ii) lumbar region, at L3 near the center of mass; (iii) knee, 3 cm above the kneecap; and (iv) ankle, 3 cm above the lateral malleolus. At both the knee and ankle, the devices were placed on the outside of the right leg on all athletes, while an anatomically designed harness was used for the upper back, and the rest were secured with a specifically designed elastic band. Before the test, participants performed a standardized 10 min warm-up that included 5 min of continuous running at 7 km/h, 3 min of joint mobility exercises, and 2 min of progressions (gentle accelerations on the treadmill). This procedure was monitored in real-time via WIMU PRO™ devices (RealTrack Systems, Almería, Spain) that transmitted data wirelessly to the SPRO™ software, ensuring the correct functioning of the sensors. The main protocol was an adaptation of the VAM (Maximal Aerobic Speed) test, designed for continuous and controlled analysis. The test began at a speed of 8.0 km/h, with increments of +0.2 km/h every 12 s. The test concluded upon the athlete's voluntary exhaustion or observation of a technical criterion (e.g., unstable stride frequency, evident fatigue). The treadmill surface was flat (1% incline). Upon completion of the main test, participants performed 5 min of recovery intensity running. To minimize interference from uncontrolled variables, all participants were instructed to maintain their habitual lifestyle and normal dietary intake before and during the study. Furthermore, tests were always performed at the same time of day (i.e., 9:00 a.m.) to avoid the possible effects of circadian rhythms, and it was ensured that they had not performed high-intensity physical activity in the 48 h prior to the tests. Environmental control was kept constant (temperature 22–24 °C, humidity < 50%). All participants used standard training footwear to homogenize conditions. The integrity of the sensors was verified at all times by two researchers.

3. Results

The results of the fixed effects omnibus tests of the Linear Mixed Model are presented in Table 1.

Table 1. Fixed effects omnibus tests for PlayerLoad in Model 1 and Model 2.

	F	df	df (res)	p	ηp^2
Model 1 (Location, Speed, and their Interaction)					
Location	3391.9	5	1607	**<0.001**	**0.912**
Speed (Km/h)	4555.5	1	1608	**<0.001**	**0.739**
Location × Speed	88.6	5	1607	**<0.001**	**0.216**
Model 2 (Location, Training Zone, and their Interaction)					
Location	497.5	5	1589	**<0.001**	**0.610**
Training Zone	744.2	4	1590	**<0.001**	**0.652**
Location × Training Zone	11.6	20	1589	**<0.001**	**0.127**

F values are rounded to two decimal places. df = degrees of freedom of the effect; df (res) = residual degrees of freedom; p = p-value. $p < 0.001$ indicates a p-value less than 0.001.

As can be observed in Table 1, statistically significant effects were found for location (Model 1: F5.1607 = 3391.9 $p < 0.001$, $\eta p^2 = 0.914$; Model 2: F5.1589 = 497.5 $p < 0.001$, $\eta p^2 = 0.610$), Speed (Model 1: F1.1608 = 455.5 $p < 0.001$, $\eta p^2 = 0.739$), and training zone (Model 2: F4.1590 = 744.2 $p < 0.001$, $\eta p^2 = 0.652$). All these effects showed a very large effect size. Additionally, significant interactions were found between location and speed (Model 1: F5.1607 = 88.6 $p < 0.001$, $\eta p^2 = 0.216$), as well as between location and training zone (Model 2: F20.1589 = 11.6 $p < 0.001$, $\eta p^2 = 0.127$). Both interactions revealed a large effect size.

Regarding individual variability, the random components of the models revealed that, in Model 1 (which included speed), the variance of the random intercept for player ID (ID_jugadora) was 0.0185 (SD = 0.136), resulting in an ICC of 0.437. This value suggests that 43.7% of the total variability in PlayerLoad (log-transformed) can be attributed to consistent differences among players in this model, and the unexplained residual variance was 0.0239 (SD = 0.154). For Model 2 (which included the training zone), the variance of the random intercept was 0.0348 (SD = 0.186) with an ICC of 0.515, indicating that 51.5% of the total variability in PlayerLoad (log-transformed) is attributable to consistent differences among players. The unexplained residual variance for Model 2 was 0.0327 (SD = 0.181).

Table 2 presents the parameter estimates for the fixed effects of Model 1.

Table 2. Fixed coefficients for PlayerLoad in Model 1.

Effect	Estimate	SE	IC 95%		df	t	p
			Lower	Upper			
Intercept	0.32	0.04	0.23	0.42	6.99	6.81	**<0.001**
Location							
LK-LA	−0.14	0.01	−0.17	−0.11	1.607.62	−10.63	**<0.001**
LS-LA	−0.85	0.01	−0.88	−0.83	1.606.99	−67.33	**<0.001**
RA-LA	0.02	0.01	0.06	0.05	1.607.62	2.01	**0.045**
RK-LA	−0.12	0.01	−0.14	−0.09	1.606.99	−9.42	**<0.001**
TS-LA	−1.26	0.01	−1.29	−1.24	1.606.99	−99.28	**<0.001**
Speed (Km/h)	0.11	0.01	0.11	0.12	1.608.17	67.49	**<0.001**
LK–LA × Speed	−0.05	0	−0.06	−0.04	1.607.05	−9.42	**<0.001**
LS-LA × Speed	−0.08	0	−0.09	−0.07	1.606.99	−15.18	**<0.001**
RA-LA × Speed	−0.01	0	−0.02	−0.01	1.607.00	−2.13	**0.003**
RK-LA × Speed	−0.06	0	−0.07	−0.05	1.606.99	−11.01	**<0.001**
TS-LA × Speed	−0.09	0	−0.10	−0.08	1.606.99	−16.89	**<0.001**

LA: left ankle; RA: right ankle; RK: right knee; LK: left knee; LS: lumbar spine; TS: toracic spine; Reference category for location: LA (left ankle). p values < 0.001 are indicated for values less than 0.001. Values are presented as estimate (standard error); 95% CI = 95% confidence interval.

The results in Table 2 show how segmental external load varies significantly with body location and running speed. The right ankle (RA) showed a significantly higher PlayerLoad than the left ankle (LA) (estimate = 0.028, $p = 0.045$), representing an approximate

2.8% increase in load. Likewise, each 1 km/h increment in speed was associated with an approximate 12.5% increase in the PlayerLoad of the left ankle (estimate = 0.117, $p < 0.001$).

Significant location × speed interactions ($p < 0.05$ for all) indicate that the percentage rate of PlayerLoad increase with speed differs among segments.

Table 3 presents the parameter estimates for the fixed effects of Model 2.

Table 3. Fixed coefficients for PlayerLoad in Model 2.

Effect	Estimate	SE	IC 95% Lower	IC 95% Upper	df	t	p
Intercept	0.08	0.07	−0.05	0.21	7.23	1.26	0.246
Location							
LK-LA	−0.02	0.03	−0.24	−0.11	1589.05	−5.32	<0.001
LS-LA	−0.08	0.03	−0.85	−0.72	1589.00	−23.94	<0.001
RA-LA	0.10	0.03	0.05	0.17	1589.09	3.51	<0.001
RK-LA	−0.02	0.03	−0.23	−0.11	1589.00	−5.23	<0.001
TS-LA	−1.17	0.03	−1.24	−1.11	1589.00	−35.82	<0.001
Training Zone							
R1-R0	0.02	0.04	0.13	0.30	1589.51	4.88	<0.001
R2-R0	0.44	0.04	0.35	0.53	1589.50	10.28	<0.001
R3-R0	0.72	0.04	0.63	0.80	1589.75	16.63	<0.001
R4-R0	0.99	0.04	0.90	1.07	1589.67	23.03	<0.001
Location × Training Zone							
LK-LA × R1-R0	0.04	0.15	−0.26	0.35	1589.00	0.29	0.765
LS-LA × R1-R0	0.01	0.15	−0.29	0.31	1589.00	0.05	0.959
RA-LA × R1-R0	−0.51	0.14	−0.79	−0.23	1589.02	−3.61	<0.001
RK-LA × R1-R0	−0.05	0.15	−0.36	0.24	1589.00	−0.38	0.702
TS-LA × R1-R0	−0.21	0.15	−0.52	0.08	1589.00	−1.39	0.162
LK-LA × R2-R0	0.21	0.15	−0.08	0.50	1589.00	1.38	0.166
LS-LA × R2-R0	−0.01	0.15	−0.30	0.28	1589.00	−0.04	0.965
RA-LA × R2-R0	−0.45	0.13	−0.72	−0.19	1589.02	−3.36	<0.001
RK-LA × R2-R0	0.14	0.15	−0.15	0.44	1589.00	0.96	0.336
TS-LA × R2-R0	−0.17	0.15	−0.47	0.11	1589.00	−1.17	0.241
LK-LA × R3-R0	0.16	0.14	−0.12	0.45	1589.00	1.09	0.273
LS-LA × R3-R0	−0.17	0.14	−0.47	0.11	1589.00	−1.18	0.235
RA-LA × R3-R0	−0.45	0.13	−0.71	−0.18	1589.03	−3.35	<0.001
RK-LA × R3-R0	0.16	0.14	−0.12	0.45	1589.00	1.11	0.267
TS-LA × R3-R0	−0.33	0.14	−0.63	−0.04	1589.00	−2.25	0.024
LK-LA × R4-R0	0.04	0.15	−0.24	0.34	1589.00	0.31	0.756
LS-LA × R4-R0	−0.32	0.14	−0.62	−0.03	1589.00	−2.19	0.028
RA-LA × R4-R0	−0.40	0.13	−0.67	−0.14	1589.03	−3.02	0.003
RK-LA × R4-R0	0.10	0.14	−0.18	0.40	1589.00	0.72	0.467
TS-LA × R4-R0	−0.44	0.14	−0.74	−0.15	1589.00	−2.99	0.003

LA: left ankle; RA: right ankle; LK: left knee; RK: right knee; LS: lumbar spine; TS: thoracic spine. Reference category for location: LA (left ankle). Reference category for training zone: R0 (50–60% HRmax). p values < 0.001 are indicated for values less than 0.001. Values are presented as estimate (standard error); 95% CI = 95% confidence interval.

The results in Table 3 show that PlayerLoad varies significantly among segments and increases with the intensity of the training zone (R4–R0: estimate = 0.992, $p < 0.001$; 170.9% increase). A significantly higher PlayerLoad was also observed in RA compared to LA (estimate = 0.107, $p < 0.001$; 11.3% increase in R0). Significant location × training zone interactions ($p < 0.05$) reveal that the percentage increment of PlayerLoad with intensity is attenuated in RA, LS, and TS compared to LA.

Figure 2 presents the fixed effects profiles for PlayerLoad as a function of the combinations of location, speed, and training zone.

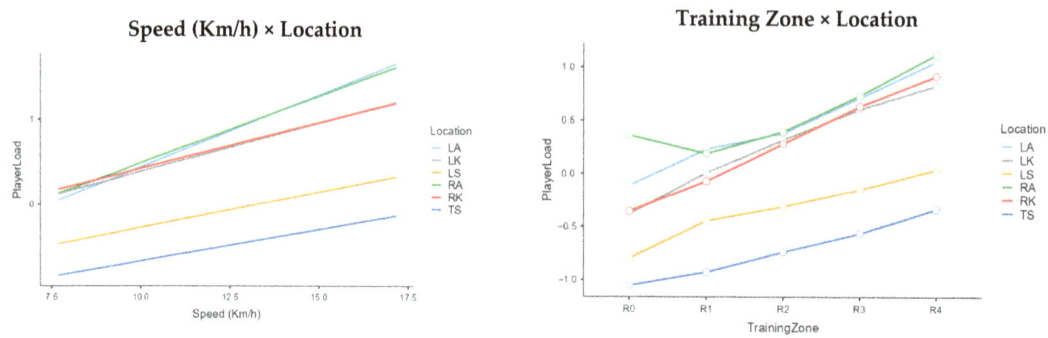

(**a**) (**b**)

Figure 2. Interaction profiles for PlayerLoad as a function of location, speed, and training zone. (**a**) Relationship between Speed (Km/h) and Location. (**b**) Relationship between Training Zone and Location. LA: left ankle; RA: right ankle; RK: right knee; LK: left knee; LS: lumbar spine; TS: toracic spine; R0: 50–60% HRmax; R1: 60–70% HRmax; 70–80% HRmax; R3: 80–90% HRmax; R4: >90% HRmax.

As observed in Figure 2a, the relationship between PlayerLoad and speed shows a non-uniform dynamic among segments, with more pronounced percentage increases in the ankles. Similarly, Figure 2b shows how the effect of the training zone on PlayerLoad differs according to location.

4. Discussion

The aim of this study was to describe and analyze the segmental external load profile in elite futsal players. An observational within-subject repeated measures model was used. Specifically, the influence of running speed, training zone, and inter-individual variability were analyzed. The findings confirm that segmental external load, measured using the PlayerLoad index [25], is significantly influenced by speed and training intensity. Individual variability in load response has also been observed. This confirms the general hypothesis of this work, and provides key information to optimize training and to individualize the effects of linear running in the observed sample.

To analyze the obtained data, two separate Linear Mixed Models (LMMs) were employed. This multivariate approach allowed for addressing the hierarchical structure of repeated measurements performed on the same futsal players [26]. The decision to use two separate LMMs allowed for controlling the high collinearity between speed and training zone. This enabled a reliable estimation of their independent effects and interactions [27]. LMMs also allowed for modeling individual variability among the athletes and understanding the interactions between body location, speed, and training zone [17].

Regarding the analysis of the results, specifically the omnibus tests for fixed effects (Table 1), it was observed that both the main effects of location, speed (Km/h) (in Model 1), training zone (in Model 2), and their interactions were highly significant ($p < 0.001$ in all cases). These findings confirm the interdependence between segmental load and speed and intensity factors. In this regard, the effect sizes (ηp^2) also revealed that location, speed, and training zone showed very large effects (ranging between $\eta p^2 = 0.610$ and 0.914), and the Location × Speed and Location × Training Zone interactions showed large effects ($\eta p^2 = 0.216$ and 0.127, respectively).

Regarding individual variability, the intraclass correlation coefficients were 0.437 for Model 1 and 0.515 for Model 2. These values show that variability in PlayerLoad is attributable to differences among players [26].

This difference in segmental load suggests that, although running speed increases, biomechanical load is not uniformly distributed across the analyzed body segments. This indicates the complexity of the process by which the body adapts to force absorption and transmission during linear running in the analyzed futsal players.

The results of Model 1, regarding the Location × Speed interaction, indicate that distal areas such as the ankles (LA, RA) exhibit a more pronounced percentage increase in PlayerLoad as speed increases. This may be due to the fact that, during the ground contact phase of running, the ankles can be one of the first joints to absorb this impact [28]. As speed increases, ground reaction forces (GRFs) acting on the body increase considerably, leading to more direct and proportional changes in acceleration and, consequently, in the PlayerLoad recorded in these joints [25].

In contrast, the knees (LK, RK) and the upper and lower trunk (LS, TS) showed a more attenuated percentage increase in PlayerLoad with increasing speed, as revealed by the interaction parameters of Model 1. This may be due to their greater ability to reduce, distribute, and balance the forces produced during running [29]. For example, the knees can dynamically adjust their flexion and stiffness to better absorb impact and generate force in later phases of running compared to the ankles, which translates into less marked changes in acceleration and, consequently, in PlayerLoad, even at higher running speeds [30].

Similarly, in the trunk (LS and TS), PlayerLoad shows a smaller percentage increase at high speeds. This may be due to a biomechanical adaptation where the trunk tends to become more rigid and stable to maintain balance during linear running. This translates into a reduction in movement and, therefore, a smaller and less proportional increase in PlayerLoad in these regions [31].

These findings on the variation in segmental load due to speed are consistent with Gómez-Carmona et al. [13], who also reported that the dynamics of accelerometric load differed across body locations and segments at various running speeds in young football players. Nevertheless, the use of Linear Mixed Models in the present study, specified in two separate models for greater precision, allowed for understanding these interactions, revealing percentage change patterns not previously described in the literature.

Along these lines, the results found in the location × training zone interaction are also relevant (Model 2: $F(20,1589) = 11.6$, $p < 0.001$, $\eta p^2 = 0.127$). With a large effect size, the results of this study show that the influence of the training zone on segmental PlayerLoad differs significantly according to body location. This also indicates specific load patterns for each intensity level.

The parameters of Model 2 detail how the PlayerLoad observed in the LA, as the reference location, progressively increases with the intensity of the training zone. For example, an increase of 24.6% from R0 to R1 was observed, reaching an increase of 170.9% from R0 to R4. However, the significant location × training zone interactions (Table 3, Figure 2b) revealed that this increasing percentage pattern differs notably for other locations.

When analyzing the significant interactions of Model 2, an atypical pattern is observed in RA in Figure 2b, as PlayerLoad decreases from zone R0 to R1. This atypical pattern can be explained by the presence of asymmetries in the limbs of Futsal players, related to the dominance of one leg [32], or with neuromuscular changes occurring when transitioning from R0 to R1 [33]. The singularity of this pattern and its potential implications for optimizing performance and preventing injuries should be addressed in new lines of research.

Unlike previous studies that analyzed load in different body parts and at various speeds [13,34], the present study is the first to describe in detail the complex relationship between body location and training zones, as defined by maximal heart rate. Our findings confirm that segmental PlayerLoad varies as a function of effort intensity, an aspect scarcely explored in the literature within the context of linear running using multimodal measurements. These results are particularly useful for planning high-intensity training loads in elite female futsal players, allowing for more precise individualization based on real segmental demands.

Another important point of this study is the individual variability found in segmental PlayerLoad. The observed intraclass correlation coefficients (ICCs), which ranged between 0.437 (Model 1) and 0.515 (Model 2), indicate that approximately between 43.7% and 51.5% of the total variation in PlayerLoad is due to differences among professional players, rather than random factors or measurement error. This demonstrates that, even in a controlled and standardized task such as linear running, the external load response is not identical for all athletes. These findings are consistent with previous studies that examined how factors such as age [32], sex [33], injuries [35], or physical condition [36] influence linear running mechanics, highlighting the need to consider the biomechanical and physiological particularities of each player.

This existing difference among the players in the present study generates valuable practical implications for designing linear running training. In this way, these findings indicate that group-level planning without individualization could even be harmful for some athletes. As observed in the sample of this study, the response to external load in linear running is highly individualized and could be related to differences in running techniques, biomechanics, body composition, or the individual neuromuscular efficiency of each athlete. Therefore, it is essential to carry out continuous and personalized monitoring of external load at the segmental level to ensure that each athlete receives training tailored to their individual needs and characteristics.

5. Practical Implications and Future Applications

A practical application of this knowledge is that, by understanding that certain body segments present asymmetrical load patterns or differential responses to intensity and speed (such as the higher basal load and the attenuated increase pattern in the right ankle, or the smaller percentage increases in the trunk at high intensities), coaches can adjust training loads or include specific exercises to compensate for these particular demands in concrete segments. These data can also aid in the design of sports equipment. In this sense, it is necessary to utilize more ergonomic equipment adapted to the anatomical and biomechanical demands of each body segment. In this regard, IMU manufacturers should consider designing miniaturized devices that allow for the simultaneous use of multiple sensors on different body parts, or that can even be integrated directly into sportswear. Similarly, conducting individualized and continuous monitoring of external load over time becomes key to optimizing performance and preventing injuries in specific body areas, thus managing load according to each athlete's intrinsic needs.

6. Study Limitations and Future Research Directions

The present study presents several limitations that should be considered. One of these limitations is that data collection was carried out on a treadmill during linear running. While this controlled environment allowed for the precise manipulation and isolation of variables such as speed and intensity, it does not fully replicate the dynamic reality of futsal. Futsal involves frequent multidirectional movements, highly intermittent efforts, and constant decision-making processes in varied game situations, such as cutting, pivoting, and acceleration/deceleration with and without the ball. This can contribute differently to segmental load, thus affecting the direct transferability of these specific load profiles to real-game situations. Nevertheless, this standardized approach was considered necessary to investigate in isolation the specific effects of speed and intensity on segmental load.

Another limitation is the sample size. Although this is common practice in studies with high-performance athletes, it implies that the results should be considered within this field and should not be generalized to broader populations. This limited sample size also restricts the complexity of random-effects structures that could be robustly estimated within the Linear Mixed Models, influencing aspects such as the individual variability of random slopes. Furthermore, while the logarithmic transformation substantially improved the normality of the residuals, the formal statistical tests for normality remained significant for Model 1, suggesting minor deviations from perfect normality; however, visual inspection of Q-Q plots indicated practical acceptability, supported by the known robustness of LMMs with large sample sizes.

For future research, it would be important to confirm these segmental load profiles and interaction patterns in competition and training situations. Specifically, it would be beneficial to deepen the understanding of atypical load patterns observed in the right ankle and differential load responses in trunk segments across intensities. Furthermore, it is necessary to replicate this research in other populations. Future studies could also benefit from the analysis of other variables, such as perceived internal load, individual players' playing profiles, and limb dominance.

7. Conclusions

The present study allows us to describe how external load affects different body parts in professional female futsal players during linear treadmill running. The results show a differentiated impact of running speed and training zones on distinct body segments. Specific and asymmetrical segmental load patterns were observed, alongside considerable individual variability among athletes. These findings are important for understanding the significance of monitoring load in different body segments. They also highlight the need to adjust training loads by considering each player's demands. This approach is key to optimizing performance and contributing to injury prevention in this elite population.

Author Contributions: Conceptualization, D.H.V.-G. and C.N.-M.; Methodology, D.H.V.-G.; Validation, C.N.-M. and J.P.-O.; Formal analysis, D.H.V.-G.; Investigation, D.H.V.-G., C.N.-M. and J.P.-O.; Data curation, D.H.V.-G. and J.P.-O.; Writing—original draft preparation, J.P.-O., D.H.V.-G., and C.N.-M.; Writing—review and editing, D.H.V.-G., C.N.-M. and J.P.-O.; Visualization, C.N.-M.; Supervision, J.P.-O. and D.H.V.-G. All authors have read and agreed to the published version of the manuscript.

Funding: This research received no external funding.

Institutional Review Board Statement: This study was conducted in accordance with the Declaration of Helsinki and was approved by the Ethics Committee of the University of Murcia (protocol code 3180/2020; date of approval: 14 December 2020).

Informed Consent Statement: Informed consent was obtained from all subjects involved in the study.

Data Availability Statement: The data supporting the findings of this study are openly available in DIGITUM, the Institutional Repository of the University of Murcia, at http://hdl.handle.net/10201/156980 (accessed on 1 July 2025).

Acknowledgments: The authors would like to thank the players and coaching staff of the participating futsal team for their cooperation and commitment during data collection. No Generative AI tools were used in the writing, analysis, or preparation of this manuscript.

Conflicts of Interest: The authors declare no conflicts of interest. The funders had no role in the design of the study; in the collection, analyses, or interpretation of data; in the writing of the manuscript; or in the decision to publish the results.

Abbreviations

The following abbreviations are used in this manuscript:

IMU	Inertial Measurement Unit
LMM	Linear Mixed Model
ICC	Intraclass Correlation Coefficient
LA	Left Ankle
RA	Right Ankle
LK	Left Knee
RK	Right Knee
LS	Lumbar Spine
TS	Thoracic Spine
SSG	Small-Sided Games
COD	Change of Direction
HR	Heart Rate
GRF	Ground Reaction Force
VAM	Maximal Aerobic Speed

References

1. Bourdon, P.C.; Cardinale, M.; Murray, A.; Gastin, P.; Kellmann, M.; Varley, M.C.; Gabbett, T.J.; Coutts, A.J.; Burgess, D.J.; Gregson, W.; et al. Monitoring athlete training loads: Consensus statement. *Int. J. Sports Physiol. Perform.* **2017**, *12* (Suppl. S2), S2161–S2170. [CrossRef]
2. Halson, S.L. Monitoring training load to understand fatigue in athletes. *Sports Med.* **2014**, *44*, 139–147. [CrossRef]
3. Oliveira, J.P.; Sampaio, T.; Marinho, D.A.; Barbosa, T.M.; Morais, J.E. Exploring injury prevention strategies for futsal players: A systematic review. *Healthcare* **2024**, *12*, 1387. [CrossRef] [PubMed]
4. Dawson, L.; McErlain-Naylor, S.A.; Devereux, G.; Beato, M. Practitioner usage, applications, and understanding of wearable GPS and accelerometer technology in team sports. *J. Strength Cond. Res.* **2024**, *38*, e373–e382. [CrossRef] [PubMed]
5. Gadea-Uribarri, H.; Lago-Fuentes, C.; Bores-Arce, A.; Villavicencio Álvarez, V.E.; López-García, S.; Calero-Morales, S.; Mainer-Pardos, E. External load evaluation in elite futsal: Influence of match results and game location with IMU technology. *J. Funct. Morphol. Kinesiol.* **2024**, *9*, 140. [CrossRef] [PubMed]
6. Spyrou, K.; Freitas, T.T.; Marín-Cascales, E.; Alcaraz, P.E. Physical and physiological match-play demands and player characteristics in futsal: A systematic review. *Front. Psychol.* **2020**, *11*, 569897. [CrossRef]
7. Ribeiro, J.N.; Gonçalves, B.; Coutinho, D.; Brito, J.; Sampaio, J.; Travassos, B. Activity profile and physical performance of match play in elite futsal players. *Front. Psychol.* **2020**, *11*, 1709. [CrossRef]
8. Serrano, C.; Felipe, J.L.; Garcia-Unanue, J.; Ibañez, E.; Hernando, E.; Gallardo, L.; Sanchez-Sanchez, J. Local positioning system analysis of physical demands during official matches in the Spanish futsal league. *Sensors* **2020**, *20*, 4860. [CrossRef]
9. Kose, M.G.; Hazir, T.; Kin-Isler, A. Metabolic power responses to different small sided games in football and futsal players. *Int. J. Perform. Anal. Sport* **2023**, *23*, 489–502. [CrossRef]
10. Ayarra, R.; Nakamura, F.Y.; Iturricastillo, A.; Castillo, D.; Yanci, J. Differences in physical performance according to the competitive level in futsal players. *J. Hum. Kinet.* **2018**, *64*, 275–285. [CrossRef]
11. Teixeira, A.S.; Arins, F.B.; De Lucas, R.D.; Carminatti, L.J.; Dittrich, N.; Nakamura, F.Y.; Guglielmo, L.G.A. Comparative effects of two interval shuttle-run training modes on physiological and performance adaptations in female professional futsal players. *J. Strength Cond. Res.* **2019**, *33*, 1416–1428. [CrossRef] [PubMed]
12. Amani-Shalamzari, S.; Khoshghadam, E.; Donyaei, A.; Parnow, A.; Bayati, M.; Clemente, F.M. Generic vs. small-sided game training in futsal: Effects on aerobic capacity, anaerobic power and agility. *Physiol. Behav.* **2019**, *204*, 347–354. [CrossRef] [PubMed]
13. Gómez-Carmona, C.D.; Bastida-Castillo, A.; Moreno-Pérez, V.; Ibáñez, S.J.; Pino-Ortega, J. Multi-location external workload profile in U-18 soccer players. *Rev. Int. Cienc. Del Deporte* **2021**, *17*, 124–139. [CrossRef]
14. Villarejo García, D.H.; González-Fernández, F.T.; Rico-González, M.; Pino-Ortega, J.; Del Rosso, S.; Puche-Ortuño, D. Technical and tactical performance in professional female futsal players: A descriptive analysis depending on teams level and playing group. *Int. J. Perform. Anal. Sport* **2025**, *25*, 47–58. [CrossRef]
15. Villarejo-García, D.H.; Puche-Ortuño, D.; Gómez-Carmona, C.D.; Pino-Ortega, J. Multivariate analysis of performance indicators in elite women's futsal: A principal component approach to understanding game dynamics. *Int. J. Sports Sci. Coach.* **2025**, 17479541251343609. [CrossRef]
16. Cid, F.M. *Estadística Avanzada Para Educación Física: Diseño de Experimentos y Estadística Multivariante*; Editorial Académica Española: London, UK, 2016.

17. Tabachnick, B.G.; Fidell, L.S. *Using Multivariate Statistics*; Pearson Education: Boston, MA, USA, 2013.
18. World Medical Association. World Medical Association Declaration of Helsinki: Ethical principles for medical research involving human subjects. *JAMA* **2013**, *310*, 2191–2194. [CrossRef]
19. RealTrack Systems. *WIMU PRO™ User Manual: Technical Documentation*; RealTrack Systems: Almería, Spain, 2023.
20. Boyd, L.J.; Ball, K.; Aughey, R.J. The reliability of MinimaxX accelerometers for measuring physical activity in Australian football. *Int. J. Sports Physiol. Perform.* **2011**, *6*, 311–321. [CrossRef]
21. Sylta, O.; Tønnessen, E.; Seiler, S. From heart-rate data to training quantification: A comparison of 3 methods of training-intensity analysis. *Int. J. Sports Physiol. Perform.* **2014**, *9*, 100–107. [CrossRef]
22. Cohen, J. *Statistical Power Analysis for the Behavioral Sciences*, 2nd ed.; Lawrence Erlbaum Associates: New York, NY, USA, 1988.
23. Jamovi Project. *Jamovi*, version 2.6; Jamovi Project: Sydney, NSW, Australia, 2024. Available online: https://www.jamovi.org (accessed on 15 March 2024).
24. R Core Team. *R: A Language and Environment for Statistical Computing*, version 4.5.0; R Foundation for Statistical Computing: Vienna, Austria, 2024. Available online: https://www.R-project.org (accessed on 15 March 2024).
25. Gadea-Uribarri, H.; Mainer-Pardos, E.; Bores-Arce, A.; Albalad-Aiguabella, R.; López-García, S.; Lago-Fuentes, C. External Load Variability in Elite Futsal: Positional Demands and Microcycle Structuring for Player Well-Being and Performance. *Sports* **2025**, *13*, 7. [CrossRef]
26. Villarejo-García, D.H.; Navarro-Martínez, C.; Pino-Ortega, J. Uso de la estadística multivariante para analizar el rendimiento en competiciones de futsal: Revisión sistemática. *Retos Nuevas Perspect. Educ. Fís. Deporte Recreación* **2025**, *66*, 539–554. [CrossRef]
27. Cid, F.M. *Estadística Básica Para Educación Física: Estadística Descriptiva e Inferencial Univariada*; Editorial Académica Española: London, UK, 2015.
28. Xu, Y.; Yuan, P.; Wang, R.; Wang, D.; Liu, J.; Zhou, H. Effects of foot strike techniques on running biomechanics: A systematic review and meta-analysis. *Sports Health* **2021**, *13*, 71–77. [CrossRef]
29. Struzik, A.; Karamanidis, K.; Lorimer, A.; Keogh, J.W.L.; Gajewski, J. Application of leg, vertical, and joint stiffness in running performance: A literature overview. *Appl. Bionics Biomech.* **2021**, *2021*, 9914278. [CrossRef] [PubMed]
30. Jaén-Carrillo, D.; Roche-Seruendo, L.E.; Felton, L.; Cartón-Llorente, A.; García-Pinillos, F. Stiffness in running: A narrative integrative review. *Strength Cond. J.* **2021**, *43*, 104–115. [CrossRef]
31. Huang, L.; Wang, X.; Wang, Z.; Wu, X. Research on optimal control of treadmill shock absorption based on ground reaction force constraint. *Appl. Sci.* **2024**, *14*, 9509. [CrossRef]
32. Fukuchi, C.A.; Fukuchi, R.K.; Duarte, M. Effects of walking speed on gait biomechanics in healthy participants: A systematic review and meta-analysis. *Syst. Rev.* **2019**, *8*, 153. [CrossRef] [PubMed]
33. Barrett, R.; Noordegraaf, M.; Vonk, M.; Morrison, S. Gender differences in the variability of lower extremity kinematics during treadmill locomotion. *J. Mot. Behav.* **2008**, *40*, 62–70. [CrossRef]
34. Pardo Albiach, J.; Mir-Jimenez, M.; Hueso Moreno, V.; Nácher Moltó, I.; Martínez-Gramage, J. The relationship between VO2max, power management, and increased running speed: Towards gait pattern recognition through clustering analysis. *Sensors* **2021**, *21*, 2422. [CrossRef]
35. Van Oeveren, B.T.; de Ruiter, C.J.; Beek, P.J.; van Dieën, J.H. The biomechanics of running and running styles: A synthesis. *Sports Biomech.* **2024**, *23*, 516–554. [CrossRef]
36. Bohannon, R.W.; Williams Andrews, A. Normal walking speed: A descriptive meta-analysis. *Physiotherapy* **2011**, *97*, 182–189. [CrossRef]

sports

MDPI

Article

Effects of a Short-Term Ballistic Training Program on Performance and Strength Deficit in Elite Youth Female Soccer Players

Irineu Loturco [1,2,3,4,5,6,*], Bernardo Requena [5], Valter P. Mercer [1], Tulio B. M. A. Moura [1], Matheus G. A. Alexandre [6], Lucas D. Tavares [6] and Lucas A. Pereira [1,2]

1 NAR—Nucleus of High Performance in Sport, São Paulo 04753-060, Brazil; valterpreis@gmail.com (V.P.M.); tuliobernardo@gmail.com (T.B.M.A.M.); lucasa_pereira@outlook.com (L.A.P.)
2 Department of Human Movement Sciences, Federal University of São Paulo, São Paulo 11015-020, Brazil
3 UCAM Research Center for High Performance Sport, UCAM—Universidad Católica de Murcia, 30107 Murcia, Spain
4 Facultad de Deporte, UCAM—Universidad Católica de Murcia, 30107 Murcia, Spain
5 FSI—Football Science Institute, 18016 Granada, Spain; bernardorequena@icloud.com
6 Scientific Department, São Paulo Football Federation, São Paulo 01141-040, Brazil; matheus.alexandre@fpf.org.br (M.G.A.A.); lucas.tavares@fpf.org.br (L.D.T.)
* Correspondence: irineu.loturco@terra.com.br

Abstract: This study examined the effects of a short-term ballistic training program on neuromuscular performance and strength-deficit (SDef) in elite youth female soccer players. Twenty-two under-20 athletes completed a 4-week intervention during the pre-season phase, comprising 12 loaded and 8 unloaded ballistic training sessions performed at maximal intended velocity. Pre- and post-intervention assessments included vertical jumps (squat jump [SJ], countermovement jump [CMJ]), sprinting speed (5, 10, and 20 m), one-repetition maximum (1RM) and peak force (PF) in the half-squat (HS), and peak power and velocity during jump squats (JS) at 30% of 1RM. SDef was calculated as the percentage difference in PF between 1RM in the HS and 30% 1RM. Significant improvements were observed in SJ, CMJ, sprint speed, 1RM-strength, and bar-derived mechanical outputs (ES = 1.18–1.66; $p < 0.05$), with no significant changes in SDef. These results indicate that elite youth female soccer players can improve strength-, power-, and speed-related capacities without compromising force production at higher movement velocities (thus maintaining their SDef). The improvements observed likely reflect the combined effect of a high-frequency, velocity-oriented training approach and a concurrent reduction in traditional technical–tactical (i.e., soccer-specific) training volume. This is the first study to demonstrate that ballistic exercises alone—when properly structured—can enhance neuromuscular performance in female soccer players without increasing SDef. These findings provide practical guidance for practitioners aiming to optimize physical development in team-sport athletes without relying on heavier training loads or extended resistance training sessions—and, especially, without compromising their ability to apply force at higher velocities.

Keywords: team sport; women athletes; football; athletic performance; resistance training; muscle strength

1. Introduction

In team sports, optimizing neuromuscular qualities such as strength, power, and speed is essential for enhancing athletic performance [1–3]. In this context, the concept of strength deficit (SDef)—defined as the difference between an athlete's maximal force production capacity and the force applied against lighter loads at higher movement velocities—has recently emerged as a meaningful performance indicator [3–5]. While previous studies have investigated the SDef in male populations (e.g., male soccer and rugby players) [5,6], its characterization and responsiveness to training in female athletes, particularly in elite team sports such as soccer, remain unexplored.

Recent evidence in male soccer players suggests that traditional resistance training programs, specifically those relying on moderate to heavy loads (i.e., 60–90% one-repetition maximum [1RM]) [6], tend to increase maximum strength but may also lead to an increase in SDef. These adaptations could potentially impair the production of force under dynamic and high-velocity conditions that define—and are critical to—most sport-specific tasks, especially in soccer (e.g., jumping, sprinting, changing direction, and kicking) [6–8]. In contrast, ballistic exercises, performed with light and very-light loads (i.e., using only body mass [BM] as overload), particularly when executed at maximal intended velocity, have been hypothesized to maintain or even reduce SDef while still improving strength- and power-related parameters [4,6,9,10].

To date, no study has directly examined whether it is possible to improve maximum strength, peak force, movement velocity (e.g., jump squat [JS] peak velocity), power, sprint speed, and vertical jump ability without concomitantly increasing SDef in athletic populations. More importantly, no investigation has evaluated this phenomenon (i.e., changes in SDef) in female athletes. Therefore, the present study aimed to analyze the effects of a 4-week strength–power training intervention, comprising only loaded and unloaded ballistic exercises (including plyometric exercises), on a wide range of performance outcomes and SDef in elite youth female soccer players.

Based on previous findings and recommendations [6,11], we hypothesized that it would be possible to enhance strength, power, and sprint performance without an associated increase in SDef. Confirming this hypothesis could have direct implications for training prescription in high-performance sport environments, supporting the implementation of targeted interventions that minimize the unnecessary use of multiple traditional (non-ballistic) exercises and heavy loading intensities, specifically in sports where explosive actions are crucial [10,12,13].

2. Materials and Methods

2.1. Subjects

Twenty-two elite under-20 female soccer players (age: 17.3 ± 1.7 years; height: 1.65 ± 0.07 m; body mass [BM]: 62.9 ± 8.9 kg), all from the same soccer club and with at least three years of experience in systematic strength–power and plyometric training, participated in this study. These athletes competed in the "São Paulo State Championship", one of the most important Brazilian under-20 soccer competitions. The study was approved by the local Ethics Committee, and all participants—and, when necessary (i.e., for players under 18 years old), their legal guardians—signed an informed consent form prior to participation.

2.2. Study Design

This quasi-experimental study investigated the effects of a ballistic-based resistance training program on strength, power, and speed performance in under-20 female soccer players. Athletes were assessed before and after a 4-week training period, always at the same time of the day, and were properly familiarized with both the training and testing procedures. A detailed overview of the team's typical weekly training schedule during the intervention is provided in Table 1. Over the course of the training program, players completed 12 loaded ballistic sessions—including JS, jump lunges, and jump deadlifts—and 8 unloaded ballistic sessions that included traditional jumps (i.e., squat jumps (SJ) and countermovement jumps (CMJ), as well as plyometric jumps (i.e., drop jumps and hurdle jumps). Due to time constraints, the height of the boxes (used for drop jumps) and the hurdles was standardized at 30 cm. However, despite the fixed height, players were instructed to jump as high as possible in both jump types, thereby exerting maximal effort in all attempts. The training program was primarily based on previous studies that highlighted the superiority of ballistic JS, especially when performed with light loads, over traditional squats for maximizing force and power output [5,12–14], as well as the interference effects (i.e., negative impact) of high volumes of aerobic-based training (e.g., soccer-specific training) on speed–power development [11,15]. Across all training sessions, players were consistently encouraged to perform all exercises at maximal intended velocity. Physical testing followed a fixed sequence: SJ, CMJ, sprinting speed (with split times at 5, 10, and 20 m), 1RM in the half-squat (HS) exercise, and JS at 30% HS 1RM. Prior to testing, players performed a standardized warm-up that included general exercises (e.g., 10 min of moderate-paced running followed by 3 min of dynamic lower-limb stretching) and specific drills (i.e., submaximal attempts of each test).

Table 1. Typical weekly training schedule followed by the female soccer team during the 4-week intervention period.

	Monday	Tuesday	Wednesday	Thursday	Friday	Saturday	Sunday
Morning	Rest	Speed warm-up (technical drills followed by 4–6× maximal short sprints of 10–15 m) Technical training	Small-sided games #	Speed warm-up (technical drills followed by 4–6× maximal short sprints of 10–15 m) Technical training	Small-sided games #	Technical training	Friendly matches ¥
Afternoon	* Ballistic training	* Ballistic training	Unloaded jump training +	* Ballistic training	Unloaded jump training +	Rest	Rest

Note: * Resistance exercises included 4–6 sets of 4–6 repetitions of (1) jump squats, (2) alternating jump lunges, and (3) jump deadlifts performed sequentially in this order at ≈ 30% 1RM, with 2–3 min of rest between sets. + Unloaded jumps consisted of 4–6 sets of 4–6 repetitions of (1) squat jumps, (2) countermovement jumps, (3) drop jumps, and (4) hurdle jumps, performed in this order, with 2–3 min of rest between sets. Regarding the sprint bouts, players started each short sprint from a standing position, with a rest interval of 2–3 min between efforts. Sprints were performed on natural grass (i.e., a soccer field), with players wearing their own soccer shoes. All physical training sessions were performed with the same volume and intensity across the 4-week intervention. # Small-sided games involved approximately 30–35 min of total playing time, comprising 4–5 drills with 4–5 min of rest between each drill. ¥ Two friendly matches were played during the study period, scheduled on alternate Sundays.

2.3. Procedures

2.3.1. Jump Performance Assessments

Vertical jump performance was evaluated through both the SJ and CMJ protocols. During the SJ, athletes adopted a static position with knees flexed at ≈ 90° for 2 s before jumping vertically, avoiding any preparatory action. For the CMJ, athletes performed a self-selected countermovement followed by full extension of the legs, ensuring natural jumping mechanics were preserved [16]. All trials were conducted with hands placed on the hips. Each athlete performed five trials, with 15 s of rest between attempts. A contact mat (Elite Jump System; S2 Sports, São Paulo, Brazil) was used to record jump height, and the highest jump was retained.

2.3.2. Sprint Speed Testing

Sprint speed was assessed on an indoor track using electronic timing systems. Four sets of photocells (Elite Speed System; S2 Sports, São Paulo, Brazil) were placed at 0, 5, 10, and 20 m along the sprinting track. Athletes performed two maximal-effort sprints from a stationary start, positioned 0.5 m behind the initial set of timing gates. Sprint speed was computed by dividing the distance covered by the time elapsed. A rest period of 5 min was provided between sprints, and the best result was retained.

2.3.3. One-Repetition Maximum in Half-Squat Exercise

Maximum strength was assessed using the HS 1RM test, as previously described [17]. Prior to testing, players completed a standardized warm-up consisting of 5 repetitions at intensities ranging from 40% to 60% of their previously estimated 1RM, based on their most recent 1RM measurements. Three minutes after the warm-up, players were allowed up to 5 trials at approximately 70%, 80%, 90%, and >95% of the estimated 1RM to accurately determine their 1RM [17]. A 3 min rest interval was provided between each successive attempt. In all trials, athletes were instructed to move the barbell as quickly as possible during the concentric phase of the lift. Peak force (PF) was measured during the heaviest load attempts (>95% of the estimated 1RM) using a linear velocity transducer (T-Force Dynamic Measurement System; Ergotech Consulting, Murcia, Spain) sampling at 1000 Hz and attached to the Smith-machine barbell. The 1RM and PF values were normalized to the players' BM.

2.3.4. Bar-Derived Variables and SDef in the Jump Squat Exercise

Peak power (PP), peak velocity (PV), and PF were assessed during the JS exercise using a load equivalent to 30% of the HS 1RM. The assessment was performed on a Smith Machine (Hammer Strength Equipment, Rosemont, IL, USA). Players completed three maximal-effort repetitions, aiming to move the bar as fast as possible, with 15 s rest intervals between each attempt. A linear velocity transducer (T-Force Dynamic Measurement System; Ergotech Consulting, Murcia, Spain), operating at a sampling frequency of 1000 Hz, was attached to the bar to record mechanical variables. The highest PV value and its corresponding PF and PP values were recorded. All values were normalized by expressing the absolute measurements relative to each athlete's BM. SDef was calculated as the percentage difference between the PF at 30% 1RM and the PF at 1RM.

2.4. Statistical Analysis

Data are presented as means ± standard deviation. Normality was assessed using the Shapiro–Wilk test. Pre- and post-assessment comparisons were conducted using paired *t*-tests. Statistical significance was established at a threshold of $p < 0.05$. Effect sizes (ES) were determined using Cohen's d [18] and interpreted based on the criteria proposed by Rhea [19] for highly trained individuals: trivial (<0.25), small (0.25–0.50), moderate (0.50–1.00), and large (>1.00). The absolute and relative reliability of the dependent variables was evaluated using the coefficient of variation (CV) and the two-way random intraclass correlation coefficient (ICC), respectively.

3. Results

All variables demonstrated high levels of absolute and relative reliability (i.e., ICC > 0.90 and CV < 10%). Significant increases were observed in SJ and CMJ performance from pre- to post-tests (ES = 1.18 and 1.66, respectively; $p < 0.05$; Figure 1). Table 2 presents the comparisons of PV, PF, and PP measured during the JS exercise with a load corresponding to 30% 1RM, as well as relative strength, PF at 1RM, and SDef at 30% 1RM, between pre- and post-assessments. Figure 2 illustrates the sprint speed comparisons between pre- and post-tests. Significant improvements were detected at all tested distances (ES = 1.21, 1.29, and 1.37 for 5, 10, and 20 m, respectively; $p < 0.05$).

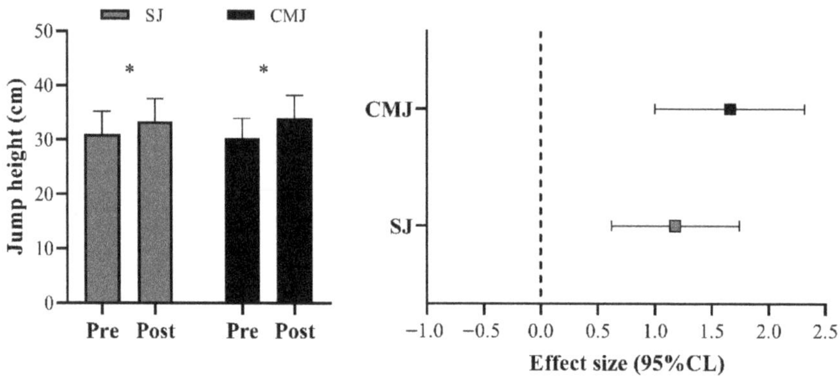

Figure 1. Comparisons of squat jump (SJ) and countermovement jump (CMJ) performance between pre- and post-tests. CL: confidence limits; * $p < 0.05$.

Table 2. Comparisons of the mechanical variables between pre- and post-intervention assessments.

	Pre	Post	p-Value	ES (95% CL)
JS PV at 30% 1RM ($m \cdot s^{-1}$)	1.96 ± 0.12	2.03 ± 0.13	<0.001	1.28 (0.69; 1.86)
JS PF at 30% 1RM ($N \cdot kg^{-1}$)	7.09 ± 0.51	7.42 ± 0.61	0.014	0.57 (0.12; 1.02)
JS PP at 30% 1RM ($W \cdot kg^{-1}$)	11.9 ± 1.4	12.9 ± 1.6	<0.001	0.90 (0.40; 1.39)
1RM rel	1.23 ± 0.13	1.39 ± 0.17	0.032	0.49 (0.04; 0.93)
PF at 1RM ($N \cdot kg^{-1}$)	47.8 ± 11.2	49.5 ± 11.2	0.076	0.40 (−0.04; 0.83)
SDef at 30% 1RM (%)	83.9 ± 6.3	83.9 ± 5.9	0.442	0.17 (−0.26; 0.59)

Note: JS: jump squat; 1RM: one-repetition maximum; PV: peak velocity; PF: peak force; PP: peak power; SDef: strength deficit; ES: effect size; CL: confidence limits.

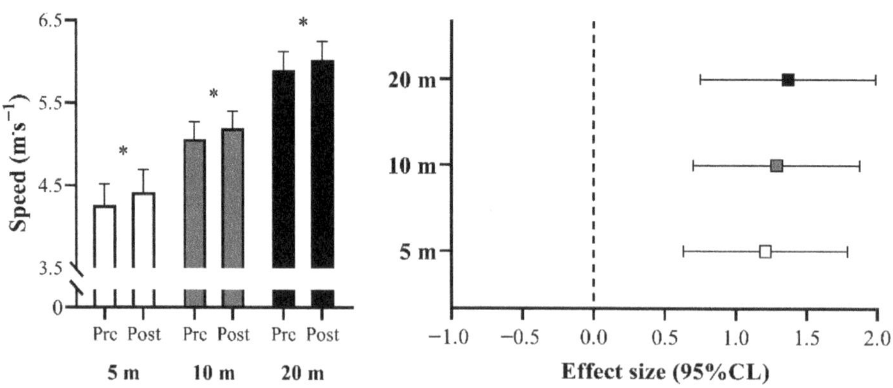

Figure 2. Comparisons of sprinting speed over the different distances tested between pre- and post-tests. CL: confidence limits; * $p < 0.05$.

4. Discussion

This study is the first to examine the effects of a short-term ballistic training program on a range of speed, power, and strength measures, as well as SDef, in elite youth female soccer players. The results demonstrate that it is indeed possible to simultaneously improve jumping ability (i.e., SJ and CMJ), sprint speed (5, 10, and 20 m), maximum strength, and force–power outputs (JS peak force, velocity, and power), without a concomitant increase in SDef during a highly demanding and congested training period such as the soccer pre-season.

Conducting intervention studies with soccer players during pre-seasons is extremely challenging due to the high volume and specific types of training required to prepare them to cope with competitive demands [6,11,15]. Additionally, the highly traditional training routines followed by coaching staff—characterized by large volumes of soccer-specific training (i.e., technical–tactical sessions) [6,11,15]—and their resistance to major or more innovative training strategies make such studies extremely rare [11]. Even rarer are those reporting consistent and meaningful improvements across a range of performance measures (especially speed and power metrics) within such short time periods (i.e., 3- to 4-week pre-seasons) [15,20–22]. Notably, during pre-seasons or other training and competitive phases (e.g., in-season), significant improvements in strength, speed, and power qualities are uncommon not only among female players but also in their male counterparts, especially under elite training conditions [15,20,23–25].

In this context, the maintenance of SDef after this 4-week intervention is particularly relevant. Previous evidence in male soccer players has shown that increases in maximum strength following traditional resistance training are frequently accompanied by an increase in SDef, suggesting that athletes tend to utilize lower percentages of their maximum force at higher velocities and against lighter loads, such as their own BM [4,6]. In contrast, the present findings demonstrate that a precise and efficient ballistic training program—emphasizing movement velocity (and lighter loads) rather than heavier loads—can improve neuromechanical performance without impairing force application at higher velocities. These results may reflect the specific design of the training protocol, which prioritized unloaded and light-loaded ballistic exercises (i.e., 20–30% 1RM), along with maximal short sprints (i.e., 10–15 m), performed at high frequency (i.e., three to four strength–power sessions and one to two sprint sessions per week).

An additional factor that likely contributed to the observed improvements in speed and power capabilities in this study was the strategic modification of the soccer-specific training schedule and volume. In close collaboration with the coaching staff, the volume of traditional soccer training (i.e., technical–tactical sessions) was deliberately reduced in favor of higher-intensity, shorter training sessions (i.e., small-sided games lasting to $\approx$ 30–35 min, divided into 4–5 drills with 4 to 5 min rest intervals between each drill). This adjustment, combined with the high frequency of speed and power training sessions, may be considered an uncommon but apparently effective strategy to adopt during soccer pre-seasons—particularly when the main purpose is to enhance neuromuscular abilities. This innovative and nontraditional training approach potentially improved most strength, speed, and power qualities in the female soccer players, without compromising their ability to apply force at higher velocities (i.e., increasing the SDef).

Although this study did not include a control group—a common limitation in investigations involving competitive athletes [23,26–28]—the consistent improvements across multiple neuromechanical variables, supported by prior intra-team seasonal data, provide compelling evidence for the efficacy of the implemented training program [11,15,23]. In previous pre-seasons or short-term studies conducted with team-sport athletes at comparable levels, performance gains—specifically in speed and power—were generally absent or even negative following standard practices characterized by high volumes of sport-specific training [11,15,23]. This marked contrast reinforces the uniqueness and practical relevance of the present findings. However, it is important to note that the current study design does not allow for the isolation of the effects resulting from reduced volumes of soccer-specific training from those associated with high-frequency ballistic training [10,11,15]. Nevertheless, these findings suggest that combining light-loaded (or even unloaded) ballistic exercises with lower volumes of technical–tactical training may be highly effective in enhancing strength, speed, and power performance in elite youth female soccer players.

This study has inherent limitations related to its quasi-experimental design. Due to the applied nature of working with elite youth female soccer players during the pre-season, it was not feasible to include a control group, as splitting the team into separate training conditions would interfere with their preparation for upcoming competitions. Although the absence of a non-training control group limits causal inferences, the significant improvements observed in neuromuscular qualities—particularly sprint speed over different distances—following a short-term ballistic training program represent highly relevant findings, as such improvements are uncommon during short soccer pre-seasons or short training phases [11,15,23,29]. In summary, this study provides valuable and practically important evidence that elite youth female soccer players can improve strength, power, speed, and jump performance without increasing SDef over a 4-week pre-season, provided that the resistance training program is strategically structured and based on ballistic- and velocity-oriented methods [6,10,13]. These results have direct implications for practitioners aiming to optimize neuromuscular capacities in elite sport settings without compromising the transfer of strength and power to sport-specific tasks. Future studies should explore the long-term effects of ballistic training across different phases of the season and compare its impact with other strength–power training strategies. Investigations including male players and employing randomized controlled designs could further support and extend the findings presented here. Additionally, examining individual response patterns may help tailor programs to optimize transfer to sport-specific performance.

5. Conclusions

This study provides novel evidence that a short-term, high-frequency ballistic training program comprising both loaded and unloaded exercises performed at maximal intended velocity can improve strength-, power-, and speed-related abilities in elite youth female soccer players without increasing SDef. From an applied perspective, these findings indicate that ballistic training strategies (e.g., JS, jump lunges, and plyometrics) using light or no external loads can be highly effective for enhancing neuromechanical qualities relevant to elite soccer performance, particularly during congested training periods such as the pre-season. When performed under these loaded (or even unloaded) conditions, ballistic exercises can improve force application at higher velocities without compromising an athlete's ability to produce force against lighter loads (i.e., increasing SDef), potentially supporting better transfer to sport-specific actions (e.g., sprinting, jumping, kicking, and dribbling). Importantly, as previously suggested [11,23], reducing the volume of traditional technical–tactical sessions in favor of shorter, high-intensity drills and speed–power-oriented sessions may optimize physical development without impairing soccer-specific preparation, provided this adjustment is well-integrated with the coaching staff. Coaches working in high-performance female soccer can effectively implement short-term ballistic training schemes to improve athletic performance, without the need for heavier loads or extended training sessions to achieve their objectives. These practical strategies may help overcome traditional barriers to neuromuscular development in elite soccer settings, where time constraints and accumulated fatigue are commonly considered limiting factors.

Supplementary Materials: The following supporting information can be downloaded at: https://www.mdpi.com/article/10.3390/sports13070237/s1.

Author Contributions: Conceptualization, I.L. and L.A.P.; Data curation, I.L. and L.A.P.; Formal analysis, I.L. and L.A.P.; Investigation, I.L., V.P.M., T.B.M.A.M., M.G.A.A., L.D.T., and L.A.P.; Methodology, I.L., V.P.M., T.B.M.A.M., M.G.A.A., L.D.T., and L.A.P.; Project administration, I.L. and L.A.P.; Supervision, I.L. and L.A.P.; Visualization, I.L., B.R., V.P.M., T.B.M.A.M., M.G.A.A., L.D.T., and L.A.P.; Writing—original draft, I.L. and L.A.P.; Writing—review and editing, I.L., B.R., and L.A.P.; All authors have read and agreed to the published version of the manuscript.

Funding: This research received no external funding.

Institutional Review Board Statement: The study was conducted in accordance with the Declaration of Helsinki and approved by the Ethics Committee of Federal University of São Paulo (protocol code 4.355.629, 22 October 2020).

Informed Consent Statement: Informed consent was obtained from all subjects involved in the study.

Data Availability Statement: The minimal dataset can be found in Supplementary Materials S1.

Conflicts of Interest: The authors declare no conflicts of interest.

References

1. McGuigan, M.R.; Wright, G.A.; Fleck, S.J. Strength training for athletes: Does it really help sports performance? *Int. J. Sports Physiol. Perform.* **2012**, *7*, 2–5. [CrossRef] [PubMed]
2. Suarez-Arrones, L.; Gonzalo-Skok, O.; Carrasquilla, I.; Asián-Clemente, J.; Santalla, A.; Lara-Lopez, P.; Núñez, F.J. Relationships between change of direction, sprint, jump, and squat power performance. *Sports* **2020**, *8*, 38. [CrossRef] [PubMed]
3. Suchomel, T.J.; Nimphius, S.; Stone, M.H. The importance of muscular strength in athletic performance. *Sports Med.* **2016**, *46*, 1419–1449. [CrossRef] [PubMed]
4. González-Badillo, J.J.; Sánchez-Medina, L.; Pareja-Blanco, F.; Rodríguez-Rosell, D. La velocidad de ejecución y el deficit de fuerza. In *Fundamentals of Velocity-Based Resistance Training*; Ergotech: Murcia, Spain, 2017; pp. 109–114.
5. Loturco, I.; Pereira, L.A.; Freitas, T.T.; Bishop, C.; Pareja-Blanco, F.; McGuigan, M.R. Maximum strength, relative strength, and strength deficit: Relationships with performance and differences between elite sprinters and professional rugby union players. *Int. J. Sports Physiol. Perform.* **2021**, *16*, 1148–1153. [CrossRef]
6. Loturco, I.; Pereira, L.A.; Bishop, C.; Zanetti, V.; Freitas, T.T.; Pareja-Blanco, F. Effects of a resistance training intervention on the strength-deficit of elite young soccer players. *Biol. Sport.* **2022**, *39*, 615–619. [CrossRef]
7. Carling, C. Interpreting physical performance in professional soccer match-play: Should we be more pragmatic in our approach? *Sports Med.* **2013**, *43*, 655–663. [CrossRef]
8. Faude, O.; Koch, T.; Meyer, T. Straight sprinting is the most frequent action in goal situations in professional football. *J. Sports Sci.* **2012**, *30*, 625–631. [CrossRef]
9. McKay, A.K.A.; Stellingwerff, T.; Smith, E.S.; Martin, D.T.; Mujika, I.; Goosey-Tolfrey, V.L.; Sheppard, J.; Burke, L.M. Defining training and performance caliber: A participant classification framework. *Int. J. Sports Physiol. Perform.* **2022**, *17*, 317–331. [CrossRef]
10. Newton, R.U.; Kraemer, W.J.; Häkkinen, K. Effects of ballistic training on preseason preparation of elite volleyball players. *Med. Sci. Sports Exerc.* **1999**, *31*, 323–330. [CrossRef]
11. Loturco, I.; Alcaraz, P.E.; Oliveira, L.P.; Tavares, L.D.; Requena, B.; Freitas, T.T.; Pereira, L.A. Challenges in speed and power development across age categories: A comparative study of female and male football players. *Biol. Sport.* **2025**, *42*, 3–9. [CrossRef]
12. Cormie, P.; McGuigan, M.R.; Newton, R.U. Developing maximal neuromuscular power: Part 2—Training considerations for improving maximal power production. *Sports Med.* **2011**, *41*, 125–146. [CrossRef]
13. McBride, J.M.; Triplett-McBride, T.; Davie, A.; Newton, R.U. The effect of heavy- vs. Light-load jump squats on the development of strength, power, and speed. *J. Strength Cond. Res.* **2002**, *16*, 75–82. [PubMed]
14. Rossetti, M.L.; Munford, S.N.; Snyder, B.W.; Davis, S.E.; Moir, G.L. The effects of multiple sets of squats and jump squats on mechanical variables. *J. Strength Cond. Res.* **2020**, *34*, 1017–1023. [CrossRef] [PubMed]
15. Loturco, I.; Pereira, L.A.; Kobal, R.; Zanetti, V.; Gil, S.; Kitamura, K.; Abad, C.C.; Nakamura, F.Y. Half-squat or jump squat training under optimum power load conditions to counteract power and speed decrements in brazilian elite soccer players during the preseason. *J. Sports Sci.* **2015**, *33*, 1283–1292. [CrossRef] [PubMed]
16. Ugrinowitsch, C.; Tricoli, V.; Rodacki, A.L.; Batista, M.; Ricard, M.D. Influence of training background on jumping height. *J. Strength Cond. Res.* **2007**, *21*, 848–852.
17. Brown, L.E.; Weir, J.P. Asep procedures recommendation i: Accurate assessment of muscular strength and power. *J. Exerc. Physiol. Online* **2001**, *4*, 1097–9751.

18. Cohen, J. (Ed.) Some issues in power analysis: Effect size. In *Statistical Power Analysis for the Behavioral Sciences*, 2nd ed.; Lawrence Erlbaum Associates: Hillsdale, NJ, USA, 1988; pp. 531–535.
19. Rhea, M.R. Determining the magnitude of treatment effects in strength training research through the use of the effect size. *J. Strength Cond. Res.* **2004**, *18*, 918–920.
20. Los Arcos, A.; Yanci, J.; Mendiguchia, J.; Salinero, J.J.; Brughelli, M.; Castagna, C. Short-term training effects of vertically and horizontally oriented exercises on neuromuscular performance in professional soccer players. *Int. J. Sports Physiol. Perform.* **2014**, *9*, 480–488. [CrossRef]
21. Meckel, Y.; Harel, U.; Michaely, Y.; Eliakim, A. Effects of a very short-term preseason training procedure on the fitness of soccer players. *J. Sports Med. Phys. Fit.* **2014**, *54*, 432–440.
22. Taylor, J.; Portas, M.D.; Wright, M.D.; Hurst, C.; Weston, M. Within-season variation of fitness in elite youth female soccer players. *J. Athl. Enhanc.* **2013**, *1*, 1–5. [CrossRef]
23. Freitas, T.T.; Pereira, L.A.; Reis, V.P.; Fernandes, V.; Alcaraz, P.E.; Azevedo, P.; Loturco, I. Effects of a congested fixture period on speed and power performance of elite young soccer players. *Int. J. Sports Physiol. Perform.* **2021**, *16*, 1120–1126. [CrossRef] [PubMed]
24. Barra-Moura, H.; Guilherme Vieira, J.; Zacaron Werneck, F.; Wilk, M.; Pascoalini, B.; Queiros, V.; Gomes de Assis, G.; Bichowska-Paweska, M.; Vianna, J.; Vilaca-Alves, J. The effect of complex contrast training with different training frequency on the physical performance of youth soccer players: A randomized study. *PeerJ* **2024**, *12*, e17103. [CrossRef] [PubMed]
25. Thomakos, P.; Spyrou, K.; Katsikas, C.; Geladas, N.D.; Bogdanis, G.C. Effects of concurrent high-intensity and strength training on muscle power and aerobic performance in young soccer players during the pre-season. *Sports* **2023**, *11*, 59. [CrossRef] [PubMed]
26. Molina, R.; Lapresa, D.; Arana, J.; Alvarez, I.; Salazar, H. Wellness and session rating of perceived exertion in professional basketball players within different weekly contexts. *J. Strength Cond. Res.* **2025**, *39*, e546–e551.
27. Carron, M.A.; Scanlan, A.T.; Doering, T.M. Quantifying the training loads and corresponding changes in physical qualities among adolescent, schoolboy rugby league players. *Sports* **2024**, *12*, 251. [CrossRef]
28. Purdom, T.M.; Levers, K.S.; Ryan, G.A.; Brown, L.; Giles, J.; McPherson, C. Female soccer periodization on anaerobic power/capacity. *J. Strength Cond. Res.* **2023**, *37*, 2405–2410. [CrossRef]
29. Oliveira, R.S.; Leicht, A.S.; Bishop, D.; Barbero-Álvarez, J.C.; Nakamura, F.Y. Seasonal changes in physical performance and heart rate variability in high level futsal players. *Int. J. Sports. Med.* **2013**, *34*, 424–430. [CrossRef]

sports

MDPI

Article

Relating Anthropometric Profile to Countermovement Jump Performance and External Match Load in Mexican National Team Soccer Players: An Exploratory Study

Israel Rios-Limas [1,2,†], Carlos Abraham Herrera-Amante [2,3,†], Wiliam Carvajal-Veitía [2,4], Rodrigo Yáñez-Sepúlveda [5], César Iván Ayala-Guzmán [2,6], Luis Ortiz-Hernández [7], Andrés López-Sagarra [8], Pol Lorente-Solá [9] and José Francisco López-Gil [10,11,*]

1 Sports Nutrition Department, Mexican Football Federation (FMF), Mexico City 50200, Mexico; irios@fmf.mx
2 Ibero-American Network of Researchers in Applied Anthropometry (RIBA), 04120 Almería, Spain; carlos.amante@academicos.udg.mx (C.A.H.-A.); wiliamcarvajal790@gmail.com (W.C.-V.); cesar.ayala@ibero.mx (C.I.A.-G.)
3 Nutritional Assessment and Nutritional Care Laboratory (LECEN), Division of Health Sciences, Tonala University Center, University of Guadalajara, Tonalá 45425, Mexico
4 Subdirectorate of Teaching and Research, Institute of Sports Medicine (IMD), Havana 10800, Cuba
5 Faculty of Education and Social Sciences, Universidad Andres Bello, Viña del Mar 252000, Chile; rodrigo.yanez.s@unab.cl
6 Health Department, Iberoamerican University, Mexico City 01219, Mexico
7 Nutrition and Physical Activity Laboratory, Metropolitan Autonomous University Campus Xochimilco, Mexico City 04960, Mexico; lortiz@correo.xoc.uam.mx
8 Sports Science Department, Mexican Football Federation (FMF), Mexico City 50200, Mexico; anlopez@fmf.mx
9 Mexico National Team, Mexican Football Federation (FMF), Mexico City 50200, Mexico; plorente@fmf.mx
10 School of Medicine, Universidad Espíritu Santo, Samborondón 092301, Ecuador
11 Vicerrectoría de Investigación y Postgrado, Universidad de Los Lagos, Osorno 5311269, Chile
* Correspondence: josefranciscolopezgil@gmail.com
† These authors contributed equally to this work.

Abstract: ***Background/Objectives:*** The role of body composition in sports performance has been widely studied, particularly in soccer. Understanding how anthropometric characteristics impact movement efficiency and neuromuscular performance is crucial for optimizing player performance. This study examined the relationship between body composition and locomotor performance in elite soccer players. ***Methods:*** Thirty-six male soccer players from the Mexican National Team participated in the study, where body composition was assessed using surface anthropometry. Players underwent tests to measure countermovement jump (CMJ) performance, sprinting speed, maximum acceleration, and distance covered during two games of the CONCACAF Nations League quarterfinals. Correlation matrices were created to identify the most significant associations, followed by generalized linear models (GLMs) to associate body composition variables with performance metrics. ***Results:*** Anthropometric profile tables were created by playing position. Higher body fat percentage (%BF) was associated with lower performance. Specifically, higher %BF was associated with slower sprint speed (B = −0.74 m/s, $p < 0.001$) and shorter distance covered (B = −4.86 m/min, $p < 0.001$). Conversely, greater muscularity, reflected by corrected girth values for the thigh and calf, was associated with improved CMJ performance. Thigh corrected girth was positively associated with concentric mean force (B = 48.85 N, $p < 0.001$), and calf corrected girth was positively associated with peak power (B = 240.50 W, $p < 0.001$). These findings underscore the importance of low body fat and high lean mass for efficient movement. ***Conclusions:*** The results highlight the critical role of body composition in enhancing soccer performance, particularly for explosive movements like jumps, sprints, and accelerations. This study suggests that monitoring and optimizing body composition should be a central focus of nutrition, training, and conditioning strategies, adapted to the specific positional demands of professional soccer.

Keywords: soccer; anthropometry; body composition; sports nutritional sciences; athletic performance

1. Introduction

The anthropometric and body composition profiles of soccer players have been widely reported across Latin American [1–4] and European samples [5–7], from youth to elite levels. These studies consistently report differences by playing position or age group. For instance, Rodríguez-Rodríguez et al. [1] and Junior et al. [2] observed that goalkeepers tend to be taller and heavier, while forwards generally present greater muscle mass. Similarly, Holway et al. [3] and Toselli et al. [5] noted that older players exhibit higher body mass, muscle mass, and bone/muscle index compared to younger counterparts. While these studies provide a comprehensive anthropometric description, to the best of our knowledge, few have directly examined the relationship between these characteristics and performance indicators such as match load or neuromuscular capacity. One exception is the work by Radzimiński et al. [6], which highlighted the relevance of further exploring how anthropometric factors may influence physical performance in competitive settings.

This gap is particularly relevant given that elite soccer is characterized by the complex interaction of physical, physiological, tactical, and contextual variables that, together, determine on-field performance. International studies developed with youth [8–10], semi-professional [11], intercollegiate [12], and professional female [13] soccer players have made significant progress in characterizing these variables. These studies reported that anthropometric parameters, body composition, and biomechanics directly influence key aspects such as sprints, vertical jumps, direction changes, power, explosive strength, metabolic capacity, and flexibility. However, the aforementioned findings were primarily observed in non-elite or female samples, and few studies have been conducted with elite soccer players [5,6]. Hence, despite these advances, many investigations lack an integrative approach incorporating indicators of functional and contextual performance, principally in elite male soccer players or during official matches. This limits a comprehensive understanding of the interactions between body structure and function.

Technologies such as the Global Positioning System (GPS) have proven essential for evaluating physical performance during training and competition. Previous studies have used this technology to analyze metrics such as total distance covered, high-intensity running, accelerations, and decelerations, as well as estimations of energy expenditure during exercise, providing a detailed and objective perspective of performance on the pitch [14–18]. Nevertheless, the relationship between body composition and speed, distance, and acceleration has not been explored in elite soccer players. In young Chilean professional soccer players [9], greater muscle mass in the lower limbs and lower body fat percentages have been associated with improved acceleration and sprint performance. In professional European soccer players [6], high-speed running distance was negatively correlated with lipid mass. In professional Greek soccer players [18], speed running was negatively related to stretch stature and body mass. In Spanish semi-professional soccer players [11], it was reported that players have morphologically distinct profiles according to playing position, which, in turn, correlates with speed, distance covered, squat jump, countermovement jump, and maximum oxygen uptake. These findings illustrate how body composition and anthropometrics relate to the competitive and positional demands of the match in non-elite athletes. Also, these findings underscore the need for further research considering a broader range of factors and their interactions with performance in elite soccer players.

International tournament data provide further context for highly trained athletes. Ju et al. [19] reported that, although no significant differences in high-intensity running distances exist between confederations such as CONCACAF, UEFA, and CONMEBOL, European players tend to outperform others in technical–tactical metrics, such as passing accuracy and line-breaking actions.

Mexico's case is especially relevant in this global context, as it is one of the top-performing teams in the CONCACAF region. Despite the recent success of the Mexican National Team—champions of the 2025 CONCACAF Nations League. The studies conducted with Mexican soccer players stem from descriptive investigations of youth [20], first division plus under 17, and under 20 [21] soccer players. Only one study was performed with Mexican National Team soccer players [4], in which anthropometric and performance indicators were studied but not correlated. Therefore, research that comprehensively addresses Mexico's club and national team's physical, physiological, and morphofunctional aspects is scarce, limiting our understanding of how these variables interact and influence performance.

This lack of integrative information has hindered the development of evidence-based training and monitoring strategies tailored to the specific characteristics of Mexican soccer players. Therefore, exploring how physical, physiological, and morphofunctional variables interact with match performance is essential to optimize sports professionals' decision-making on and off the field.

In this context, a comprehensive analysis of anthropometric, countermovement jump, and match performance variables can provide deeper insight into soccer success. Accordingly, this study addresses this knowledge gap by characterizing and analyzing the multi-dimensional relationships between these variables in elite Mexican soccer players. This will be useful in advancing scientific understanding and providing practical knowledge to enhance players' individual and collective development in an increasingly demanding competitive environment.

2. Materials and Methods

2.1. Study Design

A descriptive, cross-sectional study was conducted. Participants attended the assessment location once to collect anthropometric and countermovement jump test data. Additionally, before two FIFA match dates, players underwent performance monitoring assessments. The study followed the Strengthening Reporting of Observational Studies in Epidemiology (STROBE) guidelines [22,23].

2.2. Setting

The study was conducted during the Mexican National Soccer Team's training camp on the FIFA date heading into the Concacaf Nations League quarterfinals. The training camps took place from November 11 to 19 2024: from November 11 to 15 in San Pedro Sula, Honduras, and from November 16 to 19 at the Mexican Football Federation's (FMF) High-Performance Center (CAR, by its acronym in Spanish) in Mexico City.

The study was approved by the Research Ethics Committee of the Autonomous Metropolitan University Campus Xochimilco (code: DCBS.CD.071.21) and was registered at clinicaltrials.gov (identifier: NCT06941064). Individual information (i.e., demographic, descriptive data, and sports experience) was collected using a brief form for practical sports nutrition advice [24]. All participants provided verbal informed consent after the principal investigator thoroughly explained the study's objectives, procedures, benefits, and potential risks. Written consent could not be obtained due to personal and contractual restrictions associated with their professional clubs. Nevertheless, according to Winter and Maughan [25], the principles of informed consent may not be fully upheld in professional sports, principally when data are collected from routine measurements taken at various stages of the competition and during the off-season. However, this study was conducted using the ethical principles established in the Declaration of Helsinki [26] and international guidelines for Good Clinical Practice.

2.3. Participants

Thirty-six male soccer players from the Mexican National Team participated in the study (age: 27.3 years old [IQR: 24.2–28.4]; stretch stature: 177.9 cm [IQR: 171.3–182.9]; body mass: 77.9 kg [IQR: 71.3–82.9]; competitive sports experience: 10.4 years [IQR: 7.2–13.6]; weekly training volume: 20 h [IQR: 16.6–23.4]). All participants were members of the Mexican National Team at the time of the study and had competed in international tournaments. Specifically, 11 players (30.6%) were playing for international clubs, including England (n = 3; 8.3%), Italy (n = 2; 5.6%), Russia (n = 2; 5.6%), Belgium (n = 1; 2.8%), Greece (n = 1; 2.8%), Portugal (n = 1; 2.8%), Saudi Arabia (n = 1; 2.8%), and Denmark (n = 1; 2.8%). The remaining 25 players (69.4%) were participating in Mexico's Liga MX. Additionally, 44% of the players had competed in at least one FIFA World Cup prior to the assessment date. To determine the appropriate sample size for detecting a strong association between body composition and GPS-derived performance metrics in elite football athletes, we conducted an a priori power analysis using G*Power (version 3.1.9.7). Assuming a large effect size (Pearson's correlation coefficient, r = 0.80), a significance level (α) of 0.05, and a desired power ($1 - \beta$) of 0.80, the analysis indicated that a minimum of 25 participants would be required to detect a statistically significant correlation. This sample size is feasible within the context of a national football team cohort and ensures sufficient power to validate the hypothesized association.

Athletes who attended the assessment area during the training camps were invited to participate in the study, and those who gave verbal assent were included in the sample. Players not called up to the Mexican National Team on the above dates were excluded from the study. The timeline of the evaluations carried out is shown in Figure 1.

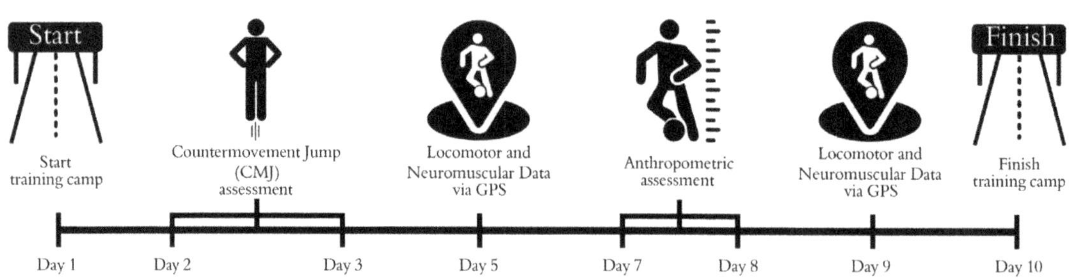

Figure 1. Timeline of assessments conducted during the 10-day training camp. The training camp began on Day 1. Countermovement jump (CMJ) assessments were conducted on Days 2 and 3 in San Pedro Sula, Honduras. Locomotor and neuromuscular data were collected via GPS during match play on Day 5 (Game 1, San Pedro Sula) and Day 9 (Game 2, Toluca, Mexico). Anthropometric assessments were performed on Days 7 and 8 at the High-Performance Center (CAR FMF), Mexico City. The camp concluded on Day 10. All assessments were scheduled to avoid interference with training and to ensure data quality and consistency.

2.4. Assessments

2.4.1. Anthropometric Measurements

Anthropometric measurements were performed by a Level 2 ISAK-certified anthropometrist, following the International Society for the Advancement of Kinanthropometry (ISAK) standards [27]. Body mass (kg) was measured using a digital scale with a precision of 50 g (SECA® 874, Hamburg, Germany). Stretch stature (cm) was assessed using a portable stadiometer with a precision of 1 mm (SECA® 217, Hamburg, Germany). Girth measurements (cm) were obtained using a non-extensible, flexible steel tape with a precision of 1 mm (Rosscraft®, Surrey, Canada). Skinfold thicknesses (mm) were measured with a skinfold caliper accurate to 1 mm (Harpenden, Holtain Ltd., Bryberian, Crymmych, Pembrokeshire). All instruments were calibrated before the measurement process.

All anthropometric variables were measured at least twice. A third measurement was taken if the difference between the first and second measurements exceeded 5% for skinfolds or 1% for any other variable. The mean value was used for data analysis when two measurements were taken. The median value was used for data analysis when three measurements were taken [27]. Intra-evaluator technical error of measurement (TEM) was calculated (25), yielding 4.06% for skinfolds and 0.89% for other variables.

2.4.2. Body Composition

Body composition was estimated using surface anthropometry. Body fat percentage (%BF), specifically lipid mass, was calculated using five predictive equations: Yuhasz [28], Sloan [29], Wilmore and Behnke [30], Durnin and Womersley [31], and Jackson and Pollock [32]. Adipose mass was then derived using the Ross and Kerr equation [33]. Meanwhile, muscle mass (MM) was estimated using two anthropometric equations: Martin et al. [34] and Lee et al. [35].

Additionally, adiposity and muscularity were analyzed using skinfold sums and corrected girths, respectively. The sum of six skin folds consisted of the triceps, subscapular, supraspinal, abdominal, thigh, and calf skinfolds. Meanwhile, the eight skinfolds' sum included the triceps, subscapular, biceps, iliac crest, supraspinal, abdominal, thigh, and calf skinfolds. Corrected girths were calculated for the arm, chest, thigh, and calf using the following equation: girth in centimeters − ($\pi \times$ skinfold in centimeters) [36]. Triceps, subscapular, anterior thigh, and calf skinfold were used to compute corrected girths. The sum of the four corrected girths was calculated.

2.4.3. Countermovement Jump

The countermovement jump (CMJ) assessments were conducted using a ForceDecks Max platform (VALD Performance, Brisbane, Australia). This allows for a detailed kinetic and temporal variables analysis through a dual high-precision platform system [37]. The assessment protocol has been previously standardized and validated [38].

After a brief warm-up, including dynamic stretches and sub-maximal jumps (five individual repetitions and two sets of five repeated CMJs), participants performed three maximum-effort CMJs at a self-selected counter-movement depth, with approximately one-minute rest intervals between each attempt. During each jump, participants were instructed to "jump as fast and as high as they could", keeping their hands on their hips. This instruction was standardized, as it influences the force-time characteristics of the CMJ.

Force data were collected at 1000 Hz and processed to obtain variables such as take-off velocity, jump height (calculated from the take-off velocity), and the modified reactive strength index (jump height divided by time to take-off). The moment of the jump was calculated as the product of take-off velocity and body mass. The average of the three attempts was used for statistical analysis.

2.4.4. Locomotor and Neuromuscular Data

Locomotor and neuromuscular external load metrics were obtained using WIMU Pro GPS tracking units operating at 10 Hz (RealTrack Systems, Almería, Spain). This system has been validated for time–motion analysis in soccer, demonstrating strong intra- and inter-unit reliability (mean velocity bias ranging from 1.18 to 1.32 km·h^{-1}; mean distance bias between 2.32 and 4.32 m; intraclass correlation coefficient > 0.93) [39]. To minimize the variability between units, each player was assigned a specific device that they used consistently throughout the data collection period. The GPS units were positioned in a vest pocket designed explicitly by the manufacturer. The devices were powered on 15 min before kickoff to ensure optimal data capture.

On average, 12.1 $\pm$ 2.4 satellites were connected during recordings, and the horizontal geometric dilution of precision was 0.57 $\pm$ 0.14—both values reflecting a high-quality GPS signal [40,41]. After each match, data were downloaded using SPro software (version 980, RealTrack Systems, Almería, Spain). All locomotor and neuromuscular variables were adjusted relative to the total match duration. The thresholds used for high-speed running and high metabolic load were >21 km·h^{-1} and >25.5 W·kg^{-1}, respectively. The variables included in the analysis were distance per minute (Distance [m/min]), maximum speed (Max speed [km/h]), number of accelerations $\geq$ 3 m·s^{-2} per minute (Acc+3/min), number of decelerations $\geq$ 3 m·s^{-2} per minute (Dec+3/min), high metabolic load distance per minute (HMLD/min), sprint distance per minute (Sprint/m), number of sprints per minute (N Sprints/m), and high-speed running per minute (HSR/min).

2.5. Study Size

A non-probabilistic convenience sampling method was used. All participants were members of the Mexican National Team at the time of the study and had competed in international tournaments. Notably, 44% had participated in at least one FIFA World Cup, and 29.7% were playing for European soccer clubs. Therefore, the sample represents Mexican elite soccer players. Moreover, according to Pituch and Stevens [42], a minimum of 15 participants is sufficient for developing reliable equation models, supporting the adequacy of the current sample size.

2.6. Statistical Methods

Statistical procedures were performed using R version 4.4.1 (R Core Team, Vienna, Austria) within the integrated development environment RStudio version 2023.06.2+561 "Mountain Hydrangea" (Posit, PBC, Boston, MA, USA).

The age, anthropometric, and body composition variables and indexes had asymmetric distributions, so the median and interquartile range (IQR) were used to describe these characteristics (Table 1). After a Kruskal–Wallis test, statistical differences between playing positions were assessed using Dunn's post hoc test with Bonferroni correction.

Due to the nature of the competition, not all participants who underwent anthropometric assessment could participate in one or both matches. This meant that the sample size differed for some analyses. Table 1 shows the information for the overall sample (n = 36), while, for subsequent analyses, only the data from active athletes during competitions were used (n = 22).

Table 1. Anthropometric characteristics of Mexican National Team soccer players for the overall sample and by playing position.

Variables	Goalkeepers (n = 4)	Lateral (Outside) Defenders (n = 5)	Central Defenders (n = 6)	Offensive Midfielders (n = 7)	Defensive Midfielders (n = 6)	Forwards (n = 8)	Overall Sample (n = 36)
	Median (IQR)	**Median (IQR)**	**Median (IQR)**	**Median (IQR)**	**Median (IQR)**	**Median (IQR)**	**Median (IQR)**
Age (y)	26.6 (24.2–31.0)	27.3 (27.2–27.9)	25.7 (23.6–27.2)	26.5 (24.8–27.7)	27.0 (24.2–29.4)	29.1 (24.2–32.8)	27.3 (24.2–28.4)
Basics							
Body Mass (kg)	83.9 * (83.5–84.9)	75.0 (72.7–76.3)	82.8 † (79.2–83.9)	69.7 *† (63.8–70.9)	74.0 (72.4–78.0)	79.5 (76.5–81.7)	77.9 (71.3–82.9)
Stretch stature (cm)	186.2 * (182.6–189.7)	177.5 (176.5–177.9)	185.7 † (183.0–189.0)	174 *† (169.5–175.1)	181.7 (177.8–184)	179.1 (176.0–184.9)	179.4 (175.4–184)
Skinfolds (mm)							
Triceps	7.1 (5.9–8.8)	6.0 (4.0–9.0)	6.0 (5.0–7.0)	5.0 (4.0–5.2)	6.5 (5.8–7.0)	5.5 (4.8–6.3)	5.6 (5.0–7.0)
Subscapular	7.1 (6.8–8.9)	8.0 (7.0–9.0)	7.5 (6.3–8.0)	7.2 (6.2–8.0)	8.5 (7.5–9.3)	8.0 (7.0–9.0)	8.0 (6.8–8.3)
Biceps	4.0 (3.8–4.0)	3.0 (3.0–4.0)	3.5 (3.0–4.0)	3.0 (3.0–3.0)	4.0 (3.8–4.3)	3.0 (3.0–3.0)	3.0 (3.0–4.0)
Iliac crest	15.0 (10.3–19.3)	8.0 (7.0–9.0)	9.5 (6.8–10.8)	8.0 (7.0–11.0)	10.0 (8.8–11.0)	9.0 (6.8–11.5)	9.0 (7.0–11.0)
Supraspinal	7.0 (6.6–8.0)	5.0 (4.0–6.0)	4.0 (3.3–5.5)	5.0 (4.0–6.0)	5.0 (4.0–5.3)	5.0 (4.8–5.2)	5.0 (4.0–6.0)
Abdominal	15.0 (11.1–18.3)	8.0 (5.8–11.0)	7.5 (6.3–8.8)	8.0 (7.0–10.2)	10.0 (9.5–11.3)	9.0 (8.0–11.0)	8.7 (7.0–11.0)
Thigh	6.2 (5.8–7.1)	6.0 (4.4–6.0)	6.0 (5.3–6.8)	5.0 (4.0–6.0)	5.5 (4.8–6.3)	5.0 (4.8–5.3)	6.0 (5.0–6.3)
Calf	4.0 (3.8–4.2)	3.2 (3.0–6.0)	5.0 (3.5–5.0)	3.2 (3.0–4.0)	6.3 (5.5–6.3)	8.5 (7.1–11.0)	4.0 (3.0–5.0)
Chest	8.7 (6.3–11.5)	5.0 (5.0–6.8)	5.0 (5.0–5.8)	6.0 (4.0–8.0)	5.5 (4.8–6.3)	6.0 (5.8–7.0)	6.0 (5.0–7.0)
Girths (cm)							
Arm (relaxed)	33.3 (32.1–34.3)	32.0 (31.5–32.5)	32.8 (32.1–33.8)	31.0 (30.5–32.0)	27.0 (26.9–27.5)	32.5 (32.0–33.1)	32.0 (31.0–33.0)
Forearm	28.8 * (28.4–29.0)	28.0 (27.5–28.2)	28.0 (27.6–28.4)	26.5 * (26.0–27.0)	27.0 (26.9–27.5)	27.8 (26.9–28.1)	27.5 (27.0–28.3)
Chest	104.0 (101.3–106.3)	100.0 (100.0–100.0)	102.8 (101.5–104.8)	98.0 (95.0–100.5)	95.3 (94.4–98.1)	103.5 (101.5–104.0)	100.8 (98.0–104.0)
Thigh (middle)	55.0 (54.9–55.4)	54.2 (53.5–55.5)	56.8 (54.9–58.6)	53.5 (52.5–54.0)	55.5 (54.3–56.4)	55.8 (55.2–58.3)	55.0 (53.9–56.1)
Calf	36.7 (36.4–37.2)	34.5 (34.5–37.0)	37.9 † (37.1–39.2)	35.2 †‡ (34.5–36.0)	36.0 (35.4–37.0)	39.0 ‡ (37.8–39.0)	37.0 (35.5–38.3)
Indexes							
BMI (kg/m^2)	24.4 (23.9–24.9)	24.1 (23.1–24.2)	23.3 (23.3–24.0)	22.4 (22.2–23.0)	23.5 (22.7–24.3)	23.9 (23.9–24.8)	23.8 (23.0–24.6)
HWR	42.6 (42.0–43.2)	42 (41.8–42.6)	43.2 (42.4–43.4)	42.4 (42.3–42.9)	42.2 (41.7–43.1)	42.4 (41.6–42.7)	42.4 (41.8–43.0)
Sum of skinfolds (mm)							
Σ 6 skinfolds §	48.0 (38.8–57.8)	37 (29.6–44.0)	36.5 (31.3–41.0)	37 (28.4–40.0)	40 (37.3–42.8)	37 (33.3–44.2)	38.5 (30.8–43.4)
Σ 8 skinfolds #	67.5 (52.8–81.5)	48.0 (39.6–57.0)	50.0 (41.3–55.0)	48.0 (38.0–54.2)	53.5 (50.8–56.5)	49 (43.0–59.7)	50.5 (39.9–59.1)
Body fat							
lipid tissue mass (%)							
Durnin and Womersley, 1974	15.4 (12.3–18.7)	10.4 (9.9–14.6)	12.1 (10.1–13.5)	11.0 (9.1–12.4)	13.4 (12.1–14.4)	11.5 (9.5–14.4)	12.3 (9.8–14.2)
Sloan, Burt, and Blyth, 1962	6.9 (6.3–7.8)	6.4 (5.7–7.2)	6.5 (5.8–6.7)	6.2 (5.1–6.7)	6.7 (6.3–7.0)	6.5 (5.9–7.9)	6.5 (5.5–7.2)
Wilmore and Behnke, 1969	12.7 (11.1–14.1)	10.1 (9.0–11.2)	10.1 (9.3–10.6)	10.1 (9.3–10.9)	10.7 (10.4–11.3)	10.3 (9.6–11.4)	10.5 (9.5–11.3)
Jackson and Pollock, 1980	8.4 (6.1–11.2)	5.3 (4.2–6.6)	5.5 (4.2–6.2)	6.3 (3.9–6.3)	6.3 (5.4–7.0)	5.4 (5.3–7.1)	5.9 (4.6–6.7)
Yuhasz, 1961	10.9 (9.5–12.3)	9.2 (8.5–10.0)	9.4 (8.6–9.9)	9.1 (8.3–9.8)	9.8 (9.5–10.0)	9.4 (8.8–10.4)	9.6 (8.5–10.3)
Adipose tissue mass (%)							
Ross and Kerr, 1991	20.5 (19.3–22.0)	17.9 (16.9–19.1)	18.2 (17.0–19.7)	18.4 (17.1–20.0)	19.4 (19.0–19.5)	18.0 (16.3–20.0)	18.8 (17.0–20.0)

Table 1. *Cont.*

Variables	Goalkeepers (n = 4)	Lateral (Outside) Defenders (n = 5)	Central Defenders (n = 6)	Offensive Midfielders (n = 7)	Defensive Midfielders (n = 6)	Forwards (n = 8)	Overall Sample (n = 36)
	Median (IQR)	Median (IQR)	Median (IQR)	Median (IQR)	Median (IQR)	Median (IQR)	Median (IQR)
Corrected girths (cm)							
Arm C.G	31.2 (30.1–31.8)	30.0 (29.7–30.2)	31.4 (30.5–31.8)	29.4 (28.6–30.7)	29.4 (28.8–30.2)	30.4 (29.8–32.0)	30.2 (29.5–31.3)
Chest C.G	100.7 (99.1–102.5)	97.8 (97.2–98.1)	100.6 (99.2–102.5)	95.7 (93.1–98.3)	92.8 (92.0–95.5)	101.2 (98.3–101.6)	98.4 (95.7–101.4)
Thigh C.G	53.3 (52.9–53.5)	52.9 (52.1–53.6)	54.9 (53.0–56.7)	51.6 (49.8–52.7)	53.8 (52.4–54.7)	54.1 (53.7–55.5)	53.5 (52.3–54.2)
Calf C.G	35.3 (35.2–35.9)	33.5 (33.1–36.1)	36.6 † (35.5–38.1)	33.9 †‡ (33.7–34.6)	35.7 (35.6–36.2)	37.7 ‡ (36.4–37.8)	35.4 (34.3–37.2)
Σ4 C.G	221.3 (217.8–224.0)	216.3 (214.5–217.4)	223.2 † (220.5–225.6)	209.5 †‡ (207.2–214.7)	211.4 (209.8–215.4)	222.2 ‡ (219.4–227.3)	217.8 (212.0–222.6)
Muscle mass (kg)							
Martin, et al., 1990	49.4 (49.2–49.8)	45.0 (43.6–47.5)	52.4 † (49.4–53.4)	42.6 †‡ (39.1–43.4)	45.5 (44.8–47.7)	49.4 ‡ (46.7–51.7)	47.5 (43.6–50.0)
Lee, et al., 2000	37.6 (36.8–37.9)	34.2 (34.0–35.0)	39.2 † (37.1–39.8)	32.6 †‡ (32.4–34.7)	34.7 (34.2–36.0)	38.2 ‡ (36.5–38.7)	35.1 (34.0–38.3)

Data are presented as the median (IQR). Statistically significant differences (adjusted $p < 0.05$) were assessed with Dunn's post hoc test (Bonferroni correction). Symbols (*, †, and ‡) denote significant differences between groups: * between goalkeepers and offensive midfielders, † between central defenders and offensive midfielders, and ‡ between offensive midfielders and forwards. § Sum of triceps, subscapular, supraspinal, abdominal, thigh, and calf skinfolds. # Sum of triceps, subscapular, biceps, iliac crest, supraspinal, abdominal, thigh, and calf skinfolds. Abbreviations: C.G, correct girth; HWR, height-to-weight ratio; BMI, body mass index.

A general exploratory correlation matrix was constructed to identify relationships among all study variables. Subsequently, draftsman plots were generated to summarize and visualize the most relevant and statistically significant correlations.

Based on the previous exploratory correlations, generalized linear models (GLMs) were developed using robust estimation methods, since the dependent variables did not follow a Gaussian distribution. The independent effect of anthropometric variables on physical performance measures, without including moderator variables, was examined with these models. Additionally, Bonferroni correction was applied across the GLMs to account for multiple comparisons. The theoretical model guiding this analytical strategy is expressed as follows:

$$Y = i_Y + \beta_1 X + \beta_2 W + \varepsilon_Y$$

where Y represents the dependent variable (e.g., jump height or energy expenditure); i_Y is the regression intercept; β_1 and β_2 are the estimated regression coefficients for the predictor variables; X is the main independent variable (e.g., stretch stature, BMI, and skinfolds sum); W represents a second predictor variable (not used as a moderator in this study); and ε_Y is the random error term.

It is worth noting that, although the model notation includes two predictors, X and W, this analysis did not incorporate interaction or moderation effects. Based on previous methodological recommendations, all models were adjusted using robust procedures to account for potential heteroscedasticity and outlier sensitivity. All models were adjusted by the athlete's age and body mass. Statistical significance was set at p-value < 0.05.

To ensure the validity of the GLMs, multicollinearity among the predictor variables was assessed using the Variance Inflation Factor (VIF). Variables with VIF values greater than 5 were carefully examined. Since no variable exceeded this threshold, multicollinearity was not considered a concern, and no further adjustments were required.

3. Results

3.1. Anthropometric Profile

Table 1 presents the anthropometric characteristics of Mexican soccer players according to their playing position.

Regarding body mass and stretch stature, goalkeepers were significantly heavier and taller than offensive midfielders ($p < 0.05$), while central defenders were also significantly taller and heavier than offensive midfielders ($p < 0.05$).

In terms of girths, goalkeepers showed significantly greater forearm girths compared to offensive midfielders ($p < 0.05$). Central defenders exhibited larger mid-calf and corrected mid-calf girths than offensive midfielders, and forwards also showed significantly higher values in these girths compared to offensive midfielders ($p < 0.05$).

As for muscularity indicators, both central defenders and forwards showed significantly greater values in the sum of four corrected girths (Σ4 C.G) and estimated muscle mass compared to offensive midfielders ($p < 0.05$).

No significant differences were found between playing positions in age; raw skinfold measurements; body mass index; waist-to-hip ratio; sum of skinfolds; body fat percentage; or corrected arm, chest, and thigh girths ($p > 0.05$).

3.2. Anthropometric Profile and CMJ Performance

The players exhibited a median jump height of 40.7 cm, with an interquartile range (IQR) of 39.8–43.9 cm. Peak power reached a median of 4434.0 W (IQR: 4028.0–4782.0), while concentric impulse was 220.9 N/s (IQR: 197.6–232.8). The median concentric force was 1619.0 N (IQR: 1531.0–1726.0), and the median concentric power was 2573.0 W (IQR: 2350.0–2679.0).

Correlations between anthropometric variables and neuromuscular performance (i.e., CMJ test data) are shown in Figure 2. Strong positive associations between body mass and all neuromuscular performance variables were observed, particularly with concentric impulse ($r = 0.92$; $p < 0.001$) and peak power ($r = 0.77$; $p < 0.001$). Additionally, the corrected calf and thigh girths and the four corrected girths sum exhibited significant positive correlations with most CMJ variables, highlighting the influence of peripheral muscle volume on force and power production. Specifically, the thigh corrected girth showed a positive and high association with concentric mean power ($r = 0.73$; $p < 0.001$) and concentric mean force ($r = 0.77$; $p < 0.001$), while the calf corrected girth had a positive and strong relationship with peak power ($r = 0.76$; $p < 0.001$) and concentric impulse ($r = 0.76$; $p < 0.001$).

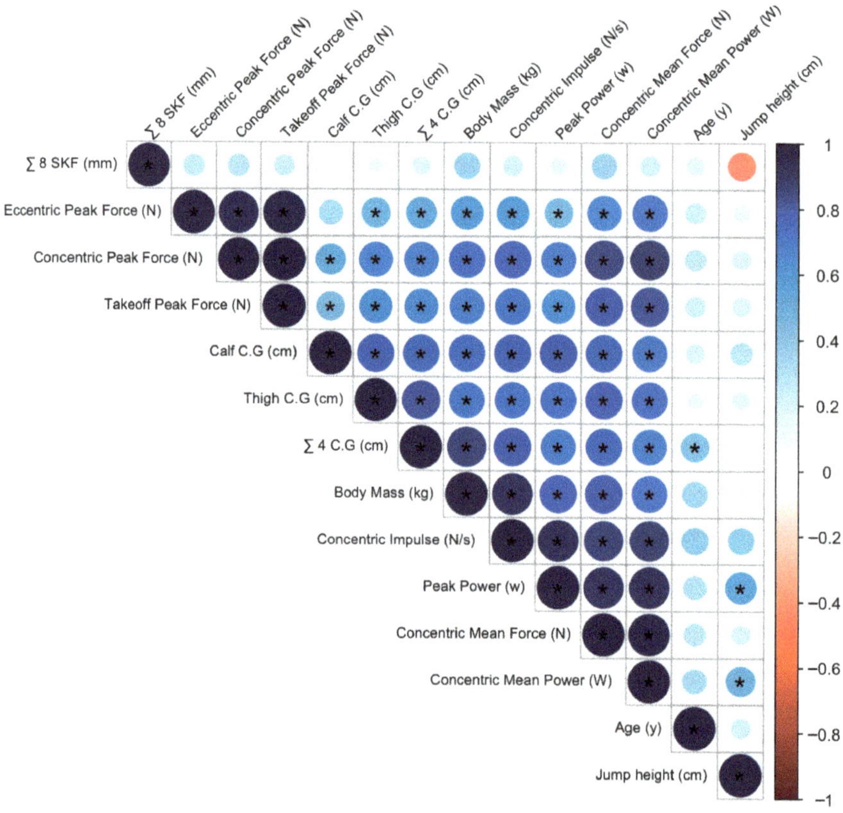

Figure 2. Draftsman correlation plot. Positive correlations are shown in blue and negative correlations in red. Color intensity and circle size are proportional to the correlation coefficients. C.G.: corrected girth; ∑: summation; SKF: skinfolds. * $p < 0.05$.

Adiposity indicators showed negative correlations with jump height. Specifically, the sum of eight skinfolds (∑8 SKF) displayed a moderate negative correlation ($r = -0.43$), which was noteworthy despite not being statistically significant ($p > 0.05$). This suggests a potential inverse relationship between subcutaneous fat and vertical jump performance, possibly due to the increased inertial load affecting explosive actions.

Finally, stretch stature also showed a positive and strong correlation with concentric impulse ($r = 0.82$; $p < 0.001$).

Given the strength and consistency of the observed correlations, particularly those involving corrected girths and neuromuscular outputs, we further explored these relationships through predictive modeling. The results of four generalized linear models (GLMs), aiming to explain CMJ performance based on key anthropometric predictors, are presented in Figure 3.

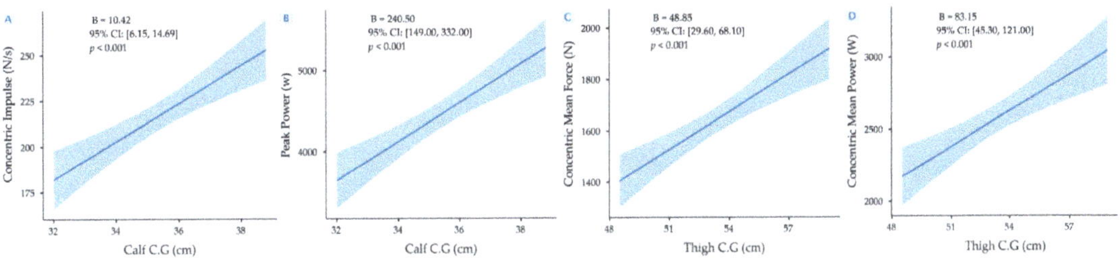

Figure 3. Generalized linear models (GLMs) showing the relationship between corrected girths (calf and thigh) and countermovement jump (CMJ) performance in players from the Mexican National Soccer Team. Models 1A and 1B use corrected calf girth as the main predictor, while Models 1C and 1D use corrected thigh girth. All models were adjusted for body mass, used robust estimation, and assumed a Gaussian distribution. Each panel displays the regression line with its 95% confidence interval (shaded area), alongside the unstandardized regression coefficient (*B*) and corresponding *p*-value. (**A**) Relationship between corrected calf girth and concentric impulse (N·s). (**B**) Relationship between corrected calf girth and peak power output (W). (**C**) Relationship between corrected thigh girth and concentric mean force (N). (**D**) Relationship between corrected thigh girth and concentric mean power (W).

Model 3A demonstrated a strong positive association between calf corrected girth (Calf C.G) and concentric impulse (N/s), indicating that greater muscle mass in the calf region may enhance force production during the jump. Specifically, each additional centimeter in calf corrected girth was associated with an increase of 10.42 N/s in concentric impulse ($B = 10.42$, 95% CI: [6.15, 14.69], $p < 0.001$).

Model 3B examined peak power (W) as the outcome variable, with calf corrected girth again emerging as a significant predictor. The results showed that each centimeter increase in this corrected girth was associated with an estimated increase of 240.50 W in peak power output ($B = 240.50$, 95% CI: [149.00, 332.00], $p < 0.001$), reinforcing the relevance of lower limb girth in explosive performance.

In Model 3C, thigh corrected girth (Thigh C.G) was significantly associated with concentric mean force, with an increase of 48.85 N per centimeter of thigh girth ($B = 48.85$, 95% CI: [29.60, 68.10], $p < 0.001$). This finding suggests that thigh musculature may also play a crucial role in force development during CMJ.

Finally, Model 3D revealed that thigh corrected girth was positively associated with concentric mean power (W), with each additional centimeter corresponding to an increase of 83.15 W ($B = 83.15$, 95% CI: [45.30, 121.00], $p < 0.001$).

3.3. Anthropometric Profile and Players' Locomotor and Neuromuscular Data

In terms of external load variables derived from GPS, players covered a median distance of 98.8 m/min (IQR: 90.1–105.2), with a maximum speed of 29.8 km/h (IQR: 28.8–30.9). The frequency of accelerations > 3 m/s^2 was 0.6 per minute (IQR: 0.4–0.7), while decelerations >3 m/s^2 occurred at a frequency of 0.7 per minute (IQR: 0.5–0.9). The distance covered at high intensity (HMLD) was 16.9 m/min (IQR: 13.8–20.0), with a median of 1.9 sprints per minute (IQR: 1.2–3.0), 0.1 sprint efforts per minute (IQR: 0.1–0.2), and 4.4 m/min of high-speed running (HSR) (IQR: 3.1–6.0). These external load metrics provide a detailed picture of the players' locomotor performance, which is crucial for understanding their neuromuscular capabilities.

Principal correlations between anthropometric profile and players' locomotor and neuromuscular data (i.e., GPS data) are shown in Figure 4. Age demonstrated a consistent and meaningful association with all eight performance variables. Specifically, older players covered less distance per minute ($r = -0.56$; $p = 0.006$), attained lower maximum speed ($r = -0.67$; $p < 0.001$), and accumulated less high metabolic load distance ($r = -0.75$; $p = 0.001$).

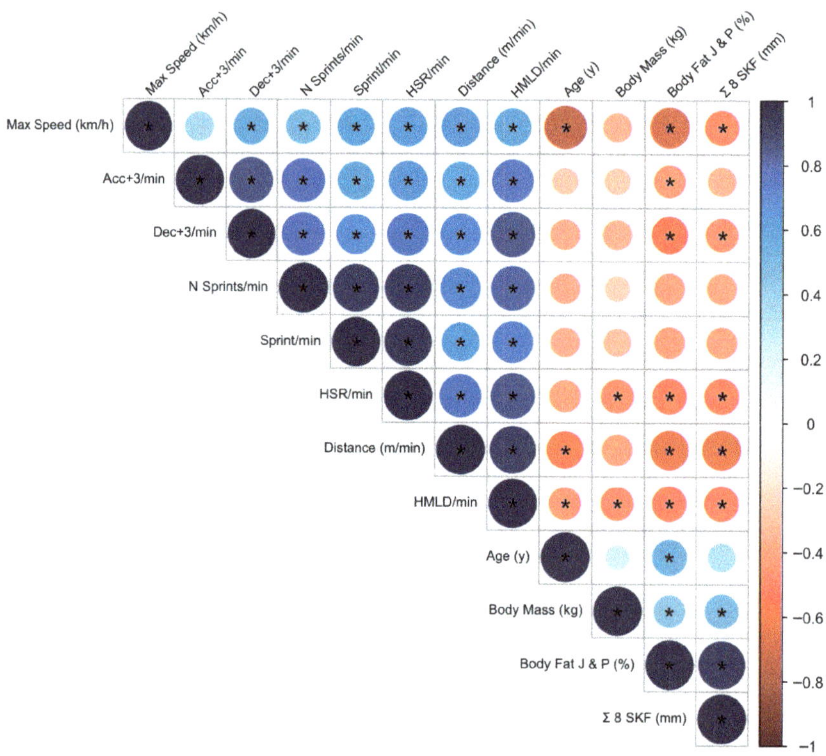

Figure 4. Draftsman correlation plot. Positive correlations are shown in blue and negative correlations in red. Color intensity and circle size are proportional to the correlation coefficients. J and P; Jackson and Pollock's predictive equation; ∑: summation; SKF: skinfolds. * p <0.05.

Anthropometric indicators of adiposity, namely, the sum of six skinfolds (∑6SKF), the sum of eight skinfolds (∑8SKF), and body fat percentage estimated via Jackson and Pollock's predictive equation [32] also exhibited relevant correlations. Among these, %BF Jackson displayed the strongest and most consistent inverse associations. For example, a higher %BF was associated with reduced match performance in distance per minute ($r = -0.63$; $p = 0.001$), maximum speed ($r = -0.62$; $p = 0.002$), decelerations ($r = -0.57$; $p = 0.005$), and high-speed running ($r = -0.53$; $p = 0.011$). Similarly, sprint-related metrics such as sprint frequency ($r = -0.47$; $p = 0.028$) and number of sprints ($r = -0.47$; $p = 0.027$) also showed significant negative correlations with %BF.

Although ∑6SKF and ∑8SKF demonstrated slightly weaker associations, notable relationships were still observed. For instance, ∑6SKF was negatively correlated with high-speed running ($r = -0.52$; $p = 0.012$) and HMLD per minute ($r = -0.49$; $p = 0.021$), while ∑8SKF showed similar trends ($r = -0.52$; $p = 0.012$ for both).

To further understand the predictive power of body fat on match performance, eight generalized linear models (GLMs) were developed, as illustrated in Figure 5.

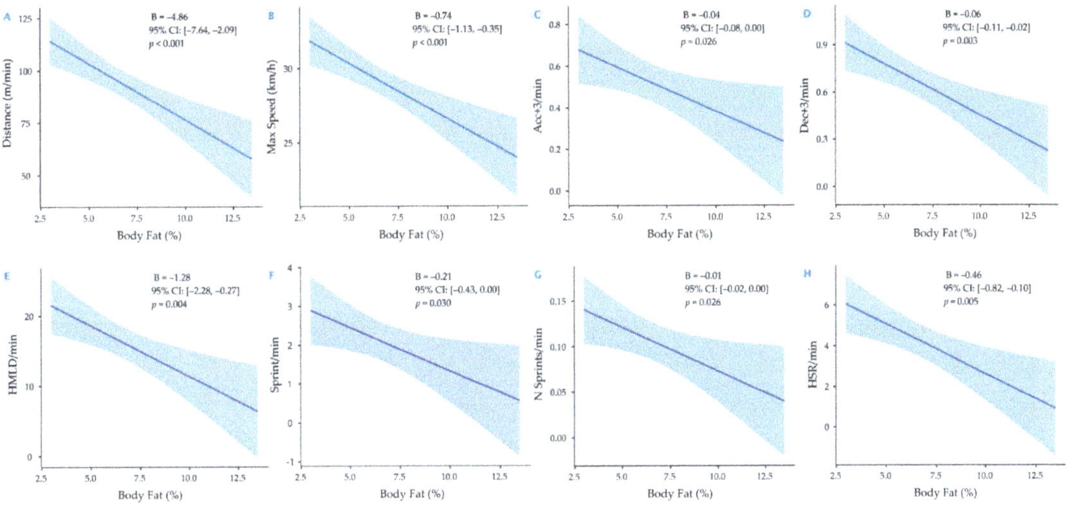

Figure 5. Generalized linear models (GLMs) showing the relationship between body fat percentage (estimated via the Jackson and Pollock equation) and GPS-derived external match load variables in Mexican National Team soccer players. All models included body fat (%) as the main predictor and were fitted using robust estimation and a Gaussian distribution. Each panel displays the regression line with its 95% confidence interval (shaded area), alongside the unstandardized regression coefficient (B) and corresponding p-value. (**A**) Distance per minute. (**B**) Maximum speed. (**C**) Number of accelerations > 3 m/s^2 per minute. (**D**) Number of decelerations > 3 m/s^2 per minute. (**E**) High metabolic load distance per minute. (**F**) Sprint distance per minute. (**G**) Number of sprints per minute. (**H**) High-speed running per minute.

Model 5A showed a strong negative association between body fat percentage and in-match distance covered per minute, indicating that higher adiposity may impair players' locomotor efficiency during a match. Specifically, each 1% increase in body fat was associated with a decrease of 4.86 m per minute ($B = -4.86$, 95% CI: [−7.64, −2.09], $p < 0.001$).

Model 5B examined maximal sprint speed as the outcome variable. Each 1% increase in body fat led to a reduction of 0.74 m/s in sprint speed ($B = -0.74$, 95% CI: [−1.13, −0.35], $p < 0.001$), suggesting that higher adiposity is linked to a lower maximal velocity capacity.

Model 5C focused on high-intensity accelerations (>3 m/s^2), with each 1% increase in body fat associated with 0.04 fewer accelerations per minute ($B = -0.04$, 95% CI: [−0.08, 0.00], $p = 0.026$).

Model 5D mirrored this trend for decelerations of similar intensity, revealing a decrease of 0.06 per minute for every 1% increase in body fat ($B = -0.06$, 95% CI: [−0.11, −0.02], $p = 0.003$). These results suggest that excessive body fat may hinder the frequency of explosive neuromuscular actions.

Model 5E showed a significant negative relationship between body fat percentage and high metabolic load distance (HMLD) per minute, with a 1.28-m reduction for every 1% increase in fat ($B = -1.28$, 95% CI: [−2.28, −0.27], $p = 0.004$).

Model 5F revealed that the number of sprints per minute declined by 0.21 with each 1% increase in lipid mass ($B = -0.21$, 95% CI: [−0.43, 0.00], $p = 0.030$), reinforcing the limiting impact of adiposity on repeated high-intensity efforts.

Model 5G addressed the total sprint frequency across the match. Each 1% rise in body fat was associated with 0.01 fewer sprints overall ($B = -0.01$, 95% CI: [−0.02, 0.00], $p = 0.026$).

Lastly, model 5H revealed a decline of 0.46 m per minute in high-speed running for each 1% increase in lipid mass ($B = -0.46$, 95% CI: [−0.82, −0.10], $p = 0.005$), further underscoring the detrimental influence of adiposity on repeated sprint and high-velocity actions.

4. Discussion

4.1. Characteristics of the Anthropometric Profile

The main findings of this study revealed significant differences in physical characteristics across positions, highlighting how these are adapted to the specific demands of each role in the game. Goalkeepers stood out due to their higher body mass, stretch stature, and girths, reflecting their need for stability and control in physical contact situations. Additionally, this group exhibited the highest body fat percentages and estimated muscle mass, attributes linked to the demands of their position. In contrast, offensive midfielders were characterized by lower body mass, stretch stature, skinfold thickness, and girths. This profile aligns with their tactical role, which requires high agility and dynamism.

The lateral and central defenders showed specific positional differences in body mass and girths, reflecting physical adaptations related to their contact and coverage functions.

A comparison between the results of this study and an anthropometric study conducted on Mexican national team players who participated in the 2002 Korea/Japan World Cup [4] highlighted the following points of comparison. The players in this study had higher average values for body mass (77.9 vs. 74.0 kg) and stretch stature (179.4 vs. 175.0 cm). Regarding body composition, the footballers in this study showed a lower body fat percentage (5.9 vs. 10.0%) compared to those evaluated 23 years ago in the pre-competitive stage leading up to the aforementioned World Cup. It is important to note that the average estimate for body fat percentage in the 2002 sample was derived from the same Jackson and Pollock equation used in this study. Therefore, based on an average extrapolation, current players have higher muscle mass and lean body mass, with an average of 3.9 kg more body mass.

The differences between the previous study and this one were significant. The previous research did not differentiate playing positions, while the current study clearly distinguishes physical characteristics by position, also incorporating specific indicators such as corrected thigh and leg girths, which emphasize the importance of peripheral muscle development in locomotor performance.

Most of the publications describing the anthropometric profile of soccer players at the international level have focused on players from lower categories at the state level [5] or from the first division in different countries [6–9,43,44]. Compared to 184 Italian players from Serie A studied by Petri et al. [9], the Mexican players in this sample had a shorter stretch stature (Mex: 179.9 cm vs. Ita: 183.9 cm), lower average body mass (Mex: 76.8 kg vs. Ita: 79.2 kg), a lower sum of eight skinfolds (Mex: 51.5 mm vs. Ita: 59 mm), and a similar BMI (Mex: 23.6 kg/m^2 vs. Ita: 23.3 kg/m^2).

In comparison to first division players from Brazil and Argentina, the Mexican soccer players showed similar characteristics in terms of average body mass and stretch stature for each playing position [7,8]. Qualitatively, goalkeepers consistently had higher body mass and stretch stature than other positions, while offensive midfielders showed the lowest values. Quantitatively, the Mexican goalkeepers in the sample analyzed (186.2 cm and 84.5 kg) were in the intermediate range compared to Brazilian goalkeepers (188.1 cm and 88.7 kg) and Argentine goalkeepers (185.4 cm and 83.7 kg). Similarly, the Mexican offensive midfielders (173.5 cm and 68.6 kg) had morphological characteristics similar to those of Brazilian players (176.4 cm and 71.9 kg) and Argentine players (173.2 cm and 71.6 kg). These findings suggest that, while there are slight differences between countries, the anthropometric dimensions of Mexican soccer players do not differ substantially from those reported in the leading South American leagues.

However, despite the clear similarities between the players studied and those from these two countries, football is one of the sports with the greatest morphological variability at the international level, even within each playing position. While there are certain trends within positions according to their function, the variability within each is considerably wide [45]. For example, among the players who participated in the 2018 World Cup in Russia, goalkeepers had stretch stature and body mass variability ranges from 178 to 201 cm and 70 to 98 kg, defenders from 167 to 200 cm and 61 to 99 kg, midfielders from 165 to 197 cm and 59 to 90 kg, and forwards from 168 to 197 cm and 61 to 98 kg. This suggests that anthropometric demands may not contribute significantly to the variance associated with success, as occurs in sports like basketball, which is more dependent on absolute stretch stature [46].

The sum of skinfolds was another variable in which Mexican players showed lower average values (38.5 mm) compared to Argentine footballers (50.9 mm), considering the sum of six skinfolds in both cases. Similarly, when analyzing the sum of eight skinfolds, the Mexican players' averages (50.5 mm) were lower than those reported for Italian players (51.3 mm), all belonging to first division teams in their respective countries. It is worth mentioning that this research not only presents the sum of skinfolds but also provides reference values obtained through various equations for estimating body fat percentage, which will allow for broader comparisons with other populations of footballers in future studies. This characteristic constitutes one of the strengths of this work [20–30].

Most of the internationally known equations in the sports field have been validated in different countries using DXA, although not all studies have yielded the same results. This highlights the principle of population specificity and the need to employ various equations in the study of population groups, as in this research [47–49]. In Mexico, the equations by Oliver, Ball, Civar, and Wilmore were the most accurate for estimating body fat percentage (BF%) compared to DXA in male professional footballers [47]. In Colombia, the body fat percentage calculation using the five-site split and the Durnin and Womersley equation most closely matched the results obtained with DXA in professional Colombian soccer players [48]. In Spanish first division players, the best field equation for assessing body fat percentage was based on iliac crest and triceps skinfolds, as well as the sum of triceps, subscapular, suprailiac, and abdominal skinfolds, since this combination also showed a good correlation with DXA [49].

4.2. Associations Between Anthropometric Profile and Neuromuscular Performance

Neuromuscular performance, particularly in tasks requiring explosiveness such as jumping, has been widely investigated in sports science. A notable example is the study by Gutiérrez and Monrroy [4], who assessed the Mexican national soccer team prior to their participation in the FIFA World Cup Korea/Japan 2002, reporting an average vertical jump height of 45 ± 8 cm. This finding highlights the relevance of explosive capacities in elite-level soccer players.

In line with this approach, the present study also evaluated neuromuscular performance in a sample of 22 soccer players using the countermovement jump (CMJ) test, yielding an average jump height of 41.65 ± 3.41 cm. It is worth noting that, due to methodological differences between tests, the values obtained via CMJ may have been higher if the traditional vertical jump protocol used in 2002 had been applied.

Beyond jump height, this study adopted a more integrative perspective of neuromuscular performance by identifying significant associations between corrected muscle girths and strength and power variables such as concentric impulse ($r = 0.92$; $p < 0.001$) and peak power ($r = 0.77$; $p < 0.001$). These results are consistent with an association between muscular development and explosive performance.

These findings align with the observations of Ramírez-Munera et al. [13], who highlighted that greater muscle volume significantly enhances performance in explosive actions. Additionally, a negative correlation was observed between the sum of eight skinfolds (Σ8 Skinfolds) and jump height ($r = -0.43$), which, although not statistically significant, provides theoretical evidence of the potential impact of adiposity on neuromuscular performance.

This result is consistent with the hypothesis that a higher lipid mass may be associated with an increased inertial load, as noted by authors such as Toro-Román et al. [11]. However, the lack of statistical significance may be due to the limited sample size or the need for more position-specific analyses.

Furthermore, a positive correlation was identified between stretch stature and concentric impulse ($r = 0.82$; $p < 0.01$), suggesting that players with greater limb length may benefit from more favorable mechanics to generate force during take-off. This association is consistent with the findings reported by Bustamante-Garrido et al. [9], reinforcing the link between biomechanics and performance in disciplines that demand explosive abilities.

4.3. Associations Between the Anthropometric Profile and Locomotor Performance

Body fat percentage (%BF) is associated with differences in the locomotor performance of soccer players, particularly when considering metrics obtained through GPS monitoring. In this study, significant negative associations were identified between %BF and key variables such as distance covered per minute ($B = -4.86$, $p < 0.001$) and maximum sprint speed ($B = -0.74$, $p < 0.001$). These results indicate that higher levels of adiposity are associated with reduced locomotor efficiency and, consequently, the players' tactical responsiveness during match play.

These findings are consistent with those reported by Enes et al. [50], who concluded that a lower proportion of body fat, together with better aerobic system development, is associated with superior sprint performance—underscoring the importance of the anthropometric profile in meeting the demands of modern soccer.

Additionally, it was observed that an increase in %BF was associated with a reduced ability to perform accelerations above 3 m/s^2 ($B = -0.04$, $p = 0.026$) and rapid decelerations ($B = -0.06$, $p = 0.003$). These results support the findings of Daly et al. [51], who reported that players with lower body fat percentages were able to sustain a higher number of high-intensity sprints during a match.

From a tactical standpoint, these limitations are especially relevant for positions such as wingers or forwards, who rely on explosive actions to gain advantages in tight spaces or rapid transitions. Consequently, body composition management emerges not only as a matter of health and fitness but also as a strategic tool for optimizing soccer performance.

4.4. Relevance of the Mathematical Model and Comparison with Other Approaches

The implementation of generalized linear models (GLMs) with robust estimation and adjustment for key variables such as body mass and age represents one of the main methodological contributions of this study. This approach not only reduces the influence of outliers and heteroscedasticity issues but also ensures that the observed associations are statistically robust and representative of the specific context of the players evaluated.

Unlike previous approaches, such as that proposed by Fields et al. [52], which incorporate mixed metrics or lack individualized adjustments, the model used in this study focuses exclusively on objective and standardized variables. This provides a framework for exploring associations between adiposity indicators (Σ8 skinfolds and %BF) and specific locomotor metrics such as HMLD/min and HSR/min. This approach yielded findings of high practical utility for monitoring and intervention in professional sports contexts.

Adjusting for age and body mass provides the model with a particular sensitivity to detect differences within a restricted and homogeneous group, such as the Mexican national team. In contrast to broader but less personalized studies, such as that of Daly et al. [50], this methodology enables the extraction of relevant individual-level patterns and the generation of specific recommendations for designing physical and nutritional interventions.

The results show that body fat percentage (%BF) has a significant negative association with various locomotor metrics. For example, the distance covered per minute yielded a coefficient of $B = -4.86$ (95% CI: [−7.64, −2.09], $p < 0.001$), indicating that, for each additional unit of %BF, players cover, on average, 4.86 m per minute. This finding underscores how higher adiposity levels compromise movement efficiency and are associated with differences in player involvement in offensive and defensive transitions.

Previous studies support this association. Varley et al. [53], for instance, reported that increased leg cell mass positively correlates with metrics such as total distance covered ($r = 0.44$), accelerations ($r = 0.45$), and decelerations ($r = 0.49$), suggesting that body composition is associated with differences in locomotor efficiency. Similarly, Şahin and Sanioğlu [54], in their analysis of 63 amateur Turkish footballers, observed that increases in %BF negatively affected 10- and 15-m sprint distances and acceleration, explaining up to 9.4% of the variance in performance.

From a tactical perspective, these locomotor limitations have clear implications. Positions such as wingers and attacking midfielders require a high capacity for sustained movement to generate passing lanes, support transitions, and apply high pressure. An elevated %BF may restrict these functions, reducing the player's tactical effectiveness. In this regard, Kapteijns et al. [55] emphasized that soccer players with more efficient body composition profiles tend to perform a greater number of high-intensity actions, particularly in roles that demand constant dynamism.

Additionally, the study showed that a higher %BF is associated with lower maximum sprint speed ($B = -0.74$, 95% CI: [−1.13, −0.35], $p < 0.001$), which is associated with a reduced ability to compete in one-on-one duels or recover defensive positions. These results are consistent with those of Ishida et al. [12], who found significant correlations between %BF and 10-m sprint times ($r = -0.45$ to -0.53) and 20-m sprint times ($r = -0.40$ to -0.49), reinforcing the notion that body fat is a limiting factor in explosive soccer performance.

4.5. Strengths and Limitations

This study presents several methodological and analytical strengths that enhance the validity of its findings. First, internationally validated methods were used to estimate body composition, including specific equations and comparative metrics according to playing position. This methodological diversity enables a more accurate, contextualized, and applicable assessment across different player profiles within soccer. Additionally, the consideration of anthropometric differences by playing position provides relevant insights into the specific physical demands imposed by each role on the field, which can inform both training program design and talent identification and development processes.

Another notable strength lies in the statistical robustness of the analytical approach employed. The mathematical model is based on generalized linear models (GLMs) with robust estimation controls for the influence of outliers and heteroscedasticity, thereby increasing the reliability of the observed associations. This type of analysis facilitates the identification of consistent and clinically meaningful patterns, even in moderate sample sizes such as the one used in this study.

However, certain limitations should also be acknowledged. The relatively small sample size and its restriction to Mexican players limit the generalizability of the results to other populations or competitive levels. This means that, although the findings are robust within the specific context analyzed, caution is required when extrapolating them to different settings, such as European leagues or youth categories. Moreover, the exclusion of interaction terms from the model limits the exploration of potential combined effects between key variables, such as the interaction between playing position and body fat percentage. This limitation reduces the model's capacity to capture the inherent complexity of soccer performance.

Lastly, the cross-sectional nature of the study prevents the observation of longitudinal changes in anthropometric profiles and performance over time. Incorporating a longitudinal analysis would enable a more comprehensive evaluation of the effects of training, competitive load, and other contextual variables on body composition and locomotor metrics.

4.6. Practical Implications

The models developed in this study suggest that optimal body composition—particularly, lower adiposity and well-developed lower limb musculature—is associated with enhanced locomotor and neuromuscular performance in soccer.

This finding highlights the importance of implementing individualized training and nutritional strategies tailored to the specific demands of each playing position. Furthermore, the use of generalized linear models (GLMs) allowed for a clear identification of these relationships, reinforcing the value of regular body composition monitoring as a potential indicator for tailoring strategies to support physical and tactical performance.

5. Conclusions

This study provides solid evidence of the influence of body composition on the athletic performance of soccer players. The results highlight position-specific differences in the anthropometric profiles of professional players. Furthermore, this exploratory analysis identified general associations between adiposity, GPS-derived metrics, and neuromuscular capacity. Although these associations were not examined by playing position due to sample size limitations, they provide valuable insights for performance monitoring and optimization. The findings emphasize the importance of tailoring dietary, training, and strategic programs to positional and tactical demands, thereby supporting a comprehensive approach to maximize individual efficiency and performance.

Author Contributions: Conceptualization, I.R.-L., C.A.H.-A. and J.F.L.-G.; Methodology, W.C.-V. and C.A.H.-A.; Software, A.L.-S. and P.L.-S.; Validation, L.O.-H.; Formal analysis, C.A.H.-A. and R.Y.-S.; Investigation, I.R.-L., C.A.H.-A., W.C.-V., R.Y.-S., A.L.-S. and P.L.-S.; Resources, A.L.-S. and P.L.-S.; Data curation, I.R.-L., C.A.H.-A. and W.C.-V.; Writing—original draft preparation, I.R.-L., C.A.H.-A., C.I.A.-G., R.Y.-S. and L.O.-H.; Writing—review and editing, I.R.-L., C.A.H.-A., W.C.-V., J.F.L.-G., C.I.A.-G. and L.O.-H.; Visualization, C.A.H.-A. and W.C.-V.; Supervision, I.R.-L. and C.A.H.-A.; Project administration, I.R.-L. and C.A.H.-A.; Funding acquisition, J.F.L.-G. All authors have read and agreed to the published version of the manuscript.

Funding: This research received no external funding.

Institutional Review Board Statement: The study was conducted in accordance with the Declaration of Helsinki and approved by the Research Ethics Committee of the Universidad Autónoma Metropolitana, Xochimilco Campus (protocol code: DCBS.CD.071.21; date: 9 March 2021).

Informed Consent Statement: Informed consent was obtained from all participants involved in the study. Due to personal and contractual restrictions with their professional clubs, written consent could not be obtained. This procedure was approved by the Research Ethics Committee, considering the occupational nature of professional sports.

Data Availability Statement: The original contributions presented in this study are included in the article. Further inquiries can be directed to the corresponding author(s).

Acknowledgments: The authors extend their heartfelt thanks to the soccer players, as well as to the coaching and medical staff, of the Mexican National Football Team for their participation and support. We are also deeply grateful to the Mexican Football Federation (FMF) for its openness and unwavering backing throughout the research process. Their confidence in our work and in the role of science in advancing the field of sports—both nationally and internationally—was essential to the completion of this study. In particular, we acknowledge Víctor Manuel Aguado, Director of Institutional Services at the FMF, for his dedication to the advancement of sports and his valuable contribution to the continued development of our national teams.

Conflicts of Interest: The authors declare no conflicts of interest. However, it is noted that I.R.-L., A.L.-S. and P.L.-S. are currently part of the coaching staff of the Mexican National Football Team. This relationship is declared to ensure transparency.

Abbreviations

The following abbreviations are used in this manuscript:

ISAK	International Society for the Advancement of Kinanthropometry
CMJ	Countermovement Jump
GPS	Global Positioning System
DXA	Dual-Energy X-ray Absorptiometry
GLM	Generalized Linear Model
%BF	Percent Body Fat
MM	Muscle Mass
HSR	High-Speed Running
HMLD	High Metabolic Load Distance
TD	Total Distance

References

1. Rodríguez-Rodríguez, F.; López-Fuenzalida, A.; Holway, F.; Jorquera-Aguilera, C. Diferencias antropométricas por posición de juego en futbolistas profesionales chilenos [Anthropometric differences per playing position in Chilean professional footballers]. *Nutr. Hosp.* **2019**, *36*, 846–853. [PubMed]
2. Junior, E.V.S.; Cavalcanti, I.F.; Santos, C.F.; Prazeres, T.M.P.; Gomes, W.S.; de Sousa Fernandes, M.S.; da Silva, J.F.; Gonçalves, J.G.; Santos, M.A.M.D.; Henrique, R.D.A. Anthropometry and Body Composition of Elite Brazilian Soccer Players according to the Playing Position. *Health Sci. J.* **2021**, *15*, 819.
3. Holway, F.; Campa, F.; Petri, C.; Pincella, M.; Ortega-Gallo, P.; Forchino, F.; Kirkendall, D. Kinanthropometry and Anatomical Body Composition of Elite Soccer Players in Argentina: The FUTREF Project. *Int. J. Kinanthrop.* **2024**, *4*, 62–71. [CrossRef]
4. Gutiérrez, C.R.; Monroy, S.E. Anthropometric and physiological characteristics in elite soccer players. *Arch. Med. Deporte* **2005**, *22*, 33–37.
5. Toselli, S.; Grigoletto, A.; Mauro, M. Anthropometric, body composition and physical performance of elite young Italian football players and differences between selected and unselected talents. *Heliyon* **2024**, *10*, e35992. [CrossRef]
6. Radzimiński, Ł.; Szwarc, A.; Padrón-Cabo, A.; Jastrzębski, Z. Correlations between body composition, aerobic capacity, speed and distance covered among professional soccer players during official matches. *J. Sports Med. Phys. Fit.* **2020**, *60*, 257–262. [CrossRef]
7. Petri, C.; Campa, F.; Holway, F.; Pengue, L.; Arrones, L.S. ISAK-Based Anthropometric Standards for Elite Male and Female Soccer Players. *Sports* **2024**, *12*, 69. [CrossRef]
8. Bongiovanni, T.; Trecroci, A.; Cavaggioni, L.; Rossi, A.; Perri, E.; Pasta, G.; Iaia, F.M.; Alberti, G. Importance of anthropometric features to predict physical performance in elite youth soccer: A machine learning approach. *Res. Sports Med.* **2021**, *29*, 213–224. [CrossRef]

9. Bustamante-Garrido, A.; Aedo-Muñoz, E.; Brito, C.; Silva-Esparza, D.; Pérez-Contreras, J.; Izquierdo-Redin, M.; Cerda-Kohler, H. Anthropometric and mechanical factors determining sprint in young soccer players: A brief report. *Front. Sports Act. Living* **2024**, *6*, 1480973. [CrossRef]
10. Pérez-López, A.; Sinovas, M.C.; Álvarez-Valverde, I.; Valades, D. Relationship between body composition and vertical jump performance in young Spanish soccer players. *J. Sport Hum. Perf.* **2015**, *3*, 1–12.
11. Toro-Román, V.; Grijota, F.J.; Muñoz, D.; Maynar-Mariño, M.; Clemente-Gil, S.; Robles-Gil, M.C. Anthropometry, Body Composition, and Physical Fitness in Semi-Professional Soccer Players: Differences between Sexes and Playing Position. *Appl. Sci.* **2023**, *13*, 1249. [CrossRef]
12. Ishida, A.; Travis, S.K.; Stone, M.H. Associations of Body Composition, Maximum Strength, Power Characteristics with Sprinting, Jumping, and Intermittent Endurance Performance in Male Intercollegiate Soccer Players. *J. Funct. Morphol. Kinesiol.* **2021**, *6*, 7. [CrossRef] [PubMed]
13. Ramírez-Munera, M.; Arcusa, R.; López-Román, F.J.; Ávila-Gandía, V.; Pérez-Piñero, S.; Muñoz-Carrillo, J.C.; Luque-Rubia, A.J.; Marhuenda, J. Relationship Between Anthropometric Profile, Body Composition, and Physical Performance in Spanish Professional Female Soccer Players at Pre-Season Onset: A Cross-Sectional Study. *J. Funct. Morphol. Kinesiol.* **2025**, *10*, 79. [CrossRef] [PubMed]
14. McEwan, G.P.; Drobnic, F.; Lizarraga, A.; Gómez-Díaz, A.; Pons, E.; Dello Iacon, A.; Unnithan, V. Changes in markers of body composition of professional male soccer players during pre-season. *Sports Med. Health Sci.* **2020**, *2*, 166–171. [CrossRef]
15. Austin, A.B.; Collins, S.M.; Huggins, R.A.; Smith, B.A.; Bowman, T.G. The Impact of Environmental Conditions on Player Loads During Preseason Training Sessions in Women's Soccer Athletes. *J. Strength Cond. Res.* **2021**, *35*, 2775–2782. [CrossRef]
16. Díez, A.; Lozano, D.; Arjol-Serrano, J.L.; Mainer-Pardos, E.; Castillo, D.; Torrontegui-Duarte, M.; Nobari, H.; Jaén-Carrillo, D.; Lampre, M. Influence of contextual factors on physical demands and technical-tactical actions regarding playing position in professional soccer players. *BMC Sports Sci. Med. Rehabil.* **2021**, *13*, 157. [CrossRef]
17. Carlos-Vivas, J.; Franco-García, J.M.; Mendoza-Muñoz, D.M.; Gómez-Pomares, S.; Pérez-Gómez, J. High-Intensity GPS-Derived Parameters in Semi-Professional Soccer: Home vs. Away Roles of the Team and Their Relationship with the Match's Final Score. *Sensors* **2024**, *24*, 4891. [CrossRef]
18. Michailidis, Y.; Vardakis, L.; Mikikis, D.; Mandroukas, A.; Metaxas, A. Match Running Performance of Elite Soccer Players and Correlations with Anthropometric and Power Indexes. *J. Sports Res.* **2019**, *6*, 44–51. [CrossRef]
19. Ju, W.; Cost, R.; Oliva-Lozano, J.M. Analysis of match performance of elite soccer players across confederations during the Men's and Women's World Cup. *Sci. Med. Footb.* **2024**, 1–13. [CrossRef]
20. Bernal-Orozco, M.F.; Posada-Falomir, M.; Quiñónez-Gastélum, C.M.; Plascencia-Aguilera, L.P.; Arana-Nuño, J.R.; Badillo-Camacho, N.; Márquez-Sandoval, F.; Holway, F.E.; Vizmanos-Lamotte, B. Anthropometric and Body Composition Profile of Young Professional Soccer Players. *J. Strength Cond. Res.* **2020**, *34*, 1911–1923. [CrossRef]
21. Osorio-Gutiérrez, A.; Zúñiga-Galaviz, U.; Gómez-Llanes, A.; Ortiz-Real, J.J.; Toledo-Domínguez, I.J.; Favela-Ramirez, C.A.; Coelho-e-Silva, M.J. Scaling corrected lower limb girths in professional male soccer players from different divisions. *JHSE* **2025**, *20*, 620–632. [CrossRef]
22. Elm, E.V.; Altman, D.G.; Egger, M.; Pocock, S.J.; Gøtzsche, P.C.; Vandenbroucke, J.P. Strengthening the reporting of observational studies in epidemiology (STROBE) statement: Guidelines for reporting observational studies. *BMJ* **2008**, *335*, 806–808. [CrossRef]
23. Vandenbroucke, J.P.; von Elm, E.; Altman, D.G.; Gøtzsche, P.C.; Mulrow, C.D.; Pocock, S.J.; Poole, C.; Schlesselman, J.J.; Egger, M.; STROBE Initiative. Strengthening the reporting of observational studies in epidemiology (STROBE): Explanation and elaboration. *Int. J. Surg.* **2014**, *12*, 1500–1524. [CrossRef]
24. Dolins, K.R. Nutrition assessment. In *Sports Nutrition: A Handbook for Professionals*, 6th ed.; Kapinski, C., Rosenbloom, C.A., Eds.; Academy of Nutrition and Dietetics: Chicago, IL, USA, 2017; pp. 156–158.
25. Winter, E.M.; Maughan, R.J. Requirements for ethics approvals. *J. Sports Sci.* **2009**, *27*, 985. [CrossRef]
26. World Medical Association. World Medical Association Declaration of Helsinki: Ethical principles for medical research involving human participants. *JAMA* **2025**, *333*, 71–74. [CrossRef]
27. Esparza Ros, F.; Vaquero-Cristóbal, R.; Marfell-Jones, M. *International Standards for Anthropometric Assessment*; International Society for the Advancement of Kinanthropometry (ISAK): Murcia, Spain, 2019; 114p.
28. Yuhasz, M.S. The Effects of Sports Training on Body Fat Man with Predictions of Optimal Body Weight. Ph.D. Dissertation, University of Illinois Urbana-Champaign, Champaign, IL, USA, 1962.
29. Sloan, A.W. Estimation of body fat in young men. *J. Appl. Physiol.* **1962**, *23*, 311–315. [CrossRef]
30. Wilmore, J.H.; Behnke, A.R. An anthropometric estimation of body density and lean body weight in young men. *J. Appl. Physiol.* **1969**, *27*, 25–31. [CrossRef]
31. Durnin, J.V.; Womersley, J. Body fat assessed from total body density and its estimation from skinfold thickness: Measurements on 481 men and women aged from 16 to 72 years. *Br. J. Nutr.* **1974**, *32*, 77–97. [CrossRef]

32. Jackson, A.S.; Pollock, M.L. Practical assessment of body composition. *Phys. Sportsmed.* **1985**, *13*, 76–90. [CrossRef]
33. Ross, W.D.; Kerr, D.A. Fraccionamiento de La Masa Corporal: Un Nuevo Método Para Utilizar en Nutrición Clínica y Medicina Deportiva. *Apunts* **1991**, *18*, 175–187.
34. Martin, A.D.; Spenst, L.F.; Drinkwater, D.T.; Clarys, J.P. Anthropometric estimation of muscle mass in men. *Med. Sci. Sports Exerc.* **1990**, *22*, 729–733. [CrossRef] [PubMed]
35. Lee, R.C.; Wang, Z.; Heo, M.; Ross, R.; Janssen, I.; Heymsfield, S.B. Total-body skeletal muscle mass: Development and cross-validation of anthropometric prediction models. *Am. J. Clin. Nutr.* **2000**, *72*, 796–803. [CrossRef] [PubMed]
36. Drinkwater, D.; Ross, W.D. Anthropometric fractionation of body mass. In *Kinanthropometry II*; Ostyn, G., Beunen, G., Simons, J., Eds.; University Park Press: Baltimore, MD, USA, 1984; pp. 177–178.
37. Collings, T.J.; Lima, Y.L.; Dutaillis, B.; Bourne, M.N. Concurrent validity and test-retest reliability of VALD ForceDecks' strength, balance, and movement assessment tests. *J. Sci. Med. Sport* **2024**, *27*, 572–580. [CrossRef] [PubMed]
38. McMahon, J.J.; Ripley, N.J.; Comfort, P. Force plate-derived countermovement jump normative data and benchmarks for professional rugby league players. *Sensors* **2022**, *22*, 8669. [CrossRef]
39. Bastida Castillo, A.; Gómez Carmona, C.D.; De la Cruz Sánchez, E.; Pino Ortega, J. Accuracy, intra- and inter-unit reliability, and comparison between GPS and UWB-based position-tracking systems used for time-motion analyses in soccer. *Eur. J. Sport Sci.* **2018**, *18*, 450–457. [CrossRef]
40. Malone, J.J.; Lovell, R.; Varley, M.C.; Coutts, A.J. Unpacking the black box: Applications and considerations for using GPS devices in sport. *Int. J. Sports Physiol. Perform.* **2017**, *12* (Suppl. S2), S218–S226. [CrossRef]
41. Rico-González, M.; Los Arcos, A.; Clemente, F.M.; Rojas-Valverde, D.; Pino-Ortega, J. Accuracy and reliability of local positioning systems for measuring sport movement patterns in stadium-scale: A systematic review. *Appl. Sci.* **2020**, *10*, 5994. [CrossRef]
42. Pituch, K.A.; Stevens, J.P. *Applied Multivariate Statistics for the Social Sciences: Analyses with SAS and IBM's SPSS*, 6th ed.; Routledge: Abingdon-on-Thames, UK, 2015.
43. Leko, B.J.; Adefisan, I.E.; Aboyewa, K.O. Anthropometric Characteristics and Somatotype Differences among Nigerian Soccer Players, in Relation to Playing Level and Playing Position. *Int. J. Kinanthrop.* **2024**, *4*, 32–43. [CrossRef]
44. Alvarado Domínguez, N.; Gutiérrez-Cruz, M. Anthropometric Characteristics, Body Composition, and Somatotype by Position in Professional Ecuadoran Soccer Players. *Cienc. Deporte* **2023**, *8*, e4310.
45. Wood, R. Anthropometry of the Players at the 2018 World Cup. Topend Sports Webside. Available online: https://www.topendsports.com/sport/soccer/anthropometry-worldcup2018.htm (accessed on 6 April 2025).
46. Zaric, I.; Kukic, F.; Jovicevic, N.; Zaric, M.; Markovic, M.; Toskic, L.; Dopsaj, M. Body Height of Elite Basketball Players: Do Taller Basketball Teams Rank Better at the FIBA World Cup? *Int. J. Environ. Res. Public Health* **2020**, *17*, 3141. [CrossRef]
47. López-Taylor, J.R.; González-Mendoza, R.G.; Gaytán-González, A.; Jiménez-Alvarado, J.A.; Villegas-Balcázar, M.; Jáuregui-Ulloa, E.E.; Torres-Naranjo, F. Accuracy of Anthropometric Equations for Estimating Body Fat in Professional Male Soccer Players Compared with DXA. *J. Sports Med.* **2018**, *7*, 6843792. [CrossRef]
48. Kammerer-López, M.; Ceballos-Feria, N.C.; Mayor-Rengifo, M.C.; Hoyos-García, H.H.; Gómez-Velásquez, S. Evaluación de la exactitud de distintas fórmulas de predicción de la composición corporal, comparadas con la absorciometría de energía dual de rayos X, en futbolistas de equipos profesionales colombianos. *Nutr. Hosp.* **2021**, *38*, 298–305.
49. Martinez-Ferran, M.; Rafei, E.; Romero-Morales, C.; Pérez-Ruiz, M.; Lam-Meléndez, A.; Munguia-Izquierdo, D.; Pareja-Galeano, H. Optimizing Field Body Fat Percentage Assessment in Professional Soccer Players. *Appl. Sci.* **2022**, *12*, 727. [CrossRef]
50. Enes, A.; Oneda, G.; Alves, D.L.; Palumbo, D.P.; Cruz, R.; Moiano-Junior, J.V.M.; Novack, L.F.; Osiecki, R. Determinant Factors of the Match-Based Internal Load in Elite Soccer Players. *Res. Q. Exerc. Sport* **2021**, *92*, 63–70. [CrossRef] [PubMed]
51. Daly, L.S.; Catháin, C.Ó.; Kelly, D.T. Do players with superior physiological attributes outwork their less-conditioned counterparts? A study in Gaelic football. *Biol. Sport* **2024**, *41*, 163–174. [CrossRef]
52. Fields, J.B.; Lameira, D.M.; Short, J.L.; Merrigan, J.M.; Gallo, S.; White, J.B.; Jones, M.T. Relationship Between External Load and Self-Reported Wellness Measures Across a Men's Collegiate Soccer Preseason. *J. Strength Cond. Res.* **2021**, *35*, 1182–1186. [CrossRef]
53. Varley, I.; Ward, M.; Thorpe, C.; Beardsley, N.; Greeves, J.; Sale, C.; Saward, C. External training load is associated with adaptation in bone and body composition over the course of a season in elite male footballers. *Bone Rep.* **2022**, *18*, 101643. [CrossRef]
54. Şahin, I.H.; Sanioğlu, A. The examination of the relationship between body composition and acceleration. *Turk. J. Kinesiol.* **2021**, *9*, 106–114. [CrossRef]
55. Kapteijns, J.A.; Caen, K.; Lievens, M.; Bourgois, J.G.; Boone, J. Positional Match Running Performance and Performance Profiles of Elite Female Field Hockey. *Int. J. Sports Physiol. Perform.* **2021**, *16*, 1295–1302. [CrossRef]

sports

MDPI

Article

Consensus of Return-to-Play Criteria After Adductor Longus Injury in Professional Soccer

José Luis Estévez Rodríguez [1,2], Jesús Rivilla García [2], Sergio L. Jiménez-Sáiz [3] and Sergio Jiménez-Rubio [3,*]

[1] Switzerland National Team, Worbstrasse 48, 3074 Muri bei Bern, Switzerland; joselu.estevez@gmail.com
[2] Faculty of Physical Activity and Sport Sciences (INEF-Sports Department), Polytechnic University of Madrid, 28040 Madrid, Spain; jesus.rivilla@upm.es
[3] Sports Science Research Studies, University Rey Juan Carlos, Fuenlabrada, 28943 Madrid, Spain; sergio.jimenez.saiz@urjc.es
* Correspondence: sergio.jimenez.rubio@urjc.es

Abstract: Return to play (RTP) decision making in professional soccer is crucial for minimising re-injury risk, reducing financial burdens on clubs, and optimising player performance. Despite its significance, there is a lack of objective criteria and consensus on RTP for adductor longus injuries, one of the most common muscle injuries in soccer. The aim of the present consensus was to validate an RTP protocol based on clinical, functional, and performance criteria through expert evaluation. This study hypothesises that a validated RTP protocol for adductor longus injuries will enhance decision making, reduce re-injury rates, and improve player performance upon return. An observational survey was designed to validate an RTP protocol through an expert panel. A total of 63 injury-management professionals (strength and conditioning coaches, physiotherapists, doctors, and rehabilitation fitness coaches) with an average experience of 12.02 ± 6.87 years participated in validating a 20-criteria RTP protocol. The protocol, divided into clinical, functional, and performance criteria, was assessed using a 5-point Likert scale. Aiken's V coefficient was calculated for content validity, with criteria validated if Aiken's V $\geq$ 0.75. Out of 20 initial RTP criteria, 14 were validated by the expert panel, with Aiken's V ranging from 0.77 to 0.94 (overall range: 0.61–0.98). Key validated criteria included pain on palpation, flexibility, imaging, athlete feedback, strength assessments, movement quality, pre-injury GPS data, and performance under simulated match conditions. Criteria such as the Copenhagen adduction exercise and specific agility tests were not validated. The expert-validated RTP protocol for adductor longus injuries provides a structured approach to decision making, potentially reducing re-injury risk, improving rehabilitation strategies, and enhancing player performance. These findings could be integrated into clinical sports-medicine practices to enhance rehabilitation effectiveness and RTP decisions in professional soccer.

Keywords: exit criteria; rehabilitation; return to performance; groin injuries; muscle injuries

1. Introduction

One of the major factors that impact the professional development and performance of the soccer player is injuries. The overall incidence of injuries in professional male soccer players was 8.1 injuries/1000 h of exposure [1]. The second most common muscle injury is that affecting the adductor [2]. In elite soccer, the season prevalence of acute adductor time-loss injuries is 14%, resulting in a mean (± SD; standard deviation) absence of 14 ± 24 days [2]. In epidemiological studies on elite European soccer, the re-injury rate over the first two months after returning from injury was reported to be 18% after acute

https://doi.org/10.3390/sports13050134

adductor injuries [2].When an injury occurs, it is essential to return quickly and with the lowest risk of recurrence to mitigate the effects on individual and team performance, as well as the implication that injuries have on the club's finances [1,3].

The decision to return to play (RTP) is a complex process based on the assessment of health and risk activity but is also influenced by the assessment of risk tolerance [4]. The combination of clinical, physiological, conditional, and performance information will be essential for optimal decision making. In addition, multidisciplinary and interdisciplinary work will be one of the keys to success, but it will be fundamental to establish criteria with solid scientific evidence due to the lack of clarity and consensus in the RTP process [5,6]. Nowadays, rehabilitation and reconditioning programmes are becoming more and more complete and holistic in their approach, seeking to address each of the phases of the injury, as well as each of the functions developed by the different professionals involved in the process [6,7].

In addition, we have found some studies related to criteria for RTP, based on the Delphi consensus, where the criteria for hamstring and groin pain injuries were established [4,8,9]. We also found a recent review on RTP criteria in hamstring injuries, where these were divided into three categories: clinical, strength, and performance criteria [8]. These were based on criteria related to functional, performance, strength, flexibility, pain, and player's confidence. Strength assessment, performance analysis, and a sport-specific skills assessment, such as sprinting in hamstring injuries, were highly valued as criteria in RTP decision making [4,9].

However, we did not find specific and objective information on the exit criteria, nor a consensus in the RTP for acute adductor injuries. The aim of this study will be to validate a protocol, composed of clinical, functional, and performance-based criteria for RTP decision making for adductor longus injuries through a panel of experts. The methodology used differs from that used in the Delphi consensus [4,9], where consensus is achieved through different rounds of anonymous questionnaires. In addition, this research focused on the adductor longus injury.

2. Methods

2.1. Study Design

An observational survey was designed to determine RTP after adductor longus injury, consisting of 20 criteria. This protocol was validated anonymously by a panel of experts and the most relevant criteria were used to determine the RTP protocol.

2.2. Participants

A total of 67 experts in the field of injuries (S&C coaches, physios, doctors, and rehab fitness coaches) were contacted to validate the RTP protocol. Four experts did not respond to the calls or/and emails, and ultimately 63 participated (age = 37.85 ± 8.17 years) as experts in the validation. In addition, all experts signed a voluntary consent form where it was explained that they had the right to withdraw from the study. They had a professional experience of 12.02 ± 6.87 years in elite clubs and national teams (Figure 1). The nationality of experts were Spanish (n = 46), Swiss (n = 5), Portuguese (n = 2), Greek (n = 3), British (n = 1), Mexican (n = 1), Argentine (n = 1), American (n = 1), Italian (n = 2), and French (n = 1).

In order to be considered eligible to participate in the study, the following inclusion criteria were established: [1] Practical experience in rehabilitation programmes for at least 3 years; [2] experience in multidisciplinary and interdisciplinary work in elite and/or pre-elite soccer of at least 3 years; [3] experience in scientific methodology and/or clinical expertise. The entire study procedure was conducted in accordance with the outlines stated in the WMA Declaration of Helsinki on the ethical principles for research involving human subjects. The study was approved by the ethical committee of the Universidad Rey Juan Carlos (registration number: 1601202303423; 9 March 2023).

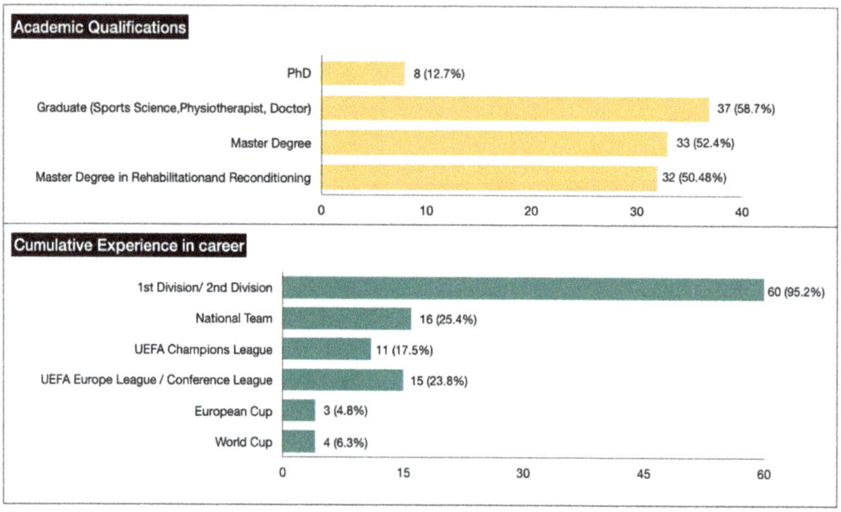

Figure 1. The profile of the panel of experts consisting of S&C coaches, physios, doctors and rehab fitness coaches.

2.3. Procedure

The RTP questionnaire was composed of twenty criteria. The criteria were divided into three categories: clinical, functional, and performance criteria, all of which were selected based on the literature with the objective of investigating each expert's assessment of the RTP process (Table 1).

Table 1. RTP questionnaire.

Criteria	Question
Clinical criteria	-Do you analyse the presence of pain on palpation when evaluating RTP in adductor longus injury? -Do you analyse flexibility when assessing RTP in adductor longus injury? -Do you use imaging to evaluate RTP in adductor longus injury? -Do you use Hip and Groin Outcome Score (HAGOS) when evaluating RTP in adductor longus injury? -Do you analyse the athlete's feedback during the RTP evaluation process in adductor longus injury?
Functional criteria	-Do you use strength testing when evaluating RTP in adductor longus injury? Hip adduction/abduction 45°/60°/90° (Ex: Force Frame Test Protocol) -Do you analyse the presence of pain on strength tests when evaluating RTP in adductor longus injury? -Do you use the pain-free Copenhagen adduction (10 repetitions) when assessing RTP in adductor longus injury? -Do you use isometric hip-adductor strength as a criterion for RTP in adductor longus injury?

Table 1. *Cont.*

Criteria	Question
	-Do you use eccentric hip-adductor strength as a criterion for RTP in adductor longus injury? -Do you analyse the presence of pain in basic strength exercises when evaluating RTP in adductor longus injury? -Do you use Counter-Movement Jump (CMJ) (presence of pain) and/or comparison with pre-injury value (Force Decks, apps or others) when evaluating RTP in adductor longus injury? -Do you use a side-to-side comparison in single-leg squat jump (Force Decks, apps or others) when evaluating RTP in adductor longus injury?
Performance criteria	-Do you analyse whether the injured athlete achieves 75–80% of pre-injury Global Positioning System (GPS) values when assessing RTP in adductor longus injury? -Do you use Repeated Sprint ability test when assessing RTP in adductor longus injury? -Do you use the L-Test/T-Test or/and Illinois agility test when evaluating RTP in adductor longus injury? -Do you use tasks in "worst case scenarios" (change in direction unplanned, sprints, High Chaos) when evaluating RTP in adductor longus injury? -Do you analyse quality of movement in planned and unplanned change in direction when evaluating RTP in adductor longus injury? -Do you use planned and unplanned kicking tasks at different distances and intensities when evaluating RTP in adductor longus injury? -Do you analyse whether the injured athlete achieves high-load team training sessions (3–5 sessions) when evaluating RTP in adductor longus injury?

The RTP questionnaire was submitted via email and collected using Google online forms. The sentence "Do you use/analyse X when evaluating RTP in adductor longus injury?" was used. It was a closed question, which had a unique response from the experts. They were asked to rate each criteria on a 5-point Likert-type scale to express their degree of agreement, with values from 1 to 5 (Strongly disagree (=1), disagree (=2), neutral (=3), agree (=4), Strongly agree (=5).

2.4. Statistical Analysis

The coefficient of content validation was calculated using Aiken's V, and its 95% confidence intervals were also determined [10]. An item was determined to be validated when the value of Aiken's V was ≥ 0.75 [10]. The calculations were carried out using Microsoft Excel 2016 software (Microsoft®, Redmond, WA, USA).

3. Results

Of the 20 RTP criteria, only 14 were considered valid, as the quantitative values given by the group of 63 experts were very high and were reflected in the Aiken V values (Table 2).

Table 2. The item content relevance score for all the twenty items as per the 63 experts, the Aiken's V and the 95% confidence intervals (CI) of Aiken's V. The ratings of the 63 experts varied on a scale from 1 to 5, where 1 corresponded to very poor relevance and 5 corresponded to very high relevance.

Ítem	1	2	3	4	5	Average	Aiken's V (95% CI)
1. Pain in palpation	1	4	7	33	18	4.00	0.75 (0.59–0.85)
2. Flexibility		1	10	28	24	4.19	0.80 (0.64–0.89)
3. Use of imaging		2	13	25	23	4.10	0.77 (0.62–0.87)
4. Hip and Groin Outcome Score	3	8	18	25	9	3.46	0.62 (0.46–0.74)
5. Athlete feedback				16	47	4.75	0.94 (0.81–0.97)
6. Strength assessment		1	5	27	30	4.37	0.84 (0.69–0.92)
7. Pain strength tests			1	21	41	4.63	0.91 (0.78–0.96)
8. Copenhagen adduction		4	24	23	12	3.68	0.67 (0.51–0.79)
9. Isometric hip adductors		1	7	31	24	4.24	0.81 (0.66–0.90)
10. Eccentric hip adductors	2	2	9	24	26	4.11	0.78 (0.62–0.87)
11. Pain in strength exercises		2	3	27	31	4.38	0.85 (0.70–0.92)
12. CMJ	1	6	17	18	21	3.83	0.71 (0.55–0.82)
13. Single-leg squat jump	1	7	16	21	18	3.76	0.69 (0.53–0.81)
14. Pre-injury GPS values	1	1	8	23	30	4.27	0.82 (0.67–0.90)
15. Repeated Sprint ability test		9	23	16	15	3.59	0.65 (0.49–0.77)
16. L-Test/T-Test or agility test	2	5	22	21	13	3.60	0.65 (0.49–0.77)
17. Worst-case scenarios	2	1	5	23	32	4.30	0.83 (0.68–0.91)
18. Planned and unplanned CoD		2	9	32	20	4.11	0.78 (0.62–0.87)
19. Planned and unplanned kicking			3	25	35	4.51	0.88 (0.74–0.94)
20. High-load team training sessions			9	27	27	4.29	0.82 (0.67–0.91)

4. Discussion

The study was designed to the validation process of a protocol to improve decision-making during RTP. The protocol was composed of 20 criteria divided into three sections (clinical, functional, and performance). Sixty-three experts (S&C coaches, physios, doctors, and rehab fitness coaches) participated in the validation of the protocol, which proved to have high validity, with high scores obtained on each of the programme items, although it should be noted that 6 of the proposed criteria were not validated by the experts. In the end, 14 criteria were validated by the experts (Figure 2).

4.1. Clinical Criteria

Pain on palpation, flexibility, use of imaging techniques, and athlete's feedback were highly rated (Aiken's V = 0.75; 0.80; 0.77; and 0.94) by the experts. Recent studies indicate that palpation pain and flexibility during clinical examinations are of great importance during the injury recovery process, in order to progress through the different phases, but they are also of great relevance as criteria in the RTP. However, we must take these results with caution, as Delphi's study [4] reported that there was no consensus among the participants regarding flexibility in adductor-related groin pain. On the other hand, previous studies related to RTP after hamstring injury observed flexibility as one of the most important criteria during RTP [11–13].

The criterion that received the highest value (Aiken's V = 0.94) from the experts was athlete's feedback. Previous studies showed the importance of this aspect in the RTP in muscle injuries [11–13]. Factors such as fear of pain, re-injury, and high motivation could have an important impact on the injured athlete and condition their RTP [8]. Moreover, the use of imaging was positively assessed by experts. It is a very useful tool to know the state of healing of the injured tissue and to have an objective assessment of the process from the clinical criterion, which can help us to identify red flags and to obtain a better diagnosis of the injury, but there are several studies that do not agree with establishing it as a criterion in the RTP [4,14,15]. As a downside, the HAGOS questionnaire was not validated by experts, although it is a very effective tool for identifying hip and/or groin problems [16], but this was perhaps insufficient to determine it as a criterion in the RTP (Aiken's V < 0.62).

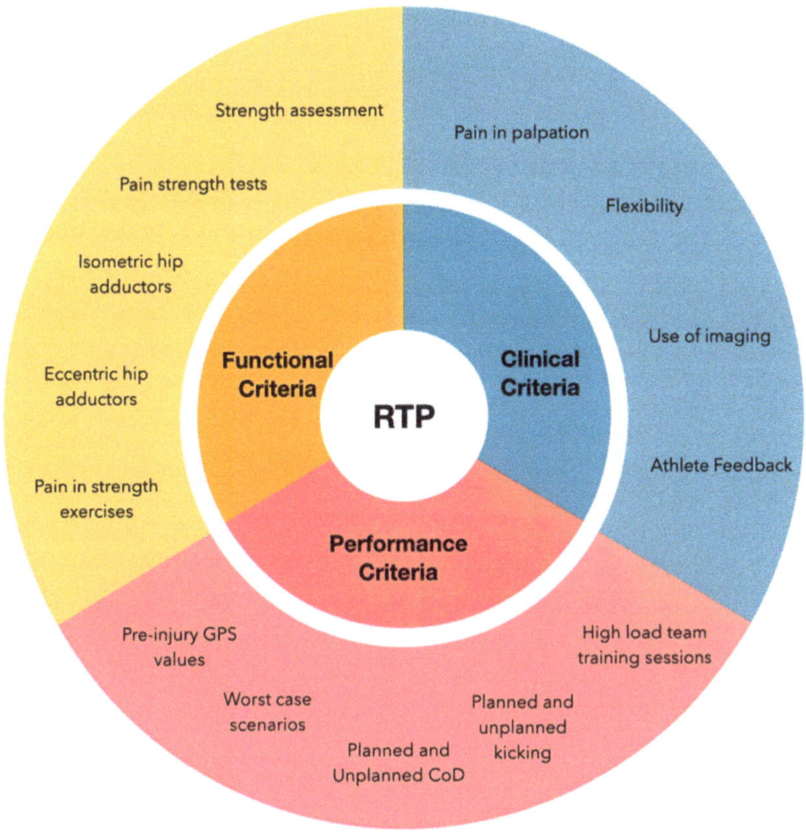

Figure 2. Validated RTP protocol. Only 14 criteria were determined as valid by the expert group.

4.2. Functional Criteria

In relation to the functional criteria for determining the RTP, it should be noted that the experts valued very confidently those criteria related to tests to measure the levels of adduction/abduction strength, pain during the execution of these and different types of contraction. In a meta-analysis [17], the most relevant factors for determining athletes with hip/groin pain were determined. It was specified that the reduction in strength levels in the adductor squeeze test can be used for such determination. A cutoff point of 465.33 N was associated with a 72% increased risk of injury [18]. In addition, there is an 83% probability of injury when force to body mass are values below 6.971 N/kg. In conclusion, this test is a simple, reliable, and cost-effective screening tool [18]. Previous studies [4,19] as well as our results agree on the importance of assessing the isometric and eccentric strength of the adductors, and evaluating the symmetry between both sides, as it seems to be an important tool for the assessment of adductor isometric and eccentric strength.

On the other hand, it should be distinguished that jumping assessments such as the Counter-Movement Jump or the single-leg squat were not validated by the experts as RTP criteria (Aiken's V < 0.70). Perhaps skills such as jumping or one-legged hopping are more closely related to knee injury, such as those affecting the ACL, as we have observed in previous studies [7,20]. Furthermore, a previous study [19] proposed the performance of 10 repetitions of the Copenhagen exercise as an RTP criterion, one of the most commonly used exercises during hip adductor injuries [21], but the experts did not validate this exercise for inclusion in the RTP protocol either (Aiken's V < 0.67). This is perhaps an interesting tool to use during the rehabilitation process, but insufficient to assess the RTP after an adductor longus injury.

4.3. Performance Criteria

It should be noted that the experts validated with great importance the performance criteria, determining them to be probably the closest to the environment of the training and competition context [4,6–8]. The specific skills that were assessed by the experts were directly related to the mechanisms of adductor longus injury (kicking, sprint, and change in direction) [4,15,19]. It seems that "kicking a ball" or change in direction are actions that are directly related to adductor longus injury, so the assessment of these skills may serve as a more relevant criterion in the RTP assessment process [4]. Nevertheless, the experts did not consider the assessment of the sprint to be of great importance (Aiken's V < 0.65), although previous studies [8,12] do justify the importance of this type of test in hamstring injury, probably because of its direct involvement in the mechanism of injury. On the other hand, they did not consider the manoeuvrability and/or agility tests (L-Test/T-Test or/and Illinois) to be of great relevance either, perhaps because they are carried out in a closed and planned environment. It should be distinguished that previous studies [22,23] have indicated the relevance of change in direction in hip/groin pain, as when an injury occurs there are kinematic and kinetic changes that can affect the correct mechanics of movement and thus increase the risk of re-injury, so the authors suggest the importance of working on the re-education of this skill during the rehabilitation process. The experts validated the evaluation of the change in direction in open and closed environments as a criterion, where uncertainty plays a fundamental role in the development of these tasks and brings the injured athlete closer to the real context of their sport [24,25].

In addition, the experts confidently valued the criteria related to the worst-case scenarios and the importance of reaching pre-injury GPS values (Aiken's V > 0.80). Several authors [26,27] have already defined the importance of these aspects during the final phase of rehabilitation in injuries. A previous study [24] shows the "control-chaos continuum" that are used in the rehabilitation programmes to simulate situations of maximum demand close to the reality of competition. On the other hand, previous studies [6,7,24] defined the RTP criterion as achieving GPS performance values during the rehabilitation process that are close to pre-injury values, with the aim of adapting the injured athlete to the conditional demand that they will encounter on his return to training with the team and return to play. Finally, the return to team training and high-demand sessions with the team was rated very clearly by the experts. It will be the last step prior to the RTP and many studies [6–8,12,19,26,27] observed this phase of the process as a fundamental criterion for returning to competition.

To conclude, one of the future lines of research could be to evaluate the efficacy of the protocol in soccer players with an adductor longus injury. Additionally, it should be noted that the sample used was representative and that they had significant professional and academic experience, but the results should perhaps be interpreted with caution, and a larger sample and greater variability in the nationality of experts or the possibility that they can add comments or extra criteria could possibly be taken into account for a future line of research.

5. Conclusions

A protocol to improve decisions during RTP following an adductor longus injury was validated by a group of experts, although 6 criteria out of the 20 proposed were discarded. The protocol was divided into three categories in order to unify the RTP criteria of the different professionals involved in a rehabilitation programme. This protocol could help clubs in their decisions during a player's return to competition after an adductor injury, in order to reduce the risk of re-injury, enhance the injured player's performance, and reduce the costs generated by injury.

Author Contributions: Conceptualization, J.L.E.R., S.J.-R. and S.L.J.-S.; methodology, J.L.E.R., S.J.-R. and J.R.G.; validation, J.L.E.R., J.R.G., S.L.J.-S. and S.J.-R.; formal analysis, J.L.E.R., J.R.G., S.L.J.-S. and S.J.-R.; investigation, J.L.E.R., and S.J.-R.; data curation, J.L.E.R., J.R.G., S.L.J.-S. and S.J.-R.; writing—original draft preparation, J.L.E.R., J.R.G., S.L.J.-S. and S.J.-R.; writing—review and editing, J.L.E.R., J.R.G., S.L.J.-S. and S.J.-R.; supervision, J.L.E.R., J.R.G., S.L.J.-S. and S.J.-R.; project administration, J.L.E.R., J.R.G., S.L.J.-S. and S.J.-R. All authors have read and agreed to the published version of the manuscript.

Funding: This research received no external funding.

Institutional Review Board Statement: The study was approved by ethical committee of the Universidad Rey Juan Carlos (registration number: 1601202303423; 9 March 2023).

Informed Consent Statement: Informed consent was obtained from the subjects involved in the study.

Data Availability Statement: The original contributions presented in the study are included in the article; further inquiries can be directed to the authors.

Conflicts of Interest: The authors declare no conflicts of interest.

References

1. López-Valenciano, A.; Ruiz-Pérez, I.; Garcia-Gómez, A.; Vera-Garcia, F.J.; Croix, M.D.S.; Myer, G.D.; Ayala, F. Epidemiology of injuries in professional football: A systematic review and meta-analysis. *Br. J. Sports Med.* **2020**, *54*, 711–718. [CrossRef] [PubMed]
2. Ekstrand, J.; Hägglund, M.; Waldén, M. Epidemiology of muscle injuries in professional football (soccer). *Am. J. Sports Med.* **2011**, *39*, 1226–1232. [CrossRef] [PubMed]
3. Eliakim, E.; Morgulev, E.; Lidor, R.; Meckel, Y. Estimation of injury costs: Financial damage of English Premier League teams' underachievement due to injuries. *BMJ Open Sport Exerc. Med.* **2020**, *6*, e000675. Erratum in *BMJ Open Sport Exerc. Med.* **2020**, *6*, e000675corr1. [CrossRef]
4. Vergani, L.; Cuniberti, M.; Zanovello, M.; Maffei, D.; Farooq, A.; Eirale, C. Return to Play in Long-Standing Adductor-Related Groin Pain: A Delphi Study Among Experts. *Sports Med.-Open* **2022**, *8*, 11. [CrossRef] [PubMed]
5. Ardern, C.L.; Glasgow, P.; Schneiders, A.; Witvrouw, E.; Clarsen, B.; Cools, A.; Gojanovic, B.; Griffin, S.; Khan, K.M.; Moksnes, H.; et al. 2016 Consensus statement on return to sport from the First World Congress in Sports Physical Therapy, Bern. *Br. J. Sports Med.* **2016**, *50*, 853–864. [CrossRef]
6. Estévez Rodríguez, J.L.; Rivilla García, J.; Jiménez-Rubio, S. Return to Performance of a Soccer Player with an Adductor Longus Injury: A Case Report. *Medicina* **2024**, *60*, 1998. [CrossRef]
7. Mitchell, A.; Waite, O.; Holding, C.; Greig, M. The Development of a Return to Performance Pathway Involving A Professional Soccer Player Returning From A Multi-Structural Knee Injury: A Case Report. *Int. J. Sports Phys. Ther.* **2023**, *18*, 450–466. [CrossRef]
8. Perna, P.; Kerin, F.; Greig, N.; Beato, M. Return-to-play criteria following a hamstring injury in professional football: A scoping review. *Res. Sports Med.* **2025**, *33*, 175–194. [CrossRef]
9. Zambaldi, M.; Beasley, I.; Rushton, A. Return to play criteria after hamstring muscle injury in professional football: A Delphi consensus study. *Br. J. Sports Med.* **2017**, *51*, 1221–1226. [CrossRef]
10. Penfield, R.D.; Giacobbi, J.P.R. Applying a Score Confidence Interval to Aiken's Item Content-Relevance Index. *Meas. Phys. Educ. Exerc. Sci.* **2004**, *8*, 213–225. [CrossRef]
11. Delvaux, F.; Rochcongar, P.; Bruyère, O.; Bourlet, G.; Daniel, C.; Diverse, P.; Reginster, J.Y.; Croisier, J.L. Return-to-play criteria after hamstring injury: Actual medicine practice in professional soccer teams. *Br. J. Sports Med.* **2013**, *47*, e3. [CrossRef]

12. Van Der Horst, N.; Backx, F.J.G.; Goedhart, E.A.; Huisstede, B.M.; on behalf of HIPS-Delphi Group. Return to play after hamstring injuries in football (soccer): A worldwide Delphi procedure regarding definition, clinical criteria and decision-making. *Br. J. Sports Med.* **2017**, *51*, 1583–1591. [CrossRef] [PubMed]
13. Dunlop, G.; Ardern, C.L.; Andersen, T.E.; Lewin, C.; Dupont, G.; Ashworth, B.; O'Driscoll, G.; Rolls, A.; Brown, S.; McCall, A. Return-to-Play Practices Following Hamstring Injury: A Worldwide Survey of 131 Premier League Football Teams. *Sports Med.* **2020**, *50*, 829–840. [CrossRef]
14. Branci, S.; Thorborg, K.; Nielsen, M.B.; Hölmich, P. Radiological findings in symphyseal and adductor-related groin pain in athletes: A critical review of the literature. *Br. J. Sports Med.* **2013**, *47*, 611–619. [CrossRef]
15. Serner, A.; Weir, A.; Tol, J.L.; Thorborg, K.; Yamashiro, E.; Guermazi, A.; Roemer, F.W.; Hölmich, P. Associations Between Initial Clinical Examination and Imaging Findings and Return-to-Sport in Male Athletes with Acute Adductor Injuries: A Prospective Cohort Study. *Am. J. Sports Med.* **2020**, *48*, 1151–1159. [CrossRef]
16. Thorborg, K.; Hölmich, P.; Christensen, R.; Petersen, J.; Roos, E.M. The Copenhagen Hip and Groin Outcome Score (HAGOS): Development and validation according to the COSMIN checklist. *Br. J. Sports Med.* **2011**, *45*, 478–491. [CrossRef]
17. Mosler, A.B.; Agricola, R.; Weir, A.; Hölmich, P.; Crossley, K.M. Which factors differentiate athletes with hip/groin pain from those without? A systematic review with meta-analysis. *Br. J. Sports Med.* **2015**, *49*, 810. [CrossRef] [PubMed]
18. Moreno-Pérez, V.; Travassos, B.; Calado, A.; Gonzalo-Skok, O.; Del Coso, J.; Mendez-Villanueva, A. Adductor squeeze test and groin injuries in elite football players: A prospective study. *Phys. Ther. Sport* **2019**, *37*, 54–59. [CrossRef]
19. Serner, A.; Weir, A.; Tol, J.L.; Thorborg, K.; Lanzinger, S.; Otten, R.; Hölmich, P. Return to Sport After Criteria-Based Rehabilitation of Acute Adductor Injuries in Male Athletes: A Prospective Cohort Study. *Orthop. J. Sports Med.* **2020**, *8*, 2325967119897247. [CrossRef]
20. Hall, M.P.; Paik, R.S.; Ware, A.J.; Mohr, K.J.; Limpisvasti, O. Neuromuscular evaluation with single-leg squat test at 6 months after Anterior Cruciate Ligament Reconstruction. *Orthop. J. Sports Med.* **2015**, *3*, 232596711557590. [CrossRef]
21. Ishøi, L.; Sørensen, C.N.; Kaae, N.M.; Jørgensen, L.B.; Hölmich, P.; Serner, A. Large eccentric strength increase using the Copenhagen Adduction exercise in football: A randomized controlled trial. *Scand. J. Med. Sci. Sports* **2016**, *26*, 1334–1342. [CrossRef] [PubMed]
22. King, E.; Franklyn-Miller, A.; Richter, C.; O'Reilly, E.; Doolan, M.; Moran, K.; Strike, S.; Falvey, É. Clinical and biomechanical outcomes of rehabilitation targeting intersegmental control in athletic groin pain: Prospective cohort of 205 patients. *Br. J. Sports Med.* **2018**, *52*, 1054–1062. [CrossRef] [PubMed]
23. Daniels, K.A.J.; King, E.; Richter, C.; Falvey, É.; Franklyn-Miller, A. Changes in the kinetics and kinematics of a reactive cut maneuver after successful athletic groin pain rehabilitation. *Scand. J. Med. Sci. Sports* **2021**, *31*, 839–847. [CrossRef]
24. Taberner, M.; Allen, T.; Cohen, D.D. Progressing rehabilitation after injury: Consider the 'control-chaos continuum'. *Br. J. Sports Med.* **2019**, *53*, 1132–1136. [CrossRef]
25. Taberner, M.; Allen, T.; O'keefe, J.; Chaput, M.; Grooms, D.; Cohen, D.D. Evolving the Control-Chaos Continuum: Part 1—Translating Knowledge to Enhance On-Pitch Rehabilitation. *J. Orthop. Sports Phys. Ther.* **2025**, *55*, 78–88. [CrossRef] [PubMed]
26. Taberner, M.; Haddad, F.S.; Dunn, A.; Newall, A.; Parker, L.; Betancur, E.; Cohen, D.D. Managing the return to sport of the elite footballer following semimembranosus reconstruction. *BMJ Open Sport Exerc. Med.* **2020**, *6*, e000898. [CrossRef]
27. Jiménez-Rubio, S.; Navandar, A.; Rivilla-García, J.; Paredes, V. Validity of an on-Field Readaptation Program Following a Hamstring Injury in Professional Soccer. *J. Sport Rehabil.* **2018**, *28*, 1–7. [CrossRef]

sports

MDPI

Article

Rule Modification's Effects on the Feedback Type Given by Coaches at Young Football Levels

Lidia Martinez-Jiménez [1,2,3], Ricardo André Birrento-Aguiar [1,2,3], Verónica Marco-Cramer [1,2,3] and Enrique Ortega-Toro [1,2,3,*]

1 Faculty of Sport Sciences, University of Murcia, 30720 Santiago de la Ribera, Spain; lidia.martinezj@um.es (L.M.-J.); ra.birrentoaguiar@um.es (R.A.B.-A.); v.marcocramer@um.es (V.M.-C.)
2 Human Movement and Sports Sciences, Faculty of Sport Sciences, University of Murcia, 30720 Santiago de la Ribera, Spain
3 Sports Performance Analysis Association, 30720 Santiago de la Ribera, Spain
* Correspondence: eortega@um.es

Abstract: Background: An adapted competition should create a favourable environment to tailor the feedback provided to the needs of young athletes. The aim of this study was to analyse the influence of rule modification on the type of feedback given by coaches to young football players. Method: The study sample consisted of four under-10 male coaches from four Spanish teams. The analysis was conducted using a quasi-experimental A-B design, in which two tournaments were played: Tournament 1 with the official Spanish Football Federation (RFEF) rules and Tournament 2 with rule modifications. All the feedback provided by the group of coaches during the two tournaments was recorded, yielding a total of 4.386 for Tournament 1 and 3.728 for Tournament 2. Results: The results showed that in both tournaments, the predominant feedback from the coaches was individual, prescriptive, affective, and non-valuable. However, they indicated that the orientation of the feedback and its autonomy positively varied during the adapted competition. The data obtained align with the results of other studies on the type of feedback given by coaches, despite some differing from scientific recommendations. Conclusions: It can be concluded that the modified rule competition promoted changes in the type of feedback provided by the coaches.

Keywords: sport initiation; competition; under-10

1. Introduction

Competition is a key component of the teaching–learning process in initiation sports, as it provides a practice that covers most of the learning situations that are essential for the training of players. At the same time, it offers massive practice if the player is active for a long time, which is the most beneficial for the training process [1,2]. Furthermore, competition promotes the transfer of learning [3,4] as it involves the construction and search for solutions to problems. Likewise, competition increases the motivation of participants and makes the teaching–learning process more attractive [5] and motivating [6] due to people's ambition to compare themselves with others. Therefore, many authors support its use in the training of athletes [7,8].

Nevertheless, the current form of competition in youth sport is not conducive to achieving the goals and formative values that should be attained in the initiation phase [9,10]. In this sense, the scientific literature argues that for competition to be truly formative and meaningful, it must be adapted to the characteristics and level of the players [4,11,12], which would also increase the development of participants' skills [13]. Various measures have been proposed to achieve the necessary adaptation, such as changing the rules or influencing the role of the coach [14]. In the case of badminton, it has been demonstrated that reducing the dimensions of the court and lowering the height of the net has a beneficial impact on the acquisition of skills among participants, encouraging the use of a greater variety of strokes [15]. In tennis, a reduction in racket size and weight, coupled with the use of larger and slower balls, has been shown to result in more accurate strokes by players [13]. Modifying the height of the net has been shown to encourage a more varied and assertive style of play, while also enhancing the motivation of the participants [16]. The alteration of the rules engenders a favourable experience for players, thereby enhancing their perception of self-efficacy [17].

Conversely, in team sports, alterations to the dimensions of the field in association football during training stages have been shown to encourage decision-making and facilitate the technical and tactical development of players [18]. The technical–tactical variability of young players in football is enhanced when aspects of the competition are modified, including the system of confrontations, the form of scoring and/or the size of the goal [19]. In beach handball, the adaptation of certain rules for trainee players up to the age of 11 and the modification of field dimensions and ball size, among other factors, has been shown to encourage player participation and adherence to the game [20]. Modifying the dimensions of the playing field to accommodate younger players, such as bringing the three-point line closer in basketball, results in alterations to the game conditions as players adapt their throwing movements, which in turn leads to a reduction in unfavourable movement patterns [21,22]. The actions of the coach have a significant impact on the learning outcomes of the players [23,24]. Nevertheless, coaches do not always conduct themselves in an appropriate manner, and they frequently exhibit negative or non-formative behaviours regarding values [25,26]. It is imperative that positive behaviours are the dominant force within the teaching–learning processes of beginner players [25]. Therefore, it is of the utmost importance that coaches receive comprehensive training and possess a clear understanding of the appropriate times and methods for providing feedback, in order to fully capitalise on its advantages [24].

Feedback can be defined as the set of information provided to an athlete or student after performing a motor execution, with the objective of influencing the same or the next action, thereby ensuring the acquisition of quality learning [27]. This process is aimed at closing the gap between current and desired learning outcomes [28]. The feedback, whether internal or external, that occurs between one action and another and that allows for modification of the execution or confirmation of the expected action is the determining factor in whether learning is meaningful [27]. Furthermore, it has been demonstrated that providing students with feedback can enhance their motivation and autonomy while also improving the classroom or team climate [29,30].

The literature offers recommendations for providing effective feedback, which are based on aspects related to the type of feedback, the timing of feedback, and the frequency of feedback [27,29]. The type of feedback can be classified in the following manner, as evidenced [22,27,31]: (a) direction (individual/group), indicating whether the information is addressed to a specific person or to several people; (b) emotional orientation (positive/negative/neutral), depending on the form and content of the feedback; and the intention of the feedback can be evaluative, descriptive, prescriptive, affective, or interrogative. Furthermore, some authors [32] have supplemented the classification of feedback types with the variable autonomy. The degree to which the type of feedback provided allows the individual to exert control over their teaching–learning process [33] has been evaluated [33].

A review of the scientific literature on the type of feedback that should be provided in competitive settings, with a particular focus on the initiation of sports, suggests a preference for the use of positive feedback [24,25]. In alignment with the intended outcome, feedback should be prescriptive, affective, and, on occasion, interrogative. The latter is recommended for guiding discovery learning [34,35]. In addition, coaches should provide feedback that is tailored to the individual [36]. Moreover, research indicates that appropriate feedback should facilitate the autonomy of the performer, thereby enhancing their experience of practice [37]. Additionally, feedback should convey values, as this is a primary objective in sport [38].

Sport constitutes an appropriate vehicle for the transmission of personal and social values to those who engage in it [39]. This is particularly salient in the context of sport initiation, where players are undergoing a process of maturational development at all levels, psychological, moral, and social [40]. These values can be further subdivided into those specifically associated with the practice of sport. For example, respect can be linked to fair play, sportsmanship, and tolerance [41,42]. While sport does not inherently possess educational value, the integration of values must be conducted through coaches, who should explicitly and concretely demonstrate the values they wish to in their athletes, and who should also utilise feedback in a manner like that employed with technical and tactical content [43]. These values are not currently evident in the competitions that take place, and the inherent competitiveness of such events has been found to result in a decrease in the inculcation of values [9]. In particular, the evidence suggests that younger football coaches are more likely to engage in negative behaviours toward their players, including the use of inappropriate language and expressions of regret, than positive behaviours [26].

The type of feedback employed by coaches varies depending on the stage of the match. Prescriptive feedback is more frequently used during the first half, whereas affective feedback is more prevalent during the second half [35]. This finding differs from another study, which found that affective feedback was the least frequently provided [27]. From an alternative perspective, some studies have indicated that most of the feedback provided by coaches is positive [44]. Regarding the direction of feedback, the literature does not indicate a clear preference for a specific type. On the one hand, coaches tend to provide group feedback more frequently [45]. On the other hand, during competitive play, they rely on individual feedback to a greater extent. The feedback provided by coaches is predominantly of a controlling nature that does not support player autonomy. Furthermore, the feedback they provide does not espouse values and does not refer to evaluative terms [32]. In alignment with the autonomy and values of feedback, it is noteworthy that many studies conducted to date have concentrated their data collection on questionnaires of coaches' perceptions, thereby failing to analyse the feedback provided by coaches.

It can be reasonably deduced that a competition designed with the specific requirements of young athletes in mind would facilitate a more conducive setting for more effective feedback. The aim of this study was to investigate the effect of a competition designed to meet the needs of young players on the type of feedback provided by coaches in the context of youth football.

2. Materials and Methods

2.1. Participants

The study sample consisted of four football coaches in four Spanish teams of boys under 10. All the coaches were male, with a mean age of 31.45 $\pm$ 11.32 and a football coaching experience of 9.32 $\pm$ 7.23 years. All four coaches had a level II federative sports qualification.

2.2. Procedure

All feedback was recorded by the coaches during two tournaments (RFEF tournament = 4386; modified tournament = 3728) involving four teams, all playing against each other. In each match, both coaches were recorded; therefore, a total of 12 matches and 24 recordings were obtained. The study followed a quasi-experimental A-B design to analyse the effects of rule modification on different types of feedback. The independent variable of the study was the rules of the game. Two tournaments were played; the first one (RFEF tournament) followed the official RFEF regulations, and in the second one (modified tournament), the following modifications were made:

- Fair play' scoring: Each team could score up to two points for "fair play". One point was the average of the rating of the players themselves, the opponents, and the parents/guardians on a scale of 0 to 1. The other point was obtained by receiving a white card from the referee (positive attitudes) or, on the contrary, by subtracting that point (negative attitudes).
- Scoring for the competition: There were 3 points for a won match, 2 points for a drawn match and 1 point for a lost match. To this final score, the 'fair play' score mentioned above was added.
- Playing time: It consisted of five 10 min periods, with a 10 min break between the third and fourth periods.
- Scoreboard: The total score of the match was the sum of the periods won by each team.
- Goalkeeper: The goalkeeper had to play at least one period as a field player.
- Headers: Headers were not allowed, unless the ball had previously bounced.
- Goal kicks: Opposing players could only cross the offside line once the ball had been put into play.

The dependent variable was the feedback provided by the coaches. The feedback was classified following an ad hoc recording sheet previously validated by a panel of experts to ensure the validity of the content and wording [46]. Specifically, the type of feedback was analysed according to the following variables (Table 1).

Table 1. Study variables occurred in the record sheet.

Variable	Category	Description	Example
Direction	Single	Targeted at a specific player.	"You have gone that move well."
	Group	Addressed to the group.	"We need to move the ball faster."
Intention	Evaluative	Provides a qualitative estimation of the performance accompanied by a justification.	"The finish on goal was correct, because the defence left us space."
	Descriptive	It involves the provision of information containing details about the execution of the movement or action performed.	"We unbalanced when you shot a goal."
	Explanatory	Seeks to give empirical reasons for the execution error. It tells you the causes. It justifies the causes of the error. Biomechanical, psychological, etc., reasons are involved.	"When you hit the ball, your body was too far away from the ball, and you didn't too far away from the ball, and you don't have enough power."
	Prescriptive	It provides information on how the next executions should be carried out.	"¡you have passed the ball in this situation!"
	Interrogative	It involves asking the player a question about the performance he/she has made, to make him/her reflect and become aware of his/her own performance.	"¿Where were your defence?"
	Emotional	Refers to information of an affective nature and is related to the emotional dimension of the player.	"Well done, Gonzalo, you are so good."
Emotional orientation	Positive	Focuses on success.	"Good shooting at goal."
	Negative	Focuses on the error.	"Don't be selfish, pass the ball to your teammate."
	Neutral	Focuses neither on the error nor on the effort.	
Autonomy	Support	Supports autonomy; empathises.	Coach's questions, reflections...
	Neutral		
	Controller	Very direct instructions; does not encourage autonomy.	"Stop that dribble"
Values		If the coach alludes to values of respect or fair play.	"Don't shot at the referee."
Other type of feedback		Not contemplated in the classification.	Coach's comments not directly addressed to the player (criticism, whispering, etc.).

The feedback data collection instrument was a microphone with a recording device (Sony ICD-PX240 4 Go, Tokyo, Japan). The microphone was placed on the coach's chest at the start of each game and removed when the referee declared the game over. In this way, the information was recorded and facilitated subsequent analysis.

Four observers (graduates in physical activity and sports science) were trained to record the categories and types of feedback. Following observer training, inter-observer and intra-observer reliability was calculated. Prior to the analysis of the feedback, the observers were trained. After the training, inter-observer and intra-observer reliability tests were performed. To analyse reliability, 5 min of feedback was analysed, reporting minimum values of 0.95 for the intention variable (Table 2).

Table 2. Training observer values.

Observation	Direction	Intention	Type	Autonomy	Values	Observers
Intra-Observation	1	0.956	0.832	0.896	1	A-A
Inter-Observation	1	0.906	0.909	0.844	1	A-B
	1	0.906	0.909	0.844	1	A-C
	1	1	1	0.844	1	A-D
	1	1	1	0.844	1	A-E

2.3. *Statistical Analysis*

Data analysis included descriptive analysis using absolute and relative frequency analysis. Then, to analyse possible relationships between the different categories of feedback and the different tournaments, an analysis was carried out using the chi-square test ($p < 0.05$). The Phi test (Phi) or Cramer's V test (V) were used to calculate the effect size. Statistical analyses were performed using SPSS, v. 28.0 for Mac; SPSS Inc., Chicago, IL, USA.

3. Results

The results show that the total amount of feedback given by coaches during the regular tournament (n = 4386) is higher than the amount of feedback given during the modified tournament (n = 3728).

Table 3 shows the amount and percentage of feedback given by coaches by direction, distinguishing between feedback given during the regular tournament and feedback given during the modified tournament.

Table 3. Descriptive values of feedback—direction variables.

Feedback Direction	Statistics	Tournament Type RFEF Tournament	Modified Tournament	Total
Single Feedback	Observed	4163	3488	7651
	Percentage	94.9%	93.6%	94.3%
Group Feedback	Observed	223	240	463
	Percentage	5.1%	6.4%	5.7%
Total *	Observed	4386	3728	8114

* Statistically significant $p < 0.05$. RFEF—Real Federación Española de Fútbol.

The data in Table 3 reflect a statistically significant relationship between the type of feedback direction and the type of tournament ($\chi 2$ (1, n = 8114) = 6860, $p < 0.05$, effect size, $p < 0.05$ Phi = 0.029), with a lower percentage of individual feedback and a higher percentage of group feedback observed in the modified tournament. Thus, it can be observed that in both tournaments, almost all feedback was of an individual nature.

Table 4 shows the number and percentage of feedback types given according to their intention. In addition, a comparison of each type of feedback can be observed depending on whether it occurs in the RFEF tournament or in the modified tournament.

Table 4. Descriptive values of feedback—intention variables.

Feedback Intention	Statistics	Tournament Type RFEF Tournament	Modified Tournament	Total
Evaluative feedback	Observed	187	124	311
	Percentage	4.3%	3.3%	3.8%
Descriptive feedback	Observed	96	242	338
	Percentage	2.2%	6.5%	4.2%
Explanatory feedback	Observed	158	0	158
	Percentage	3.6%	0.0%	1.9%
Prescriptive feedback	Observed	2633	2193	4826
	Percentage	60.0%	58.8%	59.5%
Interrogative feedback	Observed	129	91	220
	Percentage	2.9%	2.4%	2.7%
Affective feedback	Observed	1182	1078	2260
	Percentage	27.0%	28.9%	27.9%
Total *	Observed	4385	3728	8113

* Statistically significant $p < 0.05$. RFEF—Real Federación Española de Fútbol.

The results in Table 4 show statistically significant relationships between the variable feedback intention and the type of tournament ($\chi 2$ (5, n = 8113) = 233.620, $p < 0.05$; effect size, $p < 0.05$, V = 0.170), such that in the modified tournament, a statistically higher percentage of descriptive and affective feedback was observed, and lower percentages of interrogative, prescriptive, explanatory, and evaluative feedback were observed. These data also show that more than half of the feedback given by the coaches in both the RFEF and the modified tournament was of the prescriptive type and more than a quarter of the affective type, leaving the remaining four types of feedback with very low percentages.

Table 5 details the amount and percentage of the types of feedback given by coaches based on emotional orientation, distinguishing between the RFEF tournament and the modified tournament.

Table 5. Descriptive values of feedback—emotional orientation variables.

Feedback Emotional Orientation	Statistics	Tournament Type RFEF Tournament	Modified Tournament	Total
Positive feedback	Observed	963	977	1940
	Percentage	22.0%	26.2%	23.9%
Negative feedback	Observed	2381	1831	4212
	Percentage	54.3%	49.1%	51.9%
Neutral feedback	Observed	1041	920	1961
	Percentage	23.7%	24.7%	24.2%
Total *	Observed	4385	3728	8113

* Statistically significant $p < 0.05$. RFEF—Real Federación Española de Fútbol.

The results showed statistically significant relationships between the variable feedback orientation and the type of tournament ($\chi 2$ (2, n = 8113) = 26.354, $p < 0.05$; effect size, $p < 0.05$, V = 0.057). In the modified tournament, there was a higher percentage of positive and neutral feedback and a lower percentage of negative feedback. Table 6 shows that in both tournaments, approximately half of the feedback was negative, and the other half was evenly split between neutral and positive feedback. However, it is worth noting that in Tournament 2, where the rules are changed, the percentage of negative feedback decreased, while the positive feedback increased. Table 6 shows the number and percentage of feedback used by the coaches according to the degree of information autonomy, differentiating between the normal and the modified tournament.

Table 6. Descriptive values of autonomy feedback.

Autonomy Feedback	Statistics	Tournament Type RFEF Tournament	Modified Tournament	Total
Support Feedback	Observed	790	891	1681
	Percentage	18.0%	23.9%	20.7%
Neutral Feedback	Observed	248	107	355
	Percentage	5.7%	2.9%	4.4%
Controller Feedback	Observed	3345	2730	6075
	Percentage	76.3%	73.2%	74.9%
Total *	Observed	4385	3728	8113

* Statistically significant $p < 0.05$. RFEF—Real Federación Española de Fútbol.

The data in Table 6 reflect statistically significant relationships between the variable feedback autonomy and the type of tournament ($\chi 2$ (4, n = 8113) = 73.609, $p < 0.05$; effect size, $p < 0.05$, V = 0.095), so that in the modified tournament, a lower percentage of controlling and neutral feedback and a higher percentage of supportive feedback were observed. Thus, it can be observed that in both tournaments, coaches used controlling feedback three out of four times. Nevertheless, feedback tended to change when the rules were changed, with a minimal decrease in controlling feedback and an increase in supportive feedback. Table 7 details the amount and percentage of feedback given based on whether it provided value, comparing the results from the normal tournament with the modified tournament.

Table 7. Descriptive values of feedback.

Feedback Values	Statistics	Tournament Type RFEF Tournament	Modified Tournament	Total
No values	Observed	4360	3681	8041
	Percentage	99.4%	98.7%	99.1%
Values	Observed	25	47	72
	Percentage	0.6%	1.3%	0.9%
Total *	Observed	4386	3728	8114

* Statistically significant $p < 0.05$. RFEF—Real Federación Española de Fútbol.

The last set of data collected established a statistically significant relationship between the variable Feedback Values and the type of tournament ($\chi 2$ (2, n = 8114) = 10.926, $p < 0.05$; effect size, $p < 0.05$, Phi = 0.037), with a higher percentage of feedback providing values and a lower percentage of feedback not providing values in the modified tournament. Thus, the results reflect that almost all the feedback given by the coaches was non-valuative, although this contribution is considered in the result because, despite the fact that the amount of value-giving feedback increased in the modified tournament, the percentage was still minimal.

4. Discussion

An adequate teaching–learning process includes a competition adapted to the needs of the participants and feedback based on scientific recommendations. Therefore, the aim of this study was to analyse how a competition adapted to the needs of young players influences the type of feedback given by youth football coaches.

In general, the results showed that the modification of rules, such as playing time, scoreboard, competition score, and fair play score, among others, slightly changed the type of feedback given by coaches, giving feedback that is closer to the recommendations of the scientific literature. In general, it was found that coaches gave more feedback in the normal tournament than in the modified tournament.

Depending on the direction of the feedback, it was found that most of the feedback given in both the normal and the modified tournament was of an individual nature, although in the modified tournament, the percentage of group feedback increased minimally, while individual feedback decreased. In addition, this greater use of individual feedback is in line with scientific recommendations regarding the orientations that feedback should have, depending on the direction, to positively influence the teaching–learning processes of young people [27,36].

From the perspective of feedback intentions, the results reflected that the change in rules between one tournament and another did not promote major changes in the type of feedback given by coaches. It was found that almost all feedback was prescriptive and affective feedback, both in the normal tournament and in the modified tournament. In the modified tournament, the use of modified feedback increased, while interrogative feedback remained similar and evaluative feedback decreased slightly. The data from this study are in line with the recommendations of the scientific literature on the type of feedback coaches should give based on intention, and with the results obtained by other authors in previous studies, since prescriptive and affective feedback predominate [35,44]. Nevertheless, the data differ from the results obtained in other studies, where affective feedback was the least used [24]. Regarding the emotional orientation of the feedback, it was found that the type of feedback changed positively when the rules were adapted, i.e., in the second modified rule. This is reflected in a percentage increase in positive and neutral feedback, while negative feedback decreased. This change from one tournament to another may have been due to the fact that the rule change encouraged coaches to reflect on their behaviour and what may not be appropriate, and more specifically, this change may have been influenced by the inclusion of the white card, which took into account the positive attitudes of coaches and players and could be counted in the competition scoreboard [41,46]. Although this change was positive, the feedback transmitted was still mostly negative, moving away from the guidelines that determine what constitutes appropriate feedback [24,25] and in line with the results of other studies analysing coaches' feedback [47].

In line with feedback autonomy, the results showed that the percentage of supportive feedback increased in the modified tournament compared to the percentage in the normal tournament, while the opposite occurred with negative and neutral feedback, as their percentage decreased when the rules were modified. These results are positive because they reflect an influence of the rule change on the type of feedback given by the coach, which is more in line with what is considered appropriate feedback [37]. Nevertheless, it was also observed that the feedback based on autonomy that predominated in the coaches' behaviour was the controlling type, with a high percentage. These data are consistent with other studies that have analysed the autonomy of feedback from coaches and found that a high percentage of coaches used controlling feedback [32], and the data differ from the recommendations of the scientific literature, which state that appropriate and beneficial feedback for students should support their autonomy [37].

Regarding the last variable analysed, values, it was found that almost all the feedback given by the coaches did not refer to evaluative terms, this being the case in both the normal and the modified tournament. Nevertheless, it was found that the percentage of feedback that provides values increases minimally during the modified tournament, which could indicate the beginning of a change due to the change in the rules and the introduction of the white card during the competition, as it is based on the recognition of positive attitudes and fair play, among other aspects [46]. The prevalence of feedback that does not provide values is consistent with the results obtained in other studies on what coaches do [22] and is completely different from what is determined by the scientific literature on what appropriate feedback should be based on with reference to evaluative terms [38,41]. Thus, the results obtained show that in the tournament in which a rule change was implemented and adapted to the characteristics of the participants, the type of feedback given by the coaches varied, although more markedly in some variables than in others. These changes bring the feedback closer to the keys established in the scientific literature to obtain the benefits of feedback, such as a higher-quality teaching–learning process, a better team climate, and an increase in the motivation and autonomy of the participants. The modification of the rules, especially those directly related to the training of educational values, can encourage coaches to reflect on their verbal behaviour, the need to adapt to players' needs, and to consider other aspects that can benefit them in the competition, such as the white card.

Coaches are aware of the existence of this card and what they must do to get it, so they are more attentive to the type of feedback they give and try to modify it if necessary. All of this could be the reason for the results obtained and how the change in the rules influenced the type of feedback given by the coaches.

Limitations

The main limitation is that the sample was only made up of boys due to the lack of female teams. Also, the influence of biological age on the coach's feedback was not analysed. It would also be necessary to carry out studies with a wider range of teams to obtain more feedback from coaches, as well as analysing at different training levels.

5. Conclusions

The following can be concluded:

- The direction of feedback is mostly individual in both the normal and modified tournaments.
- The intention of the feedback, as well as the values it provides, does not vary across tournaments, as prescriptive, affective, non-valued feedback continues to predominate.
- The emotional orientation of the feedback changes when the fair play variable is introduced into the rules, decreasing negative feedback and increasing positive feedback.
- Coaches' feedback is less controlling and more autonomy-supportive when the rules are modified.
- Changing the rules has a positive effect on the type of feedback given by coaches, encouraging the beginning of a change in this type of feedback and moving closer to the recommendations of the scientific literature on what constitutes appropriate feedback.
- These results invite the scientific community to analyse the feedback in different experimental studies with modified competitions in individual and team sports. In this way, it will be important to analyse the variables in the type of feedback in players with different levels of maturity development.

Author Contributions: Conceptualization, L.M.-J. and E.O.-T.; methodology, L.M.-J. and E.O.-T.; software, V.M.-C.; validation, L.M.-J., R.A.B.-A. and E.O.-T.; formal analysis, L.M.-J. and E.O.-T.; investigation, L.M.-J. and E.O.-T.; resources, L.M.-J. and E.O.-T.; data curation, L.M.-J. and E.O.-T.; writing—original draft preparation, L.M.-J. and V.M.-C.; writing—review and editing, L.M.-J., R.A.B.-A. and V.M.-C.; visualisation, R.A.B.-A.; supervision, E.O.-T.; project administration, E.O.-T.; funding acquisition, E.O.-T. All authors have read and agreed to the published version of the manuscript.

Funding: This research was funded by Fundación Real Madrid, grant number FRM-UMU-36778, F.C. Cartagena SAD, grant number FCCartagena-UMU-3813, and Ministerio Ciencia, Innovación y Univerisdades, grant number PID2023-150811NB-I00 MCIN/AEI/10.13039/501100011033/FEDER, UE.

Institutional Review Board Statement: The study was conducted in accordance with the Declaration of Helsinki and approved by the Ethics Committee of University of Murcia (protocol code 2829/2020) in 14 May 2020 for studies involving humans.

Informed Consent Statement: Informed consent was obtained from all subjects involved in the study.

Data Availability Statement: Data is contained within the article.

Conflicts of Interest: The authors declare no conflit de interest.

References

1. Merino, A.; Arraiz-Pérez, A.; Sabirón-Sierra, F. Procesos formativos en el fútbol prebenjamín: El paso de la ingenuidad a la institucionalización. *Educ. Fís. Cienc.* **2016**, *18*, e013.
2. Ortega, E. Análisis de la Participación del Jugador con Balón en Etapas de Formación en Baloncesto (14–16 años) y su Relación con la Autoeficacia. Ph.D. Thesis, Universidad de Granada, Granada, Spain, 2004.
3. Ruiz, L.M. *Deporte y Aprendizaje, Procesos de Adquisición y Desarrollo de Habilidades*; Visor Distribuciones S.A: Madrid, Spain, 1997.
4. Piñar, M.I.; Cárdenas, D. La competición como herramienta formativa: Diferentes propuestas en minibasket. *Rev. Wanceulen Ef. Digit.* **2010**, *7*, 4–14.
5. Jiménez, G.; Recio, J.A.; Díaz, B.; Flórez, G. Uso de competiciones y sistemas de clasificación como metodología de evaluación de una asignatura. En Asociación de Enseñantes Universitarios de la Informática (Eds.). *Jorn. Enseñanza Informática* **2012**, *18*, 25–32.
6. Reverter, J.; Plaza, D.; Mayolas, C.; Adell, L. La competición deportiva como medio de enseñanza en los centros educativos de primaria. *Retos* **2009**, *16*, 5–8. [CrossRef]
7. Manzino, C.; Rodríguez, V. Desigualdades en el acceso a la competición deportiva: El caso de las escuelas de Montevideo (Uruguay). *Lect. Educac. Fís. Deporte* **2021**, *25*, 2–15. [CrossRef]
8. Sánchez, P. Actividad física y deportiva en las diferentes edades. *Innov. Exper. Educ.* **2008**, *11*, 1–12.
9. Buszard, T.; Farrow, D.; Reid, M. Designing Junior Sport to Maximize Potential: The Knowns, Unknowns, and Paradoxes of Scaling Sport. *Front. Psychol.* **2020**, *10*, 2878. [CrossRef]
10. Ticó, J. La competición en el deporte de base: ¿educación o perversión? *Cuad. Psicol. Deporte* **2009**, *9*, 86. Available online: https://revistas.um.es/cpd/article/view/86161 (accessed on 23 May 2024).
11. Correia, V.; Carvalho, J.; Araújo, D.; Pereira, E.; Davids, K. Principles of nonlinear pedagogy in sport practice. *Phys. Educ. Sport Pedagog.* **2019**, *24*, 117–132. [CrossRef]
12. McCarthy, J.; Bergholz, L.; Bartlett, M. *Re-Designing Youth Sport: Change the Game*; Routledge: New York, NY, USA, 2016.
13. Buszard, T.; Garofolini, A.; Reid, M.; Farrow, D.; Oppici, L.; Whiteside, D. Scaling sports equipment for children promotes functional movement variability. *Sci. Rep.* **2020**, *10*, 3111. [CrossRef]
14. Ortega, E.; Piñar, I.; Salado, J.; Palao, J.M.; Gómez, M.A. Opinión de expertos y entrenadores sobre el reglamento de la competición infantil en baloncesto. *RICYDE* **2012**, *28*, 142–150. [CrossRef]
15. Blanca, J.C. Incidencia de las Modificaciones Reglamentarias Sobre el Proceso de Aprendizaje en Badminton. Ph.D. Thesis, Universidad de Jaén, Jaén, Spain, 2021.
16. Timmerman, E.; De Water, J.; Kachel, K.; Reid, M.; Farrow, D.; Savelsbergh, G. The effect of equipment scaling on children's sport performance: The case for tennis. *J. Sports Sci.* **2015**, *33*, 1093–1100. [CrossRef] [PubMed]
17. Giménez-Egido, J.M.; Carvalho, J.; Araújo, D.; Ortega-Toro, E. Perceived self-efficacy by Under-10 tennis players when scaling the equipment and play area. *Psychol. Sport Exerc.* **2023**, *67*, 102407. [CrossRef] [PubMed]
18. Vilar, L.; Duarte, R.; Silva, P.; Chow, J.Y.; Davids, K. The influence of pitch dimensions on performance during small-sided and conditioned soccer games. *J. Sports Sci.* **2014**, *32*, 1751–1759. [CrossRef]
19. García-Angulo, A.; Palao, J.M.; Giménez-Egido, J.M.; García-Angulo, F.J.; Ortega-Toro, E. Effect of the Modification of the Number of Players, the Size of the Goal, and the Size of the Field in Competition on the Play Actions in U-12 Male Football. *Int. J. Environ. Res. Public Health* **2020**, *17*, 518. [CrossRef]
20. Sánchez-Sáez, J.A.; Morillo-Baro, J.P.; Sánchez, J.M.; Lara, D.; Arias-Estero, J.L. Estudio piloto sobre las respuestas motrices y psicológicas de jugadores y entrenadores durante la competición a la propuesta de reglas para minibalonmano playa. *Retos* **2022**, *43*, 623–633. [CrossRef]
21. Thomas, C.; Nolte, K.; Schmidt, M.; Jaitner, T. Lower Baskets and Smaller Balls Influence Mini-Basketball Players' Throwing Motions. *Biomechanics* **2023**, *3*, 71–78. [CrossRef]
22. Viciana, J.; Cervelló, E.; Ramírez, J.; San-Matías, J.; Requena, B. Influencia del feedback positivo y negativo en alumnos de secundaria sobre el clima ego-tarea percibido, la valoración de la EF y la preferencia en la complejidad de las tareas de clase. *Eur. J. Hum. Mov.* **2003**, *10*, 99–116.

23. Sánchez, D.L.; Viciana, J. Análisis del discurso de un entrenador de fútbol: Comparación entre dos situaciones diferentes de competición. *Eur. J. Hum. Mov.* **2002**, *8*, 161–173.
24. Ortín, G. Use of Feedback and Motivation in the Players. Comparison Between an Expert Coach and a New Coach. Bachelor's Thesis, Universidad de Zaragoza, Zaragoza, Spain, 2018.
25. Pinheiro, V.; Camerino, O.; Richheimer, P. Fair play in sport initiation, a study of football coaches. *Retos* **2014**, *25*, 32–35. [CrossRef]
26. Viciana, J.; Zabala, M. El papel educativo y la responsabilidad de los entrenadores deportivos. Una investigación sobre las instrucciones a escolares en fútbol de competición. *Rev. Educ.* **2004**, *335*, 163–187.
27. Mamani-Ramos, Á.A. *El Feedback Como Instrumento de Aprendizaje en Educación Física y Deporte: La Clave del Éxito*; Kinesis: Madrid, Spain, 2020.
28. Stobart, G. Fairnessin multicultural assessment systems. *Assess. Educ.* **2005**, *12*, 275–287.
29. Hattie, J.; Clarke, S. *Aprendizaje Visible: Feedback*; Ediciones Paraninfo: Madrid, Spain, 2020.
30. Huéscar, H.; Barrachina, J.; Moreno, J.A. *En Búsqueda de la Autonomía en Educación Física*; Octaedro: Barcelona, Spain, 2022. [CrossRef]
31. Palao-Andrés, J.M.; Hernández-Hernández, E.; Guerrero-Cruz, P.; Ortega-Toro, E. Efecto de distintas estrategias de presentación de feedback mediante vídeo en clases de Educación Física. *Apunts* **2011**, *106*, 26–35. [CrossRef]
32. Martínez-Jiménez, L.; Ortega-Toro, E. Estudio del feedback de entrenadores/as de voleibol a jugadoras durante la competición en etapa formativa. *JUMP* **2023**, *8*, 49–58. [CrossRef]
33. García, I.; Bustos, R.B. Desarrollo de la autonomía y la autorregulación en estudiantes universitarios: Una experiencia de investigación y mediación. *Sinéctica* **2020**, *55*, e1108. [CrossRef]
34. Fonseca-Morales, A.; Martínez-Gallego, R. Feedback y aprendizaje en el tenis: Conceptualización, clasificación e implicaciones prácticas. *ITF Coach Sport Sci. Rev.* **2022**, *30*, 49–52. [CrossRef]
35. Sánchez-Oliva, D.; Sánchez-Miguel, P.A.; Amado-Alonso, D.; Marcos, F.; García-Calvo, T. Análisis de la conducta verbal del entrenador de fútbol en función de su formación federativa y del periodo del partido en categorías inferiores. *Retos* **2010**, *18*, 24–28.
36. Boud, D.; Molloy, E. (Eds.) *Feedback in Higher and Professional Education: Understanding It and Doing It Well*; Routledge: London, UK, 2013.
37. Hernández, V.M.; Santana, P.J.; Sosa, J.J. Feedback y autorregulación del aprendizaje en educación superior. *Rev. Investig. Educ.* **2021**, *39*, 227–248. [CrossRef]
38. Unesco. *Educación de Valores a Través del Deporte*; Unesco: Paris, France, 2019.
39. Cecchini, J.A.; Montero, J.; Peña, J.V. Repercusiones del programa de intervención para desarrollar la responsabilidad personal y social de Hellison sobre los comportamientos de fair-play y el auto-control. *Psicothema* **2003**, *4*, 631–637.
40. Weinberg, R.S.; Gould, D. *Fundam Psicol Deport Ejerc Fís*, 4th ed.; Editoral Medica Panamericana: Madrid, Spain, 2010.
41. Ortega-Vila, G.; Alarcón-López, F.; Giménez Fuentes-Guerra, F.J.; Ortega-Toro, E.; Robles-Rodríguez, J.; Abad-Robles, M.T. El modelo de iniciación al fútbol y educación en valores de la Fundación Real Madrid. *JUMP* **2022**, *6*, 26–47. [CrossRef]
42. Sánchez-Alcaraz, B.J.; López, G.; Valero, A.; Gómez-Mármol, A. Los programas de educación en valores a través de la educación física y el deporte. *Act. Fís. Deport. Cienc. Prof.* **2017**, *25*, 45–58.
43. Fernández, A. *Transmitiendo Valores: El Papel de la Fundación del Real Madrid; Sesión de conferencia. In IV Jornadas de Transferencia: De la Ciencia a Los Entrenadores, Murcia, Spain*; 2023; Available online: https://www.um.es/web/agenda/actividad?id=334401&title=jornadas-de-transferencia-de-la-ciencia-a-los-entrenadores (accessed on 28 March 2024).
44. Carreras, J.C.; Fuentes-Gimenez, F.J. Methodology of education used in the education of the tennis during the stage of initiation. *Retos* **2010**, *218*, 60–65. [CrossRef]
45. Giannousi, M.; Mountaki, F.; Karamousalidis, G.; Bebetsos, G.; Kioumourtzoglou, E. Coaching Behaviors and the Type of Feedback They Provide to Young Volleyball Athletes. *J. Phys. Educ. Sport* **2016**, *16*, 1372–1380.
46. Ortega-Vila, G.; Franco, J.; Giménez, J.; Durán, J.; Jiménez, J.; Jiménez, P.J.; Lambert, J. An evaluation of the" white card" as a resource for promoting an educational sports competition. *J. Hum. Sport Exerc.* **2016**, *11*, 19–30. [CrossRef]
47. Pérez, B.L.; Seoane, A.M.; García, M.S. Differences Between Perceived and Registered Behavior of Basketball Coaches After Shot. *SAGE Open* **2015**, *53*, 215824401560251. [CrossRef]

sports

MDPI

Article

External Load Variability in Elite Futsal: Positional Demands and Microcycle Structuring for Player Well-Being and Performance

Héctor Gadea-Uribarri [1], Elena Mainer-Pardos [2,*], Ainhoa Bores-Arce [3], Rafael Albalad-Aiguabella [2], Sergio López-García [1] and Carlos Lago-Fuentes [3]

[1] Faculty of Education, Universidad Pontificia de Salamanca, 37002 Salamanca, Spain; hgadeauribarri@hotmail.com (H.G.-U.); slopezga@upsa.es (S.L.-G.)

[2] Health Sciences Faculty, Universidad San Jorge, Autov A23 km 299, Villanueva de Gállego, 50830 Zaragoza, Spain; ralbalad@usj.es

[3] Faculty of Health Sciences, Universidad Europea del Atlántico, 39011 Santander, Spain; ainhoa.bores@uneatlantico.es (A.B.-A.); carlos.lago@uneatlantico.es (C.L.-F.)

* Correspondence: epardos@usj.es

Abstract: The aim of this study was to compare the external load of each session along competitive microcycles on an elite futsal team, considering the positions and relationships of the players. The external load of 10 elite players from a First Division team in the Spanish Futsal League (age 27.5 ± 7 years, height 1.73 ± 0.05 m, weight 70.1 ± 3.8 kg) were recorded across 30 microcycles. The players' external loads were monitored using OLIVER devices. To analyse the external load, Levene's test was conducted to assess the homogeneity of variances, followed by one-way analysis of variance (ANOVA) to identify differences in dependent variables across the different microcycle days and player positions. Regarding external load during the microcycle, the day with the lowest external load was MD-1, and the days with the highest external load were MD-3 and MD-4. In addition, considering playing positions, pivots exhibited the lowest loads throughout the microcycle, whereas wingers and defenders exhibited the highest loads, depending on the variables analysed. By providing reference values from elite contexts, this study offers practical insights for S&C coaches to optimize microcycles. Furthermore, it contributes to workload management strategies within sport science and public health frameworks, promoting sustainable performance and athlete wellness in futsal.

Keywords: load monitoring; periodisation; team sport; player position

1. Introduction

Recent advances in data collection and analysis technologies have enhanced our understanding of the workload and physical demands of team sports [1]. These developments have enabled teams to refine their training programmes, thereby improving player performance and reducing injury risks in elite athletes [2,3]. Monitoring workload has become a crucial aspect of sports research, providing a solid foundation for informed decision-making and injury prevention [4,5]. Over more than two decades of study and application in various sports, the concept of training load has evolved to include both external loads (physical exertion performed during a training session or match) and internal loads (related to physical and physiological responses) [6,7].

From a multidisciplinary perspective, understanding the intricate relationships between workload, performance, and injury prevention in sport aligns with broader public health goals, such as promoting athlete wellness and longevity in sport careers. This highlights the importance of integrating sport science and public health frameworks to ensure sustainable sport development.

The global rise in futsal popularity over the past 15 years has been remarkable [8]. Despite this growth, published studies on futsal are limited [1,9–11]. For this reason, it is necessary to continue investigating the training methods employed by teams, monitoring load strategies and coaching staff strategies to better understand the physical demands of this intermittent sport [8]. In futsal, external workload monitoring is essential for tracking both training sessions and matches. Data have shown that male players cover an average distance of 4000 m per match, equivalent to approximately 120 m per minute [12], 675 m at high intensity (12–18 km/h) [1], 135 m at maximum intensity (>18 km/h) [10], 534 m in accelerations (>2 m/s^2), and 510 m in decelerations (>2 m/s^2) [13].

Training sessions across microcycles were designed to adapt player performances throughout the season. They can improve the physical attributes of players by aligning their capabilities with the sport's specific demands [8]. However, excessive training without sufficient recovery time can be detrimental, and insufficient workload can negatively impact and limit both individual and collective performance capabilities [7]. Therefore, developing strategies to monitor and control the workload during various training sessions is crucial for enhancing performance and reducing the risk of injury [8].

Furthermore, players must be well-prepared to meet the demands of the sport. Adapting training plans to adjust volume and intensity throughout competitive cycles is essential [14]. New technologies, such as global positioning systems (GPS) and inertial measurement units (IMU), have provided coaches with tools to precisely monitor the external workload experienced by players. These technologies allow for the tailoring of training sessions based on the positions of players and individual needs [10,15].

The use of advanced monitoring technologies not only improves player-specific training, but also addresses critical public health issues by reducing the prevalence of injury and promoting optimal recovery. These innovations bridge the gap between research and practice, exemplifying the multidisciplinary spirit of contemporary sports science.

Another key factor in improving performance is maintaining an appropriate balance between training and recovery. However, planning training programmes for team sports presents challenges, such as determining the appropriate workload distribution during weekly training sessions and during competitive phases [15]. To achieve a more personalised approach, considering workload data specific to players' positions would be beneficial, although such data are currently limited in futsal [14].

Knowledge of workload variations not only contributes to optimizing sport performance, but also aligns with public health priorities, ensuring the long-term health of athletes and sustainable participation in competitive sports. This underlines the importance of futsal research in the global context of sport science and health promotion.

The variation in workload metrics across microcycles has been less studied than the variability observed in competition [5,9,16,17]. Nonetheless, these variations in microcycle workloads are critical for achieving the necessary adaptations in elite team athletes [14].

Poor workload management is a primary injury risk factor in team sports and player availability [8]. To understand variations throughout a competitive season, it is essential to measure and compare workloads during microcycles. A busy schedule of matches and intense training sessions can increase fatigue, thereby elevating the risk of injury [5,14]. Therefore, workload management is vital for tailoring training to each player's individual needs, ensuring proper recovery and optimal performance on match days [7,18].

In addressing these challenges, sport science continues to evolve, offering practical strategies to improve team performance and mitigate health risks. This study contributes to examining the external loading dynamics of futsal, providing valuable information on the relationship between workload management, performance, and injury prevention.

Consequently, the aim of this study was to compare the external load of each session along competitive microcycles on an elite futsal team, considering the players' positions and relationship with competition, to provide insights that support optimised performance, injury prevention, and player well-being.

2. Materials and Methods

2.1. Participants

The external load of 10 elite players (TIER 3) [19] from a First Division team in the Spanish Futsal League was recorded (age 27.5 ± 7 years, height 1.73 ± 0.05 m, weight 70.1 ± 3.8 kg). Goalkeepers were excluded from the study. The average duration of player participation in training sessions was 1:08 ± 00:12 h:min, which included a 15 min warm-up preceding the main part of the session (Table 1).

Table 1. Duration of each training session along the microcycle.

Session	Duration (h:min) (M ± SD)
MD-5	01:11 ± 00:04
MD-4	01:20 ± 00:09
MD-3	01:16 ± 00:06
MD-2	01:10 ± 00:05
MD-1	00:50 ± 00:02

M: mean. SD: standard deviation.

2.2. Study Design

This study used a longitudinal observational design, which was conducted throughout the 2022–2023 season. A total of 30 competitive microcycles were analysed, including 125 training observations and 21 matches (146 in total) for the evaluation and analysis of external loads over a period of 30 weeks. An example of a typical microcycle is described below (Table 2).

The external load of the players was monitored using the OLIVER IMU (Barcelona, Spain) devices (Inertial Measurement Unit), which have been validated in previous studies [20,21]. All players wore the OLIVER device on their calf, with the devices being activated just before the warm-up for training sessions and immediately after the warm-up for matches [5]. The OLIVER signal frequency was set to 27 Hz. To minimise potential device variability, each player was required to consistently use the same device during all training sessions. The data were analysed using the OLIVER software platform (TryOliver Platform 2.42).

All participants were verbally informed about the purpose and procedures of the study, and each provided signed informed consent in accordance with the Declaration of Helsinki. The study was approved by the University's Research Ethics Committee (CEI-35/2022).

Table 2. Example of a typical competitive microcycle.

Session	Content	Dimension	Time
MD-5 (In the morning)	Gym		
MD-5 (In the afternoon)	Possession	28 × 20	6′
	Warming up goalkeepers	20 × 20	6′
	2 × 1 fragmented track king or every 1′30″ changes	40 × 20	6′
	Set piece + 2 × 2 link + pivot	25 × 20	8′
	Conditioned match	28 × 20	8′
	5 × 4 specific attack	20 × 20	6′
MD-4	Possession	40 × 20	6′
	2 × 2 small space with separate goalkeepers	10 × 10	5′
	3 × 3 3 teams king of the track or every 1′30″ changes	23 × 20	8′
	Conditioned match	40 × 20	8′
	Modulated match	40 × 20	2 × 4′
	5 × 4 specific defense	20 × 20	8′
MD-3	Positional game	20 × 20	5′
	Rondo + regression link	40 × 20	6′
	3 × 2 transitions	40 × 20	4′
	3 × 3 + pivots	25 × 20	6′
	Conditioned match	40 × 20	6′
	Modulated match	40 × 20	7′
MD-2	Positional game	40 × 20	7′
	Warming up goalkeepers	20 × 20	5′
	Conditioned match	40 × 20	2 × 9′
	5 × 4 specific defense	20 × 20	5′
	5 × 4 specific attack	20 × 20	5′
MD-1	Peladao	40 × 20	9′
	Match conditioned for set pieces	20 × 20	9′
	5 × 4 specific attack	20 × 20	9′
MD	Game		
MD+1	Day off		

A conditioned match refers to running time, while a modulated match refers to stopped time.

2.3. Procedure

Building on previous futsal studies [1,9,13] that analysed the conditional demands of competition, the variables examined in this study included: total distance (m), walking distance 0–6 km/h (m), jogging distance 6.1–12 km/h (m), high-intensity distance 12.1–18 km/h (m), maximum-intensity distance >18.1 km/h (m), high accuracy (m) (>2 m/s^2), High Dec (m) (>−2 m/s^2), number of accelerations (>2 m/s^2), number of decelerations (>2 m/s^2), and MAX Speed (km/h). Once the training sessions were completed, the data were categorised according to the day of the week relative to the match. MD-5 (5 days before the match), MD-4 (4 days before the match), MD-3 (3 days before the match), MD-2 (2 days before the match), MD-1 (1 day before the match), and MD (match day), based on previously published scientific studies [5,14].

2.4. Data Processing

In the pre-processing phase, a Butterworth filter was implemented to remove noise from the signals, selecting the filter parameters specifically to preserve the relevant features of our data while removing unwanted interference.

For certain analyses that require the detection of specific motion patterns, an additional smoothing process was applied using a Hanning window filter, with a window size based on our sampling frequency. No amplification of the signals is performed, as the original data provide adequate levels for our analysis.

Regarding the inherent limitations of IMUs, the accumulation of error (drift) in distance estimation by double integration of acceleration is well known. To address this limitation, pattern detection and machine learning algorithms were employed to segment the signal into discrete intervals, periodically restarting the integration process to mitigate error accumulation (i.e., detection of steps and different player actions, such as ball impact or ball driving) [20].

2.5. Statistical Analysis

The homogeneity of variances was initially assessed using Levene's test. Subsequently, one-way analysis of variance (ANOVA) was performed to identify differences in the dependent variables across the various days of the microcycle and between playing positions. When significant differences were found, Bonferroni post hoc tests were applied to analyse specific changes when variances were homogeneous; otherwise, Dunnett's T3 post hoc tests were used. The level of statistical significance was set at $p < 0.05$. Finally, the effect size (ES) was calculated to evaluate the statistical significance and to quantify the magnitude of differences between groups, utilizing Cohen's d statistic. The interpretation of Cohen's d was categorized as follows: values >0.2 indicated a small effect, >0.6 a moderate effect, and >1.2 a large effect. All statistical analyses were performed using SPSS software (version 29.0; IBM Corporation, Armonk, NY, USA).

3. Results

Table 3 presents the results obtained after comparing the recorded variables in terms of both day of the week and playing position. The competitive load was significantly higher for distances covered at various speeds greater than 6 km/h, and for the maximum speed reached during the match.

Regarding the comparison of loads across the microcycle, MD-1 showed significantly the lowest values for most variables compared with the rest of the week. Additionally, MD-5 was the second session with the lowest intensity, although it showed significantly higher distances covered at lower speeds (0–6 km/h) ($p < 0.05$). Finally, MD-4 and MD-3 were the most demanding training sessions across all variables; for instance, total distance and high accelerations (>2 m/s^2) were significantly higher in MD-3 than MD-1 ($p < 0.05$, d: 2.37; $p < 0.05$, d: 2.17, respectively) and also both variables were higher in MD-4 than MD-1 ($p < 0.05$, d: 2.08; $p < 0.05$, d: 1.85, respectively), whereas MD-2 demonstrated significant differences with MD-1 for most variables.

Table 3. Differences in external load between session of microcycle and playing position.

	Position	MD	MD-1	MD-2	MD-3	MD-4	MD-5
		M ± SD	M ± SD	M ± SD	M ± SD	M ± SD	M ± SD
Total distance (m)	Defenders	3434.57 ± 1198.55 b	2705.61 ± 344.38 ^	3787.93 ± 494.15 b,^	4087.06 ± 605.98 a,b,c,f,^	4146.3 ± 731.4 a,b,c,f,^	3587.7 ± 818.92 b,^
	Wingers	3569.08 ± 1169.04 b	2838.71 ± 309.11 °,^	3805.17 ± 635.89 b,^	4169.65 ± 526.92 a,b,c,f,^	4248.5 ± 786.28 a,b,c,f,^	3795.83 ± 662.13 b,^
	Pivots	3439.22 ± 660.25 b,c	2218.33 ± 303.17	3011.88 ± 568.8 b	3320.06 ± 566.25 b	3378.01 ± 690.36 b,c	3124.82 ± 520.57 b
	Total	3496.25 ± 1079.96 b	2659.12 ± 397.99	3615.8 ± 660.97 b	3949.11 ± 657.87 a,b,c,f	4005.41 ± 821.66 a,b,c,f	3555.1 ± 737.51 b
[0–6] km/h (m)	Defenders	1223.7 ± 388.41	1190.24 ± 163.02 ^	1630.95 ± 193.79 a,b,f,^	1591.16 ± 283.31 a,b,^	1648.78 ± 237.87 a,b,f,^	1428.98 ± 330.38 a,b,c
	Wingers	1166.65 ± 336.18	1176.36 ± 174.03 ^	1568.24 ± 201.79 a,b,f,^	1549.15 ± 226.64 a,b,f,^	1599.67 ± 238.9 a,b,f,^	1404.81 ± 239.62 a,b,c
	Pivots	1267.44 ± 282.05 b	1082.83 ± 203.99	1429.59 ± 290.21 b	1429.19 ± 275.63 b	1496.69 ± 252.66 a,b	1380.7 ± 192.12 b
	Total	1208.18 ± 343.18	1161.49 ± 181.21	1558.26 ± 234.59 a,b,f	1536.91 ± 264.87 a,b,f	1592.71 ± 247.59 a,b,f	1407.47 ± 264.96 a,b
[6.1–12] km/h (m)	Defenders	1356.27 ± 525.58 b	1103.08 ± 165.09 ^	1538.71 ± 271.84 b,^	1646.91 ± 274.97 a,b,^	1686.92 ± 352.3 a,b,c,^	1592.66 ± 328.44 b,^
	Wingers	1393.84 ± 490.04 b	1201.32 ± 139.85 °,^	1585.52 ± 270.57 a,b,^	1682.55 ± 230.96 a,b,^	1738.6 ± 368.79 a,b,c,^	1671.14 ± 353.46 a,b,^
	Pivots	1417.55 ± 260.11 b,c,d,e,f	878.67 ± 136.12	1223.5 ± 255.32 b	1345.81 ± 245.75 b	1394.11 ± 357.52 b,c	1338.19 ± 284.08 b
	Total	1387.45 ± 458.4 b	1097.49 ± 191.84	1485 ± 303.65 b	1594.11 ± 283.62 a,b,c	1638.4 ± 384.47 a,b,c	1560.44 ± 352.03 a,b
[12.1–18] km/h (m)	Defenders	676.06 ± 299.52 b,c	383.55 ± 122.48 ^	528.27 ± 145.58 b,^	697.25 ± 183.78 b,c,f,^	685.83 ± 227.73 b,c,f,^	548.93 ± 167.52
	Wingers	757.34 ± 292.57 b,c,f	413.1 ± 93.47 °,^	580.97 ± 153.64 b,°,^	761.03 ± 184.95 b,c,f,^	763.47 ± 248.38 b,c,f,^	620.07 ± 173.98
	Pivots	559.02 ± 117.64 b,c,d,e,f,°,*	228.78 ± 70.51	310.13 ± 109.69 b	449.09 ± 150.96 a,b,c	416.15 ± 184.98 a,b,c	360.20 ± 133.34
	Total	685.44 ± 275.17 b,c,f	363.34 ± 123.27	499.52 ± 177.01 b	668.28 ± 214.54 b,c,f	653.35 ± 264.53 b,c,f	530.13 ± 191.24
[18.1–3600] km/h (m)	Defenders	178.55 ± 92,36 b,c,e,f	28.74 ± 28.14	90 ± 65.45 b,^	151.73 ± 77.6 b,c,f,^	124.77 ± 84.93 a,b,^	90.36 ± 45.37 b,^
	Wingers	251.25 ± 151.39 b,c,d,e,f,°,^	47.93 ± 36.22 °,^	105.35 ± 64.15 b,^	176.91 ± 88.92 a,b,c,f,^	146.76 ± 92.2 a,b,c,f,^	99.82 ± 67.62 a,b,^
	Pivots	195.22 ± 101.21 b,c,d,e,f	28.06 ± 27.71	48.66 ± 45.79 b	95.97 ± 76.55 a,b,c,f	71.06 ± 58.64 a,b	45.74 ± 36.29 b
	Total	215.18 ± 128.02 b,c,d,e,f	36.81 ± 33.1	86.77 ± 64.55 b	149.81 ± 87.69 a,b,c,e,f	120.95 ± 87.49 a,b,c,d,f	83.02 ± 57.51 b
High Acc (m) (>2 m/s^2)	Defenders	497.6 ± 190.45 b	315.34 ± 67.06 ^	454.71 ± 91.81 b,^	541.38 ± 106.02 b,c,^	568.56 ± 141.62 b,c,^	515.72 ± 130.41 b,^
	Wingers	571.87 ± 220.84 b,c	358.43 ± 60.26 °,^	483.9 ± 124.38 b,^	604.38 ± 113.01 b,c,f,°,^	611.67 ± 150.27 b,c,f,^	545.05 ± 109.38 b,c,^
	Pivots	518.07 ± 141.49 b,c,f	268.26 ± 60.21	354.13 ± 108.49 b	447.64 ± 117.76 b,c	435.46 ± 145.27 b,c	405.67 ± 112.59 b
	Total	535.82 ± 197.27 b,c	323.79 ± 71.5	443.63 ± 120.93 b	546.87 ± 126.5 b,c,f	554.47 ± 161 b,c,f	500.09 ± 129.86 b,c
High Dec (m) (>−2 m/s^2)	Defenders	511.1 ± 212.51 b	352.4 ± 90.97	487.81 ± 107.73 b,^	562.48 ± 124.86 b,c,^	601.47 ± 143.22 b,c,^	551.36 ± 147.33 b,^
	Wingers	503.01 ± 189.79 b	366.4 ± 90.5	485.11 ± 155.32 b,^	582.17 ± 140.13 a,b,c,^	592.73 ± 162.95 a,b,c,^	563.87 ± 141.33 b,c,^
	Pivots	496.88 ± 116.98 b,c,e	262.06 ± 81.54	346.63 ± 128.57 b	426.74 ± 130.64 b,c	412.12 ± 149.86 a,b	412.56 ± 132.63 b
	Total	504.15 ± 182.87 b,c	339.21 ± 97.41	454.06 ± 145.99 b	540.21 ± 145.97 b,c	552.96 ± 171.57 b,c	522.06 ± 153.97 b,c

Table 3. *Cont.*

	Position	MD	MD-1	MD-2	MD-3	MD-4	MD-5
		M ± SD	M ± SD	M ± SD	M ± SD	M ± SD	M ± SD
High accuracy (>2 m/s²)	Defenders	128.92 ± 49.97 b	85.44 ± 16.81 ^	119.6 ± 22.71 b,^	140.43 ± 27.18 b,c,^	148.24 ± 35.37 b,c,^	134.44 ± 33.25 b,^
	Wingers	141.63 ± 53.48 b	94.06 ± 15.21 ^	125.27 ± 31.1 b,^	152.48 ± 28.45 b,c,°,^	155.63 ± 36.94 b,c,f,^	139.69 ± 25.99 b,c,^
	Pivots	134.45 ± 34.92 b,c,f	72.19 ± 15.73	94.92 ± 27.49 b	117.29 ± 27.86 b,c	116.75 ± 36.75 b,c	110.06 ± 28.73 b
	Total	135.93 ± 48.72 b,c	86.32 ± 17.89	116.26 ± 29.95 b	140.31 ± 30.86 b,c	143.77 ± 39.34 b,c,f	130.49 ± 31.6 b,c
High Dec quantity (>−2 m/s²)	Defenders	141.08 ± 62.12 b	102.12 ± 26.83 ^	138.86 ± 30.98 b,^	156.24 ± 37.31 b,c,^	168.49 ± 39.39 a,b,c,^	154.12 ± 40.18 b,^
	Wingers	131.41 ± 49.19 b	104.26 ± 27.28 ^	134.99 ± 43.58 b,^	158.54 ± 40.04 a,b,c,^	162.42 ± 44.32 a,b,c,^	156.09 ± 39.75 a,b,c,^
	Pivots	131.94 ± 29.86 b,c	74.27 ± 24.68	98.38 ± 37.84 b	117.44 ± 36.26 b	113.63 ± 41.52 b	116.03 ± 38.85 b
	Total	134.59 ± 50.17 b	97.13 ± 29.05	127.89 ± 41.42 b	148.47 ± 41.63 a,b,c	153 ± 47.29 a,b,c	145.51 ± 42.89 b,c
MAX Speed (km/h)	Defenders	24.62 ± 1.92 b,c,e,f	20.7 ± 2.71	22.75 ± 2.33 b,^	24.09 ± 1.62 b,c,f,^	23.28 ± 2.27 a,b,^	22.83 ± 1.95 b,^
	Wingers	24.64 ± 1.85 b,c,e,f	20.97 ± 2.42	22.6 ± 2.24 b,^	23.8 ± 2.14 b,c,e,f,^	22.6 ± 2.24 a,b,d	22.47 ± 2.27 b,^
	Pivots	25.14 ± 1.71 b,c,d,e,f	20.45 ± 2.73	20.94 ± 2.93	22.2 ± 2.72 a,b	22.03 ± 2.54 a,b	21.26 ± 2.43
	Total	24.75 ± 1.85 b,c,d,e,f	20.76 ± 2.59	22.27 ± 2.55 b	23.54 ± 2.24 a,b,c,e,f	22.71 ± 2.36 a,b,d	22.3 ± 2.27 b

M: mean. SD: standard deviation. a: >MD; b: >MD-1; c: >MD-2; d: >MD-3; e: >MD-4; f: >MD-5; °: >CI, *: >AL, ^: >PV.

Concerning specific positions, pivots accumulated significantly lower loads across most variables, including distances ($p < 0.05$, d: 2.03), accelerations ($p < 0.05$, d: 2.03), and deceleration ($p < 0.05$, d: 1.21), regardless of the session analysed. During competition, they covered less distance at high speeds (12–18 km/h and >18 km/h) ($p < 0.05$ for both, d: 1.51 and 0.98, respectively). Throughout the rest of the microcycle, pivots exhibited significantly lower performance for all variables during MD-5, MD-4, MD-3, and MD-2 (see Table 3). However, for MD-1, significant differences were observed only in accelerations ($p < 0.05$, d: 0.74) and deceleration ($p < 0.05$, d: 1.05).

4. Discussion

The aim of this study was to compare the external load of each session along competitive microcycles on an elite futsal team, considering the players' positions and relationships with competition. A novel aspect of this study was the analysis of the distribution of the absolute training load based on the match day and specific positions across various variables. The main findings were as follows: (a) MD-1 was the day with the lowest load, consistent with its purpose of recovery and tapering, while MD-4 and MD-3 were the days with the highest loads, reflecting their role in physical conditioning and tactical-technical development. (b) Pivots experienced the lowest loads during the microcycle, likely due to their positional role with less total distance covered, whereas wingers and defenders showed the highest loads across the different variables analysed, indicative of their higher physical demands during both defensive and offensive phases of play. These findings underscore the importance of adapting training and recovery strategies not only to optimize performance, but also to reduce the risk of overtraining and injury by addressing critical aspects of an athlete's well-being and long-term health.

Although research has been conducted in sports such as football [14], volleyball [16], basketball [22], and handball [23], regarding the distribution of training load in relation to match days and specific positions, this approach remains limited in futsal. Previous studies have mainly focused on high-intensity variables [9] or tactical aspects with and without the ball [24], but they have not thoroughly addressed how these variables fluctuate throughout the microcycle based on player positions. This highlights the need for interdisciplinary approaches that bridge the gap between sport science and applied practice and provide practical information to optimize performance and reduce the risk of injury.

The external load data obtained on the matchday were consistent with the values reported in previous futsal studies. The total distance covered in our study (3496.25 $\pm$ 1079.96 m) falls within the range reported by earlier research, which varies between 3052 $\pm$ 804 m and 3749 $\pm$ 1123 m [1,10,11,13]. Similarly, the high-intensity distance (12.1–18 km/h) in this study was 685.44 $\pm$ 275.17 m, close to the values recorded during the Final Eight of the Portuguese Cup 2018 (675.3 $\pm$ 298.1 m) [1]. Furthermore, the maximum intensity distance (>18 km/h) of 215.18 $\pm$ 128.02 m is comparable with previously reported ranges, from 254 $\pm$ 101 m [10] to 134.9 $\pm$ 54.1 m [1]. These findings demonstrate a consistent profile of external load demands across competitive futsal contexts, underscoring their relevance for broader applications in team management and player conditioning.

These similarities in metrics suggest that despite potential differences in playing style, team structure, and competitive level, the fundamental physical demands in elite futsal matches are fairly consistent. Such consistency provides a solid foundation for evidence-based strategies aimed at improving player performance and promoting long-term health in high-performance environments. It also demonstrates how standardized workload metrics can serve as a critical tool for aligning training and recovery programs with competitive demands. Regarding accelerations (>2 m/s^2) and decelerations (<−2 m/s^2), our findings (535.82 $\pm$ 197.27 m and 504.15 $\pm$ 182.87 m, respectively) also align with values observed in studies conducted on elite teams [13]. Moreover, the number of acceleration (135.93 ± 48.72) and deceleration (134.59 ± 50.17) is almost identical to that reported by teams from the National Futsal League (135 ± 41 and 129 ± 39, respectively) [10]. This finding is particularly significant because it highlights that these high-intensity actions are important to futsal dynamics and should be a focal point in the design of training and recovery programmes. For instance, prioritising exercises that simulate frequent acceleration and deceleration could enhance players' physical responsiveness during competition, especially during critical moments such as rapid transitions or counterattacks.

These data suggest that competitive loads in futsal exhibit notable consistency among elite Spanish teams and similar leagues, such as the Portuguese league [1]. However, it is essential to note that these metrics could vary depending on contextual factors, such as match duration, tactical approaches, and opposition intensity. Future research that incorporates these contextual elements may provide a more complete and nuanced understanding of external workload patterns, which could lead to advances in team performance management and injury prevention.

Regarding the structuring of the microcycle in our study, MD-1 was the day with the lowest load across all variables ($p < 0.05$). MD-4 was the day with the greatest distance covered, while MD-3 recorded the highest metres covered at high intensity (12.1–18 km/h) and maximum intensity (18.1–3600 km/h). In addition, the day on which the highest meters covered in acceleration and deceleration was MD-4. These results reflect a competitive microcycle profile aligned with common practises in other team sports, where a post-competition recovery session of low to moderate intensity is planned, alongside tapering programming [8]. Such structured approaches highlight the importance of balancing performance optimisation and recovery, reflecting a holistic strategy to manage athletes' physical and psychological readiness for competition. This strategy aims at progressive reduction of the load from MD-4 to MD-1, thereby optimising recovery and ensuring that athletes arrive in the best possible condition for the next match [25–27]. The finding that MD-1 is the day with the lowest load is consistent with previous futsal studies [9], reinforcing the idea of structuring this day as an activation session focused on preparing players for the match day.

When comparing our results with those of other sports, similarities can be found. In handball, the day with the greatest covered distance is typically MD-4, with the highest maximum-intensity runs occurring on the same day [23]. In football, the day with the greatest distance covered during training is MD-3, which differs from our article, which states MD-4 [14,28]. However, our study aligns with soccer research in that the highest distances for maximum-intensity runs were recorded on MD-3 [28]. These inter-sport comparisons not only enhance our understanding of common principles of load management, but also underscore the adaptability of microcycle structuring strategies to the unique demands of each sport. These findings contribute to a multidisciplinary understanding of workload distribution that advances sport science and public health frameworks.

The playing style influences the performance demands of each role, as observed in other sports [14]. In futsal, this research shows that pivots are the players with the lowest loads across different training days and matches, except for MD-1, where the load is similar across all positions. This finding is consistent with those of previous futsal studies [10,29]. This may be attributed to the anthropometric profile of pivots, who tend to have the highest body fat percentage compared with other positions [30].

Wingers are the players who record the highest values in variables such as distance covered, high intensity (12.1–18 km/h), maximum intensity (18.1–3600 km/h), High Acc (m) (>2 m/s^2), and High Acc count (>2 m/s^2), results that align with previous research [10]. However, for the variables of High Dec count (>−2 m/s^2) and High Dec (m) (>−2 m/s^2), depending on the training day, higher values were observed for both defenders and wingers. In matches, defenders carry the highest load on these variables, although no statistically significant differences were found. These findings emphasise the importance of considering the specific demands of each position when designing training programmes, which has already been proposed in other sports [31].

Nonetheless, in futsal, this study is the first to quantify the magnitude of efforts across the competitive microcycle according to playing position. Future research is therefore needed to confirm whether conditional profiles vary, showing pivots as the players with the lowest workload and wingers and defenders with similar workloads, with minor variations depending on the session. Moreover, based on the findings of this study, it is evident that more personalised and specific training should be developed according to the conditional demands of each position.

In handball, compared with other sports, right-wing players registered the lowest total distance covered and the shortest high-intensity distances during matches, while pivots covered the least distance and performed the fewest high-intensity efforts during training sessions [23]. In football, midfielders and attacking midfielders cover the greatest distances during the microcycle, while central defenders and forwards cover the least. However, the highest maximum-intensity distances during training are recorded by fullbacks, with midfielders covering the least [14]. Lastly, in basketball, pivots recorded the highest number of accelerations, while small forwards executed the greatest number of decelerations [32]. These inter-sport analyses highlight the importance of a multidisciplinary and comparative approach to load management, which not only benefits performance in specific sports but also informs broader sport science and athlete health frameworks. While futsal shares similarities with sports such as handball, football, and basketball, the specific demands of each discipline require further investigation to identify tailored training strategies that maximise the desired adaptations. Such an approach would not only enhance player performance but also reduce the risk of injury, particularly in highly intermittent sports like futsal.

One of the main limitations of this study is the small sample size, as only 10 players from one elite futsal team were included. This may limit the generalizability of the findings to other teams or competitive levels. Additionally, goalkeepers were not considered, thereby excluding a crucial component of the team whose physical and conditional demands are unique. Furthermore, although data from 21 official matches were collected, it was not possible to evaluate the entire 30-match season due to logistical and permission constraints, which may have affected the representativeness of the competitive demands recorded. Another limitation is the lack of contextual analysis considering factors such as match outcome, opponent quality and players' physical condition, all of which could significantly influence the observed external loads. Finally, the absence of internal load measurements, such as heart rate profiles or ratings of perceived exertion, which would provide a more comprehensive understanding of futsal match-related demands. Future studies should incorporate these parameters to gain deeper insights into the physiological responses during matches [33].

In future research, it would be advisable to expand the sample size to include more teams, competitive levels, and positions such as goalkeepers to enhance the generalizability and relevance of the findings. An extended longitudinal analysis covering multiple seasons could also be valuable, allowing the identification of consistent patterns or variations associated with tactical and physical changes over time. Moreover, incorporating contextual factors such as opponent level, match outcome, and season phase would enrich the understanding of conditional demands. Finally, exploring the relationship between monitored external load patterns during the microcycle and injury risk could help develop more effective prevention strategies.

5. Conclusions

The findings of this study highlight that the microcycle structure in an elite futsal team follows a clear pattern, where the day with the lowest external load is MD-1, used as a pre-match activation session, while the days with the highest load are MD-3 and MD-4, depending on the variables analysed. This structured approach reflects the importance of balancing recovery and preparation, ensuring that players are physically, tactically, and mentally optimised for competition. Such strategies align with holistic frameworks in sports science, aimed at sustaining high performance while minimising injury risks. Additionally, the metrics for total distance, intensity, and the number of acceleration and deceleration obtained in this study underline the importance of monitoring these variables to adjust the loads throughout the microcycle.

Regarding positions, the results reveal significant differences in conditional demands. Pivots display the lowest loads during the microcycle, while wingers stand out in variables such as high- and maximum-intensity distance, as well as accelerations, indicating greater physical demands for this position. Defenders exhibit higher loads during decelerations, particularly during matches. These insights emphasize the necessity of designing position-specific training programmes that account for these conditional differences, enhancing player readiness and reducing the risk of overuse injuries.

By offering reference values derived from elite contexts, this study provides practical guidance for S&C coaches, enabling them to plan, adjust, and optimise training programmes in futsal. Moreover, the findings contribute to the broader discourse in sport sciences and public health by addressing critical issues such as workload management, injury prevention, and player well-being. Such multidisciplinary insights are essential for advancing sustainable performance in highly intermittent sports like futsal.

Author Contributions: Conceptualization, H.G.-U., C.L.-F. and E.M.-P.; methodology, H.G.-U., C.L.-F., R.A.-A. and E.M.-P.; validation, H.G.-U., S.L.-G. and A.B.-A.; formal analysis, A.B.-A. and C.L.-F.; investigation, H.G.-U., S.L.-G., R.A.-A. and C.L.-F.; resources, H.G.-U., C.L.-F. and E.M.-P.; data curation, A.B.-A. and C.L.-F. writing—original draft preparation, H.G.-U., A.B.-A., C.L.-F. and E.M.-P.; writing—review and editing, R.A.-A. and C.L.-F.; supervision, S.L.-G., C.L.-F. and E.M.-P. All authors have read and agreed to the published version of the manuscript.

Funding: This research received no external funding.

Institutional Review Board Statement: This study was conducted in accordance with the Declaration of Helsinki and approved by the Institutional Review Board of Universidad Europea del Atlántico (CEI-35/2022) in September 2022.

Informed Consent Statement: Informed consent was obtained from all participants.

Data Availability Statement: The data from this research can be made available by the corresponding author upon reasonable request. Due to privacy concerns, the data are not accessible to the public.

Conflicts of Interest: The authors declare no conflicts of interest.

References

1. Ribeiro, J.; Gonçalves, B.; Coutinho, D.; Brito, J.; Sampaio, J.; Travassos, B. Activity Profile and Physical Performance of Match Play in Elite Futsal Players. *Front. Psychol.* **2020**, *11*, 1709. [CrossRef] [PubMed]
2. Ehrmann, F.E.; Duncan, C.S.; Sindhusake, D.; Franzsen, W.N.; Greene, D.A. GPS and Injury Prevention in Professional Soccer. *J. Strength Cond. Res.* **2016**, *30*, 360–367. [CrossRef]
3. Colby, M.J.; Dawson, B.; Heasman, J.; Rogalski, B.; Gabbett, T.J. Accelerometer- and GPS-Derived Running Loads and Injury Risk in Elite Australian Footballers. *J. Strength Cond. Res.* **2014**, *28*, 2244–2252. [CrossRef]

4. Rossi, A.; Pappalardo, L.; Cintia, P.; Iaia, F.; Fernández, J.; Medina, D. Effective injury prediction in professional soccer using GPS data and machine learning. *Stat* **2017**, *1050*, 23.
5. de Dios, V.; Alkain, P.; Castellano, J.; Rey, E. Accumulative Weekly External and Internal Load Relative to Match Load in Elite Male Youth Soccer Players. *Paediatr. Exerc. Sci.* **2021**, *34*, 119–124. [CrossRef] [PubMed]
6. Franceschi, A.; Robinson, M.; Owens, D.; Brownlee, T.; Bampouras, T.; Ferrari Bravo, D.; Enright, K. Training loads and microcycle periodisation in Italian Serie A youth soccer players. *J. Sports Sci.* **2024**, *42*, 1410–1420. [CrossRef] [PubMed]
7. Oliveira, R.; Brito, J.; Martins, A.; Mendes, B.; Calvete, F.; Carriço, S.; Ferraz, R.; Marques, M.C. In-season training load quantification of one-, two-, and three-game week schedules in a top European professional soccer team. *Physiol. Behav.* **2018**, *201*, 146–156. [CrossRef]
8. Lago Fuentes, C.; Jiménez-Loaisa, A.; Padrón Cabo, A.; Fernández-Villarino, M.; Mecías, M.; Travassos, B.; Rey, E. Monitoring the workloads of a Professional Female Futsal Team over a Season: A Case Study. *Sports* **2020**, *8*, 69. [CrossRef]
9. Illa, J.; Fernández, D.; Reche, X.; Carmona Dalmases, G.; Tarragó, J. Quantification of an Elite Futsal Team's Microcycle External Load Using High and Very High Demanding Scenarios. *Front. Psychol.* **2020**, *11*, 577624. [CrossRef]
10. Illa, J.; Alonso, Ò.; Serpiello, F.; Hodder, R.; Reche, X. Demandas de carga externa y diferencias posicionales en fútbol sala de élite mediante tecnología UWB. *Apunt. Educ. Física Y Deportes* **2021**, *3*, 53–59. [CrossRef]
11. Spyrou, K.; Freitas, T.; Marín Cascales, E.; Herrero-Carrasco, R.; Alcaraz, P. External Match Load and Influence of Contextual Factors in Elite Futsal. *Biol. Sport* **2021**, *39*, 349–354. [CrossRef]
12. Gomes, S.; Travassos, B.; Ribeiro, J.; Castro, H.; Lume Gomes, L.; Ernesto, C. Space and players' number constrain the external and internal load demands in youth futsal. *Front. Sports Act. Living* **2024**, *6*, 1376024. [CrossRef]
13. Gadea-Uribarri, H.; Lago-Fuentes, C.; Bores-Arce, A.; Villavicencio Álvarez, V.E.; López-García, S.; Calero-Morales, S.; Mainer-Pardos, E. External Load Evaluation in Elite Futsal: Influence of Match Results and Game Location with IMU Technology. *J. Funct. Morphol. Kinesiol.* **2024**, *9*, 140. [CrossRef]
14. García, A.; Gómez-Díaz, A.; Bradley, P.; Morera, F.; Casamichana, D. Quantification of a Professional soccer Team's External Load Using a Microcycle Structure. *J. Strength Cond. Res.* **2018**, *32*, 1.
15. Miguel, M.; Cortez, A.; Romero, F.; Loureiro, N.; García, J.; Ibáñez, S. Daily and weekly external loads in the microcycle: Characterisation and comparison of playing positions on amateur soccer. *Front. Sports Act. Living* **2022**, *4*, 943367. [CrossRef] [PubMed]
16. Akyildiz, Z.; Castro, H.; Cene, E.; Laporta, L.; Parim, C.; Altundağ, E.; Akarçeşme, C.; Guidetti, G.; Miale, G.; Silva, A.F.; et al. Within-week differences in external training load demands in elite volleyball players. *BMC Sports Sci. Med. Rehabil.* **2022**, *14*, 188. [CrossRef]
17. Fernandes, R.; Ceylan, H.; Clemente, F.; Brito, J.; Martins, A.; Nobari, H.; Reis, V.M.; Oliveira, R. In-Season Microcycle Quantification of Professional Women Soccer Players—External, Internal, and Wellness Measures. *Healthcare* **2022**, *10*, 695. [CrossRef] [PubMed]
18. Clemente, F.; Owen, A.; Olivares, J.; Nikolaidis, P.; Linden, C.; Mendes, B. Characterisation of the Weekly External Load Profile of Professional Soccer Teams in Portugal and the Netherlands. *J. Hum. Kinet.* **2019**, *66*, 155–164. [CrossRef] [PubMed]
19. McKay, A.; Stellingwerff, T.; Smith, E.; Martin, D.; Mujika, I.; Goosey-Tolfrey, V.; Sheppard, J.; Burke, L.M. Training and Performance Calibre: A Participant Classification Framework. *Int. J. Sports Physiol. Perform.* **2021**, *17*, 1–15.
20. Gadea Uribarri, H.; Lago-Fuentes, C.; Bores-Arce, A.; López-García, S.; Ibáñez, E.; Serrano, C.; Mainer-Pardos, E. Validity of a new tracking device for futsal match. *Acta Kinesiol.* **2024**, *17*, 17–21.
21. Gadea-Uribarri, H.; Lago-Fuentes, C.; Bores-Arce, A.; López-García, S.; Ibáñez, E.; Serrano, C.; Mainer-Pardos, E. Concordance between the new IMU and different small-sided games and real-game tasks in indoor sports: A new IMU is valid for real-game situations in indoor sports. *Acta Kinesiol.* **2024**, *18*, 53–60. [CrossRef]
22. Reina, M.; Mancha, D.; Ibáñez, S. Monitorización de un microciclo competitivo en baloncesto femenino profesional mediante dispositivos inerciales. *Rev. Int. Med. Cienc. Act. Física Deporte* **2022**, *22*, 663–685. [CrossRef]
23. Font, R.; Karcher, C.; Loscos-Fabregas, E.; Altarriba-Bartés, A.; Peña, J.; Vicens-Bordas, J.; Mesas, J.A.; Irurtia, A. The effect of training schedule and playing positions on the training load and game demands of professional handball players. *Biol. Sport* **2022**, *43*, 857–866. [CrossRef]
24. Ribeiro, J.; Yousefian, F.; Monteiro, D.; Illa, J.; Couceiro, M.; Sampaio, J.; Travassos, B. Relating external load variables with individual tactical actions with reference to playing position: An integrated analysis for elite futsal. *Int. J. Perform. Anal. Sport* **2023**, *24*, 1–16. [CrossRef]
25. Vachon, A.; Berryman, N.; Mujika, I.; Paquet, J.-B.; Arvisais, D.; Bosquet, L. Effects of tapering on neuromuscular and metabolic fitness in team sports: A systematic review and meta-analysis. *Eur. J. Sport Sci.* **2020**, *21*, 300–311. [CrossRef]
26. Mujika, I.; Halson, S.; Burke, L.; Balague, G.; Farrow, D. An Integrated, Multifactorial Approach to Optimal Performance in Individual and Team Sports. *Int. J. Sports Physiol. Perform.* **2018**, *13*, 538–561. [CrossRef] [PubMed]

27. Oliva Lozano, J.; Muyor, J.; Pérez-Guerra, A.; Gómez, D.; García-Unanue, J.; Sánchez-Sánchez, J.; Felipe, J.L. Effect of Microcycle Length on Daily External Load, Fatigue, Sleep Quality, Stress, and Muscle Soreness in Professional Soccer Players: A Full-Season Study. *Sports Health A Multidiscip. Approach* **2022**, *15*, 1–5. [CrossRef]
28. Oliva Lozano, J.; Gómez-Carmona, C.; Fortes, V.; Pino Ortega, J. Effects of training days, matches, and microcycle length on workload periodization in professional soccer players: A full-season study. *Biol. Sport* **2021**, *39*, 397–406. [CrossRef]
29. Ohmuro, T.; Iso, Y.; Tobita, A.; Hirose, S.; Ishizaki, S.; Sakaue, K.; Yasumatsu, M. Physical match performance of top Japanese futsal players in different categories and playing positions. *Biol. Sport* **2020**, *37*, 359–365. [CrossRef] [PubMed]
30. Ramos-Campo, D.J.; Martínez Sánchez, F.; Esteban García, P.; Rubio Arias, J.Á.; Bores Cerezal, A.; Clemente-Suarez, V.J.; Jiménez Díaz, J.F. Body Composition Features in Different Positions of Indoor Professional Team Players: Basketball, Handball and Futsal *Int. J. Morphol.* **2014**, *32*, 1316–1324. [CrossRef]
31. Modric, T.; Versic, S.; Sekulic, D. Playing position specifics of running performance during training and matches in male soccer players. *Acta Gymnica* **2020**, *50*, 51–60. [CrossRef]
32. Svilar, L.; Castellano, J.; Jukic, I.; Casamichana, D. Positional Differences in Elite Basketball: Selecting Appropriate Training-Load Measures. *Int. J. Sports Physiol. Perform.* **2018**, *13*, 1–24. [CrossRef]
33. Rago, V.; Brito, J.; Figueiredo, P.; Costa, J.; Krustrup, P.; Rebelo, A. I nternal training load monitoring in professional football: A systematic review of methods using rating of perceived exertion. *J. Sports Med. Phys. Fit.* **2019**, *60*, 160–171.

sports

MDPI

Article

Temperature-Related Variations in Physical Performance During Elite Soccer Matches

Vladimir Pavlinovic [1], Ryland Morgans [2] and Toni Modric [1,3,*]

[1] Faculty of Kinesiology, University of Split, 21000 Split, Croatia; vladimirpavlinovic@gmail.com
[2] School of Sport and Health Sciences, Cardiff Metropolitan University, Cardiff CF23 6XD, UK; rmorgans@cardiffmet.ac.uk
[3] High Performance Sport Center, Croatian Olympic Committee, 10000 Zagreb, Croatia
* Correspondence: toni.modric@kifst.hr; Tel.: +385-21-302-440

Abstract: The aim of this study was to examine the differences in match running performance (MRP) according to the ambient temperature during UEFA Champions League (UCL) matches. Data were collected using an optical tracking system from all teams (n = 32) in all UCL matches (n = 125) during the 2022/23 season, and classified according to the ambient temperature at which matches were played: <5 °C, 6–10 °C, 11–20 °C, and >21 °C. The results revealed the following: (i) less total distance was covered in matches played at ≥21 °C compared to the matches played at 6–10 °C (d = 0.58), (ii) less high-speed running and high-intensity running were covered in matches played at ≥21 °C compared to the matches played at 11–20 °C (d = 0.54 and 0.43, respectively), 6–10 °C (d = 0.89 and 0.8, respectively), and ≤5 °C (d = 0.62 and 0.57, respectively), and (iii) less sprinting was covered in matches played at ≥21 °C compared to the matches played at 6–10 °C (d = 0.22). These findings indicated the significant differences in MRP when UCL matches were played at different ambient temperatures, with notable reductions in overall and high-intensity efforts in warmer conditions.

Keywords: running performance; ambient temperature; soccer; environmental factors

1. Introduction

Soccer is a complex sport characterized by high physical demands, including covering large total distances and performing repeated high-intensity sprints and explosive efforts [1,2]. The most common technique to evaluate physical demands during soccer match-play is an analysis of the players' match running performance (MRP) [3,4]. The MRP typically includes total distance covered, distance covered in different speed zones, accelerations, and decelerations [5,6]. The data on MRP are used by sports scientists primarily to help practitioners in decision-making processes for structuring the elements of training and subsequent match preparation [7]. However, soccer is subject to various situational and environmental factors that affect MRP [8–10], hampering its interpretation and application in practice [11]. Specifically, situational factors within a game, such as a match outcome, match location, and opponent quality have been evaluated with differing results [12–15]. Because of physiological constraints when working in certain settings, environmental elements such as ambient temperature have also been shown to have an impact on MRP [16,17].

Specifically, when working in a hot environment, the body's thermoregulatory system activates mechanisms such as increased sweating to dissipate the heat [18]. This can cause electrolyte imbalances and dehydration, which can harm the heart and lower one's ability to do continuous physical exertion [19]. Also, working in a hot environment raises metabolic stress, prompting faster glycogen breakdown and a higher reliance on anaerobic energy sources, which can lead to early fatigue [20,21]. Conversely, prolonged exposure to cold conditions can affect the body's shivering response and cause peripheral blood vessels to constrict, potentially leading to quicker fatigue and diminished exercise performance over time [19,22].

Research suggests a decline in MRP when temperatures exceed 29 °C [23]. Reports indicate a significant increase in low-intensity demands and exercise time below 85% of maximal heart rate compared to moderate temperatures [23]. Consistent with these findings, another study reported significant effects of hot temperatures on running speed, high-speed runs, and high-intensity and explosive distance covered [24]. When considering FIFA 2014 games, the comparison between low and high temperatures did not reveal significant differences in total distance covered [25]. However, it did show that more intense actions such as the number of sprints were decreased in hotter temperatures, as well as the distance covered at high intensity [26]. Examining the impact of cold temperatures, a study involving professional soccer players generally suggested that physical performance in professional soccer does not decrease in colder conditions [26]. This contrasts with another study which found that at sub-zero temperatures, every 1 °C decrease reduced the team's sprint distance by 19.2 m [27]. However, the study also revealed that total, running, and high-speed running distances showed no significant differences across temperatures up to 10 °C [27].

While ample research exists regarding the influence of ambient temperature on the MRP of soccer players [3,4], this body of research has yet to explore multilevel mixed modeling as an alternative approach for examining the results. This approach offers the capability to assess the independent effects of a variable on an outcome while accounting for all other variables that could affect results (i.e., situational factors), allowing the true differences to be elucidated. Furthermore, although various competitions have been studied [8,28], no studies so far have analyzed the entire number of matches within high-elite competitions such as the UEFA Champions League (UCL) in the context of ambient temperature. This analysis has the potential to enhance the generalizability of evidence while providing a benchmark for elite practitioners. Thus, this study contributes to the existing body of knowledge by addressing two critical gaps: (1) the application of advanced statistical modeling to account for situational factors and (2) the comprehensive analysis of all UCL matches to provide insights specific to the highest levels of elite soccer. Therefore, the aim of the study was to examine the differences in MRP according to the ambient temperature during the UCL matches while controlling for situational factors.

2. Materials and Methods

2.1. Design

An observational study design was employed to examine the influence of ambient temperature on MRP during matches in the 2022/23 UCL season.

2.2. The Match Data

The MRP data were collected using an optical tracking system (Player & Ball Tracking System, Hawk-Eye Innovations Limited, Basingstoke, England). The system's reliability has previously been tested and reported [29]. Measurements of ambient temperature prior to kick-off in matches are systematically taken by match-day officials belonging to the UEFA. For the purpose of this study, the measurements were subsequently obtained from the official UEFA match reports. As suggested previously [26,27], the following temperature classification was employed: ≤5 °C = very cold, 6–10 °C = cold, 11–20 °C = moderate, and ≥21 °C = warm.

2.3. Match Analysis

The MRP was obtained from all teams (n = 32) playing in all matches (n = 125) matches of the UCL in the 2022/23 season. Three matches were initially excluded due to poor data quality, resulting in a final sample of 122 matches. For each match, two observations (one per team) were analyzed, yielding a total of 244 team observations for analysis. These observations were classified into four groups according to the ambient temperature at which matches were played: <5 °C (8 observations), 6–10 °C (28 observations), 11–20 °C (144 observations), and ≥21 °C (66 observations). To avoid the influence of situational factors which were shown to influence MRP [8–10], match outcome and location, quality of opponent, ball-in-play time, and red cards were noted in all matches. All data were anonymized in accordance with the principles of the Declaration of Helsinki to ensure confidentiality. The investigation was approved by the local university ethics board. The descriptive statistics of MRP according to the ambient temperature is presented in Table 1.

Table 1. Match running performance at different ambient temperatures (data are given as mean ± SE).

	≤5 °C	6–10 °C	11–20 °C	≥21 °C
Total distance (km)	111.67 ± 1.73	112.13 ± 1.09	110.35 ± 0.7	108.96 ± 0.83
Low-intensity running (km)	83.37 ± 1.2	84.42 ± 0.74	84.59 ± 0.44	84.56 ± 0.54
Moderate-intensity running (km)	18.39 ± 0.61	18.03 ± 0.38	16.87 ± 0.24	15.88 ± 0.28
High-speed running (km)	7.4 ± 0.31	7.3 ± 0.19	6.73 ± 0.11	6.37 ± 0.14
Sprinting (km)	2.62 ± 0.18	2.57 ± 0.1	2.37 ± 0.05	2.29 ± 0.07
High-intensity running (km)	10.03 ± 0.45	9.86 ± 0.27	9.1 ± 0.15	8.67 ± 0.19

2.4. Variables

Dependent variables (i.e., MRP) included total distance covered (TD) (m), low-intensity running (LIR) (m) (≤15 km/h), moderate-intensity running (MIR) (m) (15–20 km/h), high-intensity running (HSR) (m) (20–25 km/h), sprinting (SPR) (m) (≥25 km/h), and high-intensity running (HIR) (m) (≥20 km/h) [30]. The independent variables were a four-level categorical variable "ambient temperature", the three-level categorical variables "match outcome", two-level categorical variables "match location", and "red card", and the continuous variables "opponent quality" and "ball-in-play". Match outcome was categorized as win, draw, or loss, while match location was recorded as either home or away. The presence of a red card was noted with a "yes" or "no" based on whether a red card was issued during the match. Opponent quality was evaluated using the UEFA 5-year club coefficients. Ball-in-play time, as defined by the data provider, refers to the duration when the ball is actively possessed by players or available for either team to contest. Periods when the referee stops play are considered out of play and do not count towards ball-in-play time [31].

2.5. Statistical Analysis

The differences in MRP according to ambient temperature were examined using linear mixed models (LMM). Matches and teams were included as random effects. A "step-up" model construction strategy was employed, beginning with the null model. Independent variables were included if they improved model information criteria and showed statistical significance ($p \leq 0.05$) over the previous model. Model selection relied on the Akaike information criterion (AIC), with lower values indicating a better fit, and on the chi-square likelihood ratio test. Specifically, models were compared by calculating the difference in log-likelihood values between the new and previous models, with degrees of freedom based on the difference in parameters. The final models were selected based on improved AIC, log-likelihood, and significant variable effects. Model fit was evaluated using residuals versus fitted plots and Q–Q plots [32,33]. T-statistics from the LMM were transformed into effect sizes (Cohen's d) with corresponding 95% confidence intervals (CIs). These effect sizes were interpreted as follows: less than 0.2 as trivial, 0.2–0.5 as small, 0.5–0.8 as medium, and greater than 0.8 as large (8). All analyses were conducted using SPSS software, version 25.0 for Windows (IBM, Armonk, NY, USA), with a significance level set at 0.05.

3. Results

Visual inspections of residual plots for models 1, 2, 4, 5, and 6 showed no noticeable deviations from homoscedasticity or normality, with Q–Q plots indicating a good data fit. However, model 3 did not effectively represent the data structure, so the effect of ambient temperature on MIR was not further analyzed.

Examining the explained variance attributed to fixed effects alone, the models showed marginal r^2 values as follows: 0.22 for TD, 0.56 for LIR, 0.09 for HSR, 0.08 for SPR, and 0.10 for HIR. When including both fixed and random effects, conditional r^2 values were 0.95 for TD and LIR, 0.90 for HSR, 0.92 for SPR, and 0.94 for HIR (Tables 2 and 3).

Table 2 shows that ambient temperature influenced TD ($f = 3.34$, $p < 0.001$). Specifically, less TD was covered in matches played at ≥21 °C (108.96 km) compared to the matches played at 11–20 °C (110.35 km, trivial ES) and 6–10 °C (112.13 km, medium ES). As covariates, match outcome ($f = 18.46$, $p < 0.001$), ball-in-play ($f = 23.89$, $p < 0.001$), and red cards ($f = 9.34$, $p = 0.003$) influenced TD. No effect of ambient temperature on LIR was found ($f = 0.36$, $p = 0.758$).

Table 3 shows that ambient temperature influenced HSR ($f = 8.91$, $p < 0.001$), SPR ($f = 9.01$, $p < 0.001$), and HIR ($f = 7.26$, $p < 0.001$). Specifically, less HSR was covered in matches played at ≥21 °C (6.37 km) compared to the matches played at 11–20 °C (6.73 km, medium ES), 6–10 °C (7.3 km, large ES), and ≤5 °C (7.4 km, medium ES). Also, less SPR was covered in matches played at ≥21 °C (2.20 km) compared to the matches played at 6–10 °C (2.57 km, medium ES). Finally, less HIR was covered in matches played at ≥21 °C (8.67 km) compared to the matches played at 11–20 °C (9.1 km, small ES), 6–10 °C (9.86 km, large ES), and ≤5 °C (10.03 km, medium ES). As covariates, match location had an influence on SPR ($f = 21.77$, $p < 0.001$) and HIR ($f = 13.57$, $p < 0.001$).

Table 2. The effect of ambient temperature on total distance and distances covered at lower speeds while controlling for situational factors.

	Total Distance (Model 1)			Low-Intensity Running (Model 2)			Moderate-Intensity Running (Model 3) *		
Fixed Effects	**Coef (SE)**	**95%CI**	**Effect Size**	**Coef (SE)**	**95% CI**	**Effect Size**	**Coef (SE)**	**95%CI**	**Effect Size**
Intercept	86.76 (4.24)	78.37–95.15		63.24 (2.99)	57.33–69.16		-	-	
TEMP: ≤5 °C	2.71 (1.75)	−0.76–6.19	0.15 (−0.04–0.34)	−1.19 (1.24)	−3.64–1.27	−0.19 (−0.57–0.2)	-	-	-
TEMP: 6–10 °C	3.17 (1.07)	1.04–5.29	0.58 (0.19–0.97)	−0.14 (0.76)	−1.64–1.36	−0.04 (−0.42–0.35)	-	-	-
TEMP: 11–20 °C	1.39 (0.69)	0.02–2.75	0.01 (−0.37–0.39)	0.03 (0.49)	−0.93–0.99	−0.11 (−0.5–0.27)	-	-	-
MO: Loss	−1.73 (0.33)	−2.38–−1.09	−1 (−1.4–−0.61)	−1.58 (0.25)	−2.09–−1.08	−1.17 (−1.56–−0.77)	-	-	-
MO: Draw	1.42 (0.78)	−0.14–2.97	0.35 (−0.03–0.73)	1.16 (0.56)	0.06–2.26	0.4 (0.02–0.78)	-	-	-
ML: Home	-	-	-	-	-	-	-	-	-
OQ	-	-	-	-	-	-	-	-	-
BP	0.36 (0.07)	0.21–0.5	0.94 (0.54–1.33)	0.35 (0.05)	0.25–0.45	1.28 (0.87–1.69)	-	-	-
RC: No	2.55 (0.83)	0.9–4.21	0.6 (0.21–1)	1.82 (0.59)	0.65–2.99	0.6 (0.21–0.99)	-	-	-
Random effects	Coef (SE)	95%CI	*p*	Coef (SE)	95%CI	*p*	Coef (SE)	95%CI	*p*
Match	8.3 (1.49)	5.84–11.81	<0.001	3.92 (0.73)	2.72–5.65	<0.001	-	-	-
Team	8.5 (2.48)	4.79–15.05	0.001	2.65 (0.83)	1.44–4.89	0.001	-	-	-
Residuals	3.17 (0.47)	2.38–4.23	<0.001	2.04 (0.29)	1.54–2.7	<0.001	-	-	-
$R^2_{marginal}$		0.22			0.56			-	
$R^2_{conditional}$		0.95			0.95			-	
AIC		1268			1116			-	

Coef: coefficient, SE: standard error, CI: confidence interval, TEMP: temperature, MO: match outcome, ML: match location, OQ: opponent quality, BP: ball in play, RC: red cards, AIC: Akaike information criterion; * denotes inadequate model fit.

Table 3. The effect of ambient temperature on the distance covered at higher speeds while controlling for situational factors.

	High-Speed Running (Model 4)			Sprinting (Model 5)			High-Intensity Running (Model 6)		
Fixed Effects	**Coef (SE)**	**95%CI**	**Effect Size**	**Coef (SE)**	**95% CI**	**Effect Size**	**Coef (SE)**	**95%CI**	**Effect Size**
Intercept	6.37 (0.13)	6.11–6.64		2.24 (0.07)	2.11–2.38		8.56 (0.19)	8.19–8.94	
TEMP: ≤5 °C	1.03 (0.32)	0.39–1.67	0.62 (0.23–1.01)	0.33 (0.18)	−0.04–0.7	0.34 (−0.04–0.73)	1.36 (0.46)	0.44–2.28	0.57 (0.18–0.96)
TEMP: 6–10 °C	0.92 (0.2)	0.52–1.32	0.89 (0.49–1.29)	0.27 (0.12)	0.05–0.5	0.22 (0.04–0.4)	1.2 (0.29)	0.62–1.77	0.8 (0.4–1.19)
TEMP: 11–20 °C	0.35 (0.13)	0.1–0.61	0.54 (0.15–0.93)	0.08 (0.07)	−0.07–0.22	0.2 (−0.18–0.58)	0.43 (0.18)	0.07–0.8	0.45 (0.07–0.84)
MO: Loss	-	-	-	-	-	-	-	-	-
MO: Draw	-	-	-	-	-	-	-	-	-
ML: Home	-	-	-	0.1 (0.02)	0.06–0.15	0.93 (0.52–1.34)	0.21 (0.06)	0.1–0.32	0.74 (0.33–1.15)
OQ	-	-	-	-	-		-	-	-
BP	-	-	-	-	-		-	-	-
RC: No	-	-	-	-	-		-	-	-
Random effects	Coef (SE)	95%CI	*p*	Coef (SE)	95%CI	*p*	Coef (SE)	95%CI	*p*
Match	0.28 (0.05)	0.19–0.4	<0.001	0.1 (0.02)	0.08–0.14	<0.001	0.19 (0.03)	0.14–0.25	<0.001
Team	0.23 (0.07)	0.13–0.41	0.001	0.03 (0.01)	0.02–0.06	0.002	0.65 (0.11)	0.47–0.89	0.001
Residuals	0.14 (0.02)	0.11–0.19	<0.001	0.03 (0)	0.02–0.04	<0.001	0.36 (0.11)	0.2–0.66	<0.001
$R^2_{marginal}$		0.09			0.08			0.10	
$R^2_{conditional}$		0.90			0.92			0.94	
AIC		487			157			614	

Coef: coefficient, SE: standard error, CI: confidence interval, TEMP: temperature, MO: match outcome, ML: match location, OQ: opponent quality, BP: ball in play, RC: red cards, AIC: Akaike information criterion.

4. Discussion

The aim of this study was to examine differences in MRP according to the ambient temperature during UCL matches while controlling statistically for the influence of situational factors. The results revealed decreased TD, HSR, SPR, and HIR in matches played in a warm environment. On the other hand, a similar distance covered at a lower speed was found irrespective of the ambient temperature. These findings may be of great interest to support practitioners entrusted with safeguarding the players' well-being.

Previous studies examining the differences in MRP according to the ambient temperature in soccer mostly examined findings from a single country [27,34] or a single team [24]. Such findings were undoubtedly influenced by the specificities (i.e., geographical, cultural, historical, and/or social) of observed competitions and teams [35]. There are also several studies using limited samples [24] or data that can be currently considered outdated [26] due to the tremendous increases in MRP in the last decade [36]. Finally, studies have rarely controlled for the situational factors that have been repeatedly demonstrated to influence physical performance during soccer matches [8]. Consequently, it has been difficult to determine the actual differences in MRP according to the ambient temperature. To address the relevant literature gaps, the current study examined these differences by investigating teams playing in multiple countries while also controlling for several potential situational factors. The results showed that less TD was covered in UCL matches played at ≥21 °C compared to the matches played at 6–10 °C (medium ES). In addition, less HSR and HIR were covered in matches played at ≥21 °C compared to the matches played at 11–20 °C (medium and small ES, respectively), 6–10 °C (both large ES), and ≤5 °C (both medium ES). Also, less SPR was covered in matches played at ≥21 °C compared to the matches played at 6–10 °C (medium ES).

These findings clearly indicated a decrease in overall and intensive efforts in warm compared to cold environments. It has been speculated that this may be the result of pacing strategies for players to preserve their technical skills and peak running speed [25]. However, we are of the opinion that the unique feature of the observed competition (i.e., UCL) has affected our findings. As a top soccer club tournament involving the world's best players, the UCL is distinguished by highly professional and driven athletes who maintain consistently high running performance regardless of opponent or match outcome [12]. This may indicate a low reliance on pacing tactics. Therefore, decreased overall and intensive efforts in warm compared to cold environments may rather be a consequence of the body's efforts to dissipate the heat.

Specifically, when exposed to high temperatures, the body's thermoregulatory systems activate, causing reactions such as increased perspiration to aid heat [18]. Excessive sweating can cause dehydration and electrolyte imbalances, impairing cardiovascular homeostasis [19]. This might reduce the capacity for prolonged physical exertion, resulting in reduced overall efforts. Increased temperatures, on the other hand, worsen metabolic strain during exercise, resulting in rapid glycogen depletion and increased dependence on anaerobic energy pathways, ultimately leading to early exhaustion [20,21]. As the anaerobic system is associated with high-intensity efforts [37], such overload most likely resulted in reduced intensive efforts.

Our findings are generally consistent with previous studies investigating the French League 1, Russian Premier League, and German Bundesliga 1 [26,27,34,38]. However, these studies lacked data related to situational variables that have been repeatedly demonstrated to affect MRP in soccer [8]. Failure to do so brings into question any conclusions drawn from the data. Therefore, in the current study, the differences in MRP according to the ambient temperature were investigated while accounting for match outcome and location, quality of opposition, ball-in-play time, and red cards. This approach strengthens the true impact of ambient temperature on MRP in elite soccer players while eliminating the likelihood that the findings are merely due to natural match-to-match variability [39]. Indeed, our results demonstrated a substantial impact of match outcome, effective playing time, and red cards on TD, whereas match location had an influence on SPR and HIR.

It is particularly important to highlight that high-intensity efforts (i.e., HSR, SPR, and HIR), a metric commonly deemed critical to match outcome [40,41], in UCL matches played in warm environments were reduced by approximately 15%. Therefore, when confronted with high ambient temperature (over 20 °C), (i) coaches should consider adopting alternative strategies rather than striving to maintain HIR levels equivalent to those in colder environments, and (ii) practitioners entrusted with safeguarding the players' well-being should consider implementing structured hydration plans before, during, and after matches. When competing in the UCL, this is paramount for sustaining players' performance throughout a match and reducing the risk of injury or heat-related illnesses. The practical relevance of these conclusions is confirmed by the medium-to-large effect sizes [40].

Several limitations should be noted when interpreting the findings of this study. Firstly, the potential temperature variations throughout the matches were not taken into account, which would have affected the results. Secondly, match observations were classified into four groups according to the ambient temperature at which matches were played. However, groups were unequal in their sample sizes and such discrepancy likely influenced the findings. Thirdly, although the most influential factors that can affect MRP were considered, future studies should control for other match-related factors that may be impact results such as stage effect (i.e., group vs. knockout), playing position or team formation. For a more comprehensive understanding of environmental conditions effects, additional environmental factors such as relative humidity, atmospheric pressure, wind, and precipitation should be investigated in future studies. Also, there should be some attempt to account for differences in accelerations and decelerations according to ambient temperature. This may enable a more detailed understating of the physical demands required when playing in specific environmental conditions.

5. Conclusions

As far as we know, this study represents the inaugural large-scale investigation aimed at examining how the ambient temperature impacts the MRP of elite soccer teams, enhancing the generalizability of evidence while providing a benchmark for elite practitioners competing in UCL. The results indicated significant differences in MRP when matches were played at different ambient temperatures, with significant reductions in overall (e.g.,

TD) and high-intensity efforts (e.g., HSR, SPR, HIR) in warmer conditions (≥21 °C). It is therefore imperative for practitioners to account for ambient temperature when preparing for UCL matches. Specifically, when ambient temperature is forecasted to be over 20 °C, (i) soccer coaches could explore using different playing styles to achieve tactical goals while reducing physical strain, (ii) medical staff could consider structured hydration before the match and cooling techniques during half-time, and (iii) strength and conditioning coaches could reduce external training loads in the trainings preceding such matches. This is especially important for teams from northern Europe accustomed to cooler temperatures, which might experience more significant MRP declines when playing in warmer conditions.

Author Contributions: Conceptualization, T.M.; methodology, T.M.; software, V.P.; validation, R.M.; formal analysis, V.P.; investigation, V.P. and R.M.; resources, V.P.; data curation, V.P.; writing—original draft preparation, V.P. and T.M.; writing—review and editing, T.M. and R.M.; visualization, V.P.; supervision, T.M.; project administration, T.M. All authors have read and agreed to the published version of the manuscript.

Funding: This research received no external funding.

Institutional Review Board Statement: The study was conducted in accordance with the Declaration of Helsinki, and approved by the Institutional Review Board (or Ethics Committee) of the Faculty of Kinesiology, University of Split (approval number: 2181-205-02-05-19-0020).

Informed Consent Statement: As the data used in this study were collected as part of players' routine monitoring, informed consent was not required.

Data Availability Statement: The raw data supporting the conclusions of this article will be made available by the authors on request.

Conflicts of Interest: The authors declare no conflicts of interest.

References

1. De Albuquerque Freire, L.; Brito, M.A.; Muñoz, P.M.; Pérez, D.I.V.; Kohler, H.C.; Aedo-Muñoz, E.A.; Slimani, M.; Brito, C.J.; Bragazzi, N.L.; Znazen, H. Match Running Performance of Brazilian Professional Soccer Players according to Tournament Types. *Montenegrin J. Sports Sci. Med.* **2022**, *11*, 53–58. [CrossRef]
2. Castellano, J.; Huarte, X.; Casamichana, D. Match physical performance profiles in professional football: A comparative analysis among players' positions in the European five top leagues. *Int. J. Perform. Anal. Sport* **2024**, 1–21. [CrossRef]
3. García-Aliaga, A.; Martín-Castellanos, A.; Marquina Nieto, M.; Muriarte Solana, D.; Resta, R.; López del Campo, R.; Mon-López, D.; Refoyo, I. Effect of Increasing the Number of Substitutions on Physical Performance during Periods of Congested Fixtures in Football. *Sports* **2023**, *11*, 25. [CrossRef]
4. Ponce-Bordón, J.; López-Gajardo, M.; Lobo-Triviño, D.; Pulido, J.; García-Calvo, T. Longitudinal match running performance analysis of soccer in professional European leagues: A systematic review. *Int. J. Perform. Anal. Sport* **2024**, 1–25. [CrossRef]
5. Kádár, L.; Géczi, G.; Bognár, J.; Csáki, I. Movement analysis of match play in U16-U21 youth Hungarian soccer players—The influence of age, position, and contextual variables. *Int. J. Perform. Anal. Sport* **2023**, *23*, 213–231. [CrossRef]
6. Harper, D.J.; Carling, C.; Kiely, J. High-intensity acceleration and deceleration demands in elite team sports competitive match play: A systematic review and meta-analysis of observational studies. *Sports Med.* **2019**, *49*, 1923–1947. [CrossRef]
7. Aquino, R.; Vieira, L.H.P.; Carling, C.; Martins, G.H.; Alves, I.S.; Puggina, E.F. Effects of competitive standard, team formation and playing position on match running performance of Brazilian professional soccer players. *Int. J. Perform. Anal. Sport* **2017**, *17*, 695–705. [CrossRef]
8. Trewin, J.; Meylan, C.; Varley, M.C.; Cronin, J. The influence of situational and environmental factors on match-running in soccer: A systematic review. *Sci. Med. Footb.* **2017**, *1*, 183–194. [CrossRef]
9. Plakias, S.; Michailidis, Y. Factors Affecting the Running Performance of Soccer Teams in the Turkish Super League. *Sports* **2024**, *12*, 196. [CrossRef]
10. Savoia, C.; Laterza, F.; Lucadamo, A.; Manzi, V.; Azzone, V.; Pullinger, S.A.; Beattie, C.E.; Bertollo, M.; Pompa, D. The Relationship Between Playing Formations, Team Ranking, and Physical Performance in the Serie A Soccer League. *Sports* **2024**, *12*, 286. [CrossRef]
11. Šunjić, I.; Veršić, Š.; Modrić, T.; Marin, Ć.; Zalatel, P. The Comparison of Position-Specific Match Performance between the Group and Knockout Stage of the UEFA Champions League. *Sport Mont* **2024**, *22*, 9–17. [CrossRef]
12. Modric, T.; Versic, S.; Stojanovic, M.; Chmura, P.; Andrzejewski, M.; Konefał, M.; Sekulic, D. Factors affecting match running performance in elite soccer: Analysis of UEFA Champions League matches. *Biol. Sport* **2022**, *40*, 409–416. [CrossRef] [PubMed]

13. Magni, M.; Zago, M.; Vago, P.; Vandoni, M.; Carnevale Pellino, V.; Lovecchio, N. Technical Differences over the Course of the Match: An Analysis of Three Elite Teams in the UEFA Champions League. *Sports* **2023**, *11*, 46. [CrossRef]
14. Martín-Castellanos, A.; Flores, M.R.; Solana, D.M.; Del Campo, R.L.; Garrosa, F.N.; Mon-López, D. How do the football teams play in LaLiga? Analysis and comparison of playing styles according to the outcome. *Int. J. Perform. Anal. Sport* **2024**, *24*, 18–30. [CrossRef]
15. Jiménez, S.L.; Bustamante-Sánchez, Á.; Kelly, A.L.; Pareja-Galeano, H.; Lago-Penas, C. Influence of the situational variables on the performance of the teams competing in the Chinese Super League. *Int. J. Perform. Anal. Sport* **2022**, *22*, 455–466. [CrossRef]
16. de Korte, J.Q.; Eijsvogels, T.M.H.; Hopman, M.T.E.; Bongers, C.C.W.G. Thermoregulatory, Cardiovascular and Perceptual Responses of Spectators of a Simulated Football Match in Hot and Humid Environmental Conditions. *Sports* **2023**, *11*, 78. [CrossRef] [PubMed]
17. Branquinho, L.; Forte, P.; Thomatieli-Santos, R.V.; de França, E.; Marinho, D.A.; Teixeira, J.E.; Ferraz, R. Perspectives on Player Performance during FIFA World Cup Qatar 2022: A Brief Report. *Sports* **2023**, *11*, 174. [CrossRef]
18. Nybo, L. Hyperthermia and fatigue. *J. Appl. Physiol.* **2008**, *104*, 871–878. [CrossRef] [PubMed]
19. No, M.; Kwak, H.-B. Effects of environmental temperature on physiological responses during submaximal and maximal exercises in soccer players. *Integr. Med. Res.* **2016**, *5*, 216–222. [CrossRef]
20. Morris, J.G.; Nevill, M.E.; Williams, C. Physiological and metabolic responses of female games and endurance athletes to prolonged, intermittent, high-intensity running at 30° and 16° C ambient temperatures. *Eur. J. Appl. Physiol.* **2000**, *81*, 84–92. [CrossRef]
21. Mohr, M.; Mujika, I.; Santisteban, J.; Randers, M.B.; Bischoff, R.; Solano, R.; Hewitt, A.; Zubillaga, A.; Peltola, E.; Krustrup, P. Examination of fatigue development in elite soccer in a hot environment: A multi-experimental approach. *Scand. J. Med. Sci. Sports* **2010**, *20* (Suppl. 3), 125–132. [CrossRef] [PubMed]
22. Hong, J.H.; Kim, H.J.; Kim, K.J.; Suzuki, K.; Lee, I.S. Comparison of metabolic substrates between exercise and cold exposure in skaters. *J. Physiol. Anthropol.* **2008**, *27*, 273–281. [CrossRef] [PubMed]
23. Coker, N.A.; Wells, A.J.; Gepner, Y. Effect of Heat Stress on Measures of Running Performance and Heart Rate Responses During a Competitive Season in Male Soccer Players. *J. Strength Cond. Res.* **2020**, *34*, 1141–1149. [CrossRef]
24. Loxston, C.; Lawson, M.; Unnithan, V. Does environmental heat stress impact physical and technical match-play characteristics in football? *Sci. Med. Footb.* **2019**, *3*, 191–197. [CrossRef]
25. Nassis, G.P.; Brito, J.; Dvorak, J.; Chalabi, H.; Racinais, S. The association of environmental heat stress with performance: Analysis of the 2014 FIFA World Cup Brazil. *Br. J. Sports Med.* **2015**, *49*, 609–613. [CrossRef]
26. Carling, C.; Dupont, G.; Le Gall, F. The effect of a cold environment on physical activity profiles in elite soccer match-play. *Int. J. Sports Med.* **2011**, *32*, 542–545. [CrossRef]
27. Morgans, R.; Bezuglov, E.; Rhodes, D.; Teixeira, J.; Modric, T.; Versic, S.; Di Michele, R.; Oliveira, R. The relationship between ambient temperature and match running performance of elite soccer players. *PLoS ONE* **2023**, *18*, e0288494. [CrossRef] [PubMed]
28. Aquino, R.; Carling, C.; Maia, J.; Vieira, L.H.P.; Wilson, R.S.; Smith, N.; Almeida, R.; Gonçalves, L.G.C.; Kalva-Filho, C.A.; Garganta, J. Relationships between running demands in soccer match-play, anthropometric, and physical fitness characteristics: A systematic review. *Int. J. Perform. Anal. Sport* **2020**, *20*, 534–555. [CrossRef]
29. FIFA. Test Report. Available online: https://inside.fifa.com/api/resource-hub/test-report?id=a50993dbc57440dab1b606abc5717e00 (accessed on 15 June 2024).
30. Bradley, P.S. 'Setting the Benchmark' Part 1: The Contextualised Physical Demands of Positional Roles in the FIFA World Cup Qatar 2022. *Biol. Sport* **2023**, *41*, 261–270. [CrossRef]
31. Williams, J.; Hughes, M.; O'Donoghue, P. The effect of rule changes on match and ball in play time in rugby union. *Int. J. Perform. Anal. Sport* **2005**, *5*, 1–11. [CrossRef]
32. Lovell, T.; Bocking, C.; Fransen, J.; Kempton, T.; Coutts, A. Factors affecting physical match activity and skill involvement in youth soccer. *Sci. Med. Footb.* **2018**, *2*, 58–65. [CrossRef]
33. Henderson, M.J.; Fransen, J.; McGrath, J.J.; Harries, S.K.; Poulos, N.; Coutts, A.J. Situational factors affecting rugby sevens match performance. *Sci. Med. Footb.* **2019**, *3*, 275–280. [CrossRef]
34. Chmura, P.; Liu, H.; Andrzejewski, M.; Chmura, J.; Kowalczuk, E.; Rokita, A.; Konefał, M. Is there meaningful influence from situational and environmental factors on the physical and technical activity of elite football players? Evidence from the data of 5 consecutive seasons of the German Bundesliga. *PLoS ONE* **2021**, *16*, e0247771. [CrossRef]
35. Sarmento, H.; Pereira, A.; Matos, N.; Campaniço, J.; Anguera, T.M.; Leitão, J. English Premier League, Spaińs La Liga and Italýs Seriés A–What's Different? *Int. J. Perform. Anal. Sport* **2013**, *13*, 773–789. [CrossRef]
36. Barnes, C.; Archer, D.; Bush, M.; Hogg, R.; Bradley, P. The evolution of physical and technical performance parameters in the English Premier League. *Int. J. Sports Med.* **2014**, *35*, 1–6. [CrossRef]
37. Modric, T.; Versic, S.; Sekulic, D. Does aerobic performance define match running performance among professional soccer players? A position-specific analysis. *Res. Sports Med.* **2021**, *29*, 336–348. [CrossRef]
38. Link, D.; Weber, H. Effect of ambient temperature on pacing in soccer depends on skill level. *J. Strength Cond. Res.* **2017**, *31*, 1766–1770. [CrossRef]
39. Carling, C.; Bradley, P.; McCall, A.; Dupont, G. Match-to-match variability in high-speed running activity in a professional soccer team. *J. Sports Sci.* **2016**, *34*, 2215–2223. [CrossRef]

40. Di Salvo, V.; Gregson, W.; Atkinson, G.; Tordoff, P.; Drust, B. Analysis of high intensity activity in Premier League soccer. *Int. J. Sports Med.* **2009**, *30*, 205–212. [CrossRef]
41. Chmura, P.; Konefał, M.; Chmura, J.; Kowalczuk, E.; Zając, T.; Rokita, A.; Andrzejewski, M. Match outcome and running performance in different intensity ranges among elite soccer players. *Biol. Sport* **2018**, *35*, 197. [CrossRef]

sports MDPI

Article

Predictors of Risk of Muscle Injury in Non-Professional Soccer Players: An Ambispective Cohort Study

Ismael Iraqui-Rato [1] and Rubén Cuesta-Barriuso [1,2,*]

[1] Department of Surgery and Medical-Surgical Specialties, University of Oviedo, 33003 Oviedo, Spain; ismaeliraqui@gmail.com
[2] InHeFis Research Group, Instituto Asturiano de Investigación Sanitaria (ISPA), 33011 Oviedo, Spain
* Correspondence: cuestaruben@uniovi.es; Tel.: +34-985-10-33-86

Abstract: (1) Background: Soccer accounts for 30% of all sports injuries. Muscle injuries in soccer, not caused by trauma or contact, are the most common. The objective was to assess the risk of injury based on the footwear used by soccer players and the playing field and to identify the best predictive model of muscle injuries; (2) Methods: An ambispective cohort study. The primary variable was the number of muscle injuries in the last three seasons. The secondary variables were age, body mass index, type of soccer shoes and turf, training load and position on the field. The possible confounding variables were motivation for the choice of footwear, date of injuries, time playing and regular first-team player status; (3) Results: 156 players were recruited. The risk of injury is 1.03 (95% CI: 0.83; 1.27) times more frequent in players competing on artificial turf. The risk of injury is slightly higher in first-team players than in substitutes (RR = 1.02; 95% CI: 0.79; 1.32). There was no statistically significant relationship between the position on the field ($p = 0.91$), the type of shoe ($p = 0.69$) and the motivation to buy the shoes ($p = 0.82$), regarding the risk of muscle injury in these athletes. The best model to estimate risk of injury includes age, training load and soccer shoe type as confounding variables (AIC = 190.5; $p = 0.10$; $\chi^2_{(3)} = 10.14$; $p = 0.02$); (4) Conclusions: The risk of muscle injury is higher in non-professional soccer players competing on artificial pitches and in those who are regular starters on their teams. Field position, soccer shoe and motivation to purchase the soccer shoe are variables that do not increase the risk of muscle injury in these athletes. The best predictive model of injury includes age, training load and shoe type.

Keywords: soccer; muscle injury; risk; secondary prevention; physiotherapy

1. Introduction

Both professional and amateur soccer subject players to physical demands that increase the risk of musculoskeletal injuries [1]. The injury rates are varied in the literature, showing a fluctuation, during matches, from 12 to 66 injuries per 1000 h of play. During the workouts, the described rates vary from 1.5 to 7.6 injuries per 1000 h [2,3]. The incidence of injuries during competition is significantly higher, being approximately 4–6 times higher than during training [4].

Ankle, knee, hamstring, and groin injuries are the most common, accounting for more than 50% of all injuries in soccer, although more than 65% are classified as minor [5,6].

The biomechanics of soccer and its interaction with the pitch are crucial aspects that can influence the incidence of injuries in these athletes. Muscle and tendon injuries are more prevalent in amateur soccer players than in professionals (4.78%). Likewise, moderate, and serious injuries are more frequent in amateur players than in professional athletes, by 9.60% [5,6]. The maintenance of soccer pitches, which varies between professional and amateur sport mainly for reasons of financial resources, must be taken into account. This may suggest that different playing surfaces may have a significant impact on the biomechanical load experienced by players. In this regard, artificial turf, despite its technological improvements, is still associated with an increased risk of musculoskeletal injuries, such as sprains and strains [7]. A recent study [8] has described the relationship between players' positions on the field and knee pain, with forwards experiencing more pain, and found no association between players' body mass index and the occurrence of sports injuries. Variables such as age, time spent in strenuous activity, timing of puberty and overweight/obesity have been associated with an increased risk of anterior cruciate ligament injury in young adults and adolescents [9]. However, in non-professional soccer players, the variables that affect the risk of muscle injury have not yet been described beyond fatigue, overload, and intensity variables.

A proper choice of footwear is essential to prevent injuries in soccer players and improve their performance on the pitch [10]. The type of footwear, including the design of the cleats and the sole, can influence the biomechanics of the players and their susceptibility to the development of injuries [11]. In this regard, shoes with round cleats have been shown to be safer than blade-type cleats with respect to the development of torsion injuries [12]. However, in non-professional soccer players, the choice of footwear is not determined by sponsors, as the cost is borne by the player himself, and often the choice of footwear is based on price, comfort or the model of boot. It has been described how the incidence of injuries on natural grass is 57.78%, higher than the 42.22% registered on artificial turf [13]. However, despite the relevance of this choice, players may not adequately consider these factors when selecting their footwear, which may increase the risk of muscle injuries.

The aim of this study was to evaluate the risk of muscle injuries in non-professional soccer players and identify the best predictive model of muscle injuries based on anthropometric and sports variables.

2. Materials and Methods

2.1. Study Design

An ambispective cohort study.

2.2. Participants

The inclusion criteria were soccer players that (i) were non-professional, who competed in a regional territorial area (Principality of Asturias, Spain); (ii) had not undergone musculoskeletal surgery in the three seasons prior to the study; and (iii) had federated at least one year before the study period. The exclusion criteria were (i) those who had not competed, during the study seasons, for a period of more than 6 months due to a musculoskeletal injury.

2.3. Ethical Considerations

This study took into account the ethical aspects contained in the Declaration of Helsinki. The research project was approved by the Research Ethics Committee of the Principality of Asturias (CEImPA code 2024.107). The study was registered in the international database of clinical records, www.clinicaltrials.gov (NCT06425809).

2.4. Study Variables

Data collection was carried out in May 2024. This was conducted through a closed-question format interview. Data collection was carried out at the regional soccer federation using a self-reported closed-response survey model, with all interviews taking place in the same week. The primary variable was the number of lower limb muscle injuries in the last three seasons.

The secondary and modifying variables were age (years), body mass index (kg/m^2), type of training and competition shoe (rubber/metal cleat), training and competition playing field (sand/artificial turf/natural turf), type of muscle injury (fibrillar rupture/tendon muscle/strain), weekly training load (hours) and position on the field (goalkeeper/defender/midfielder/forward). The possible confounding variables were the motivation for the choice of footwear (comfort/aesthetics/price/other), the date of muscle injuries, the time competing in the category (in completed months) and the usual presence on the starting team (yes/no). These confounding variables were selected because of their influence on a possible misinterpretation of the results due to a false association between injury risk and possible modifying variables

2.5. Sample Size

The calculation of the sample size was carried out using the statistical program Stata IC16 (StataCorp LLC, College Station, TX, USA). This analysis estimated a prevalence of muscle injuries of 0.05 (5%). By calculating for amplitudes from 0.05 to 0.80 (delta = 0.02), a percentage of 5% of injury cases was expected. Using the proportion 0.05 (SD = 0.50), the sample size was calculated for effects between 0.01 and 0.8 (delta = 0.02). With these criteria, the sample size to estimate this prevalence with an accuracy of ±2% was 97 non-professional soccer players from the Principality of Asturias. The estimation of the external validity of the predictive model required a 40% larger sample. Thus, a sample size of at least 137 soccer players was estimated.

2.6. Statistical Analysis

The statistical analysis was performed with the statistical program Stata IC16 (StataCorp LLC). The statistical significance was estimated at $\alpha = 0.05$. Using a double-entry table (2 × 2), the prevalence of adverse effects in soccer players with muscle injuries in the study period was calculated. The relative risk (RR), the risk difference (RD) and the risk difference in the population (RDp) of muscle injuries in these athletes were also calculated.

The influence of possible confounding factors was also calculated by discarding those whose RR was in the range 0.67–1.50. Any variable that, when adjusted, caused changes in RR > 10% was considered a confounding factor.

Through a logistic regression analysis, the best predictive model was selected based on the AIC index and the reclassification indices, selecting the most parsimonious model, calculating the Mantel–Haenszel weighting (RRMH). The multicollinearity of the predictor variables was calculated using the variance inflation factor (VIF). The Wald test was used to check if the estimated RRs in the strata of the possible confounding factors were homogeneous.

The predictive capacity was calculated with the validity indices (area under the curve—AUC, sensitivity and specificity). With the probability of suffering a muscle injury, calculated with the logistic regression model for the athletes included in the study, the risk of injury for four athletes was calculated from the OR of the estimated model.

3. Results

3.1. Descriptive Analysis

The study included 156 soccer players. The mean age was 24.03 (SD: 4.29) years, referring to an average of 1.46 (SD: 1.66) muscle injuries throughout the three evaluation seasons. Most of the players had suffered a previous muscle injury (68.59%). Artificial turf soccer fields were the most common in training (90.38%) and in competition (52.56%). Rubber cleats were the most used (76.92%) by the players. Table 1 shows all the results of the descriptive analysis of the sociodemographic, anthropometric and sports variables of the players included in the study.

3.2. Analysis of the Risk of Muscle Injury

The risk of injury is 1.03 times more frequent in players who compete on an artificial field than in those who train on natural turf fields (RR = 1.03 [0.83; 1.27]). Players who compete on artificial fields exhibit 2% more injuries than those who usually play on natural grass (RD = 0.02). For every 1000 injuries in federated soccer players, 10 injuries occur due to competing on artificial turf fields (RDp = 0.01). Three percent of all injuries of soccer players playing on artificial turf are due to this circumstance (AFe = 0.03). One percent of the total muscle injuries that occur in federated soccer players are caused by competing on artificial fields on a regular basis (AFp = 0.01).

Table 1. Descriptive analysis (mean, standard deviation and 95% confidence interval) of the characteristics of the soccer players included in the study.

	Variables	Mean (Standard Deviation)	[95% CI]
	Age (years)	24.03 (4.29)	[23.35; 23.47]
Anthropometrics	Weight (kg)	73.73 (8.05)	[72.46; 75.01]
	Height (cm)	177.96 (7.06)	[176.84; 179.08]
	Body mass index (kg/m^2)	23.22 (1.56)	[22.98; 23.47]
Injuries	Total injuries (number)	1.46 (1.66)	[1.20; 1.72]
	Quadriceps (number)	0.33 (0.61)	[0.23; 0.42]
	Hamstrings (number)	0.70 (1.04)	[0.53; 0.86]
	Gastrocnemius (number)	0.16 (0.43)	[0.09; 0.23]
Sports	Weekly training (hours)	6.75 (2.17)	[6.41; 7.10]
	Individual training (hours)	3.10 (2.76)	[2.64; 3.52]
	Time competing in the category (months)	14.39 (4.56)	[13.67; 15.11]
		n (%)	
Previous muscle injuries	Yes	107 (68.59)	
	No	49 (31.41)	
Type of muscle injury	Fibrillar rupture	99 (63.46)	
	Tendon muscle	51 (32.69)	
	Strain	6 (3.85)	
Usual presence on the starting team	Yes	123 (78.85)	
	No	33 (21.15)	
Position on the field	Goalkeeper	12 (7.69)	
	Defender	63 (40.38)	
	Midfielder	53 (33.97)	
	Forward	28 (17.95)	
Training playing field	Natural turf	15 (9.62)	
	Artificial turf	141 (90.38)	
Competition playing field	Natural turf	74 (47.44)	
	Artificial turf	82 (52.56)	
Type of training and competition shoe	Rubber cleat	120 (76.92)	
	Multi-cleat	34 (21.79)	
	Metal cleat	2 (1.28)	
Motivation for choosing a football boot	Comfort	87 (55.77)	
	Price	24 (15.38)	
	Playing field	45 (28.85)	

The risk of injury is 1.02 times higher in starting players than in substitutes (RR = 1.02 [0.79; 1.32]). There are 1.4% more injuries in first-team players than in those who do not usually play (RD = 0.014). For every 1000 injuries in federated soccer players, there are four injuries due to playing as first-team players (RDp = 0.004). Two percent of all injuries of regular starting soccer players are due to this circumstance (AFe = 0.02). Only 0.6% of the total muscle injuries in federated soccer players are due to the presence on the starting team on a regular basis (AFp = 0.006).

Lastly, there was no statistically significant relationship between the position on the field ($p = 0.91$), the type of shoe ($p = 0.69$) and the motivation to buy the shoes ($p = 0.82$), regarding the risk of muscle injury in these athletes. Table 2 shows the results of the risk analysis depending on the training and competition field, regular presence as first-team player and the nominal qualitative variables.

Table 2. Injury risk analysis in the soccer players included in the study.

Variables		Injury Yes	Injury No	R [95% CI]	RR	RD	RDp	AFe	AFp
Usual presence on the starting team	Starting players	84	39	0.70 [0.54; 0.85]	1.02 [0.79; 1.32]	−0.014	−0.004	0.02	0.006
	Substitutes	23	10	0.68 [0.60; 0.76]					
Training playing field	Natural turf	12	3	0.80 [0.60;1.00]	0.84 [0.64; 1.11]	0.13	0.04	0.16	0.05
	Artificial turf	95	46	0.67 [0.59; 0.75]					
Competition playing field	Natural turf	50	24	0.68 [0.56; 0.77]	1.03 [0.83; 1.27]	−0.02	−0.006	0.03	0.01
	Artificial turf	57	25	0.70 [0.58; 0.78]					
Position on the field	Goalkeeper	8	4	0.67 [0.39; 0.86]	z = 0.12; *p* = 0.91				
	Defender	43	20	0.68 [0.56; 0.78]					
	Midfielder	35	18	0.66 [0.53; 0.77]					
	Forward	21	7	0.75 [0.57; 0.87]					
Type of training and competition shoe	Rubber cleat	84	36	0.70 [0.61; 0.77]	z = −0.40; *p* = 0.69				
	Multi-cleat	21	13	0.61 [0.45; 0.76]					
	Metal cleat	2	0	1.00 [0.34; 1.00]					
Motivation for choosing a football boot	Comfort	59	28	0.68 [0.57; 0.77]	z = −0.23; *p* = 0.82				
	Price	19	5	0.79 [0.60; 0.91]					
	Playing field	29	16	0.64 [0.50; 0.77]					

R: risk; 95% CI: 95% confidence interval; RR: relative risk; RD: risk difference; RDp: risk difference in the population; AFe: attributable fraction to the exposed; AFp: attributable fraction in the population.

3.3. Analysis of the Association Between the Type of Turf and First-Team Player Status

The association analysis shows that first-team player status is not a modifier of the effect of the type of soccer pitch (natural or artificial) on the development of muscle injuries. There are no statistically significant differences for the type of training turf ($\chi^2_{(1)} = 2.75$; $p = 0.09$) and competition turf ($\chi^2_{(1)} = 0.50$; $p = 0.48$), depending on whether or not the athlete is a regular first-team player. Thus, first-team player status in the soccer team is not a modifier of the effect. Table 3 shows the analysis of the association between the development of injuries and first-team player status, stratified by the regular presence on the team.

Table 3. Association between the development of muscle injuries and the playing field in training and competition, stratified by presence on the regular team.

Action	Usual Presence on the Starting Team	R [95% CI]	RR	IS	ES	RR_{wV}	$RR_{M\text{-}H}$
Training	Yes	0.85 [0.63; 1.15]	0.84	0.81	0.84	0.74	0.84
	No	0.69 [0.54; 0.87]					
Competition	Yes	1.07 [0.84; 1.36]	1.03	1.02	1.03	1.02	1.03
	No	0.89 [0.57; 1.39]					

R: risk; 95% CI: 95% confidence interval; RR: relative risk; IS: internal standardization; ES: external standardization; RR_{wV}: weighting by the inverse of the variance; $RR_{M\text{-}H}$: weighting of Mantel–Haenszel.

3.4. Building the Best Predictive Model

The selected model (AIC = 190.5) contains three predictors of muscle injury in soccer players: age, training load and shoe type. The predictive capacity of this model was compared with the following model that included one more predictor by means of reclassification indices (IDI = 0.02%; $p = 0.10$; NRI = 0.04%; $p = 0.11$). The analysis showed no differences in the results, choosing the selected model, being more parsimonious, as the best predictive model of risk of injury.

The capacity of the predictive model was estimated ($\chi^2_{(3)} = 10.14$; $p = 0.02$). When performing the multicollinearity analysis of the predictor variables, we observed how the variables are moderately correlated with each other (mean VIF = 1.12). The odds ratios obtained in the predictive model reflect that the risk of injury increases with age (OR = 1.11). As for the type of soccer shoe used, the use of rubber cleats presents the greatest risk, as well as aluminum cleats (OR = 1), while the use of multi-cleat boots presents a protective effect against suffering muscle injury (OR = 0.44; 95% CI = 0.08; 1.10). The training load does not increase the risk of injury (OR = 0.85; 95% CI = 0.72; 1.00). The results of the analysis of the predictive model with a linear regression model are shown in Table 4.

Table 4. Analysis of the predictive model with a linear regression model.

Injury		OR	SE	z	p	95% CI
	Age	1.11	0.06	2.06	0.04	1.01; 1.23
	Weekly training	0.85	0.07	−1.91	0.06	0.72; 1.00
Soccer shoe						
	Multi-cleat	0.44	0.20	−1.77	0.08	0.18; 1.10
	Metal cleat	1				
	_const	0.65	0.87	−0.32	0.75	0.05; 8.81

OR: odds ratio; SE: standard error; 95% CI: 95% confidence interval.

3.5. Validity Indices of the Selected Model

After calculating the validity indices of the model, a moderate overall predictive capacity was revealed (AUC = 0.66). For the cut-off point $p = 0.5$, it has a high predictive capacity to detect athletes with muscle injury (sensitivity [Se] of 94.3%), but a low capacity to detect subjects without injury (specificity [Sp] = 14.3%). To obtain a given sensitivity and specificity of the model, the most indicated cut-off point was estimated as closely as possible ($p = 0.66$; Se = 73.33%; Sp = 55.10%). Figure 1 shows the area under the curve calculated in the selected predictive model.

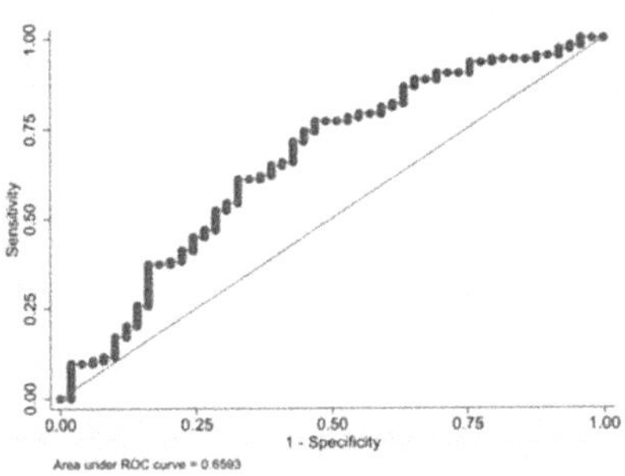

Figure 1. Area under the curve calculated in the predictive model.

3.6. Assessment of Interaction and Confusion

Evaluation of the interaction was carried out to quantify the effect of the type of training turf on the risk of injury, with the three predictors of the model (age, training load and type of soccer shoe), using the likelihood ratio test. There was statistical significance of the set of interactions (−2ln LR = 11.83; $p = 0.003$). The result indicates that the interactions between the type of training turf and the type of soccer shoe and the training load are statistically significant ($p < 0.01$). When assessing confusion, there are changes of more than 10% in all the reduced models. When analyzing the interaction to quantify the effect of the type of competition turf on the risk of injury, with the three predictors of the model (age, training load and type of soccer shoe), there was no statistical significance of the set of interactions (−2ln LR = 2.17; $p = 0.54$). Thus, the best model to estimate the effect of the competition turf on the development of injuries includes age, training load and shoe type as confounding variables.

4. Discussion

The present study aimed to evaluate the risk of muscle injuries in non-professional soccer players and identify the best predictive model of muscle injuries. Likewise, the risk of developing muscle injuries in soccer players was analyzed depending on the footwear, the playing field, age, body mass index, weekly training load and position on the field.

Although the risk of muscle injury is more frequent in players who train on artificial turf and those who are usually starters in their respective teams, there are hardly any statistically significant differences. The best predictive model of muscle injuries in these athletes determined how age, weekly training load and shoe type are the most significant predictive variables of risk of injury. These findings underline the complexity of the factors that contribute to injuries in soccer, suggesting that both environmental conditions and the individual characteristics of players should be considered when designing injury prevention programs.

The analysis of the risk of injury depending on the type of turf showed how players competing on artificial turf have 13% fewer injuries compared to those playing on natural grass. This finding could be explained by the uniformity and consistency of artificial turf, thereby being able to reduce unexpected variations of the surface. This could justify the decrease in injuries resulting from sudden changes in the terrain. Artificial surfaces provide more constant traction and cushioning, which can reduce joint and muscle stress during the execution of rapid movements and changes of direction. These results coincide with previous studies where a lower incidence of injuries has been reported in sports practice on artificial turf due to its uniform design and greater durability [14,15]. However, the results of other studies should be considered [16–18] where an association has been observed between playing on artificial turf and certain types of injuries, such as skin abrasions and specific muscle problems.

Our results found no association between the risk of muscle injuries and regular first-team player status. The training load and exposure to risk during matches is similar in starters and substitutes, regardless of how frequently they play [19]. Our results are consistent with what was observed in previous studies [15,20] reporting that first-team player status is not a determining factor in the incidence of injuries in soccer players. In addition, other factors such as adequate post-match recovery, fatigue management and player rotation strategies can play a relevant role that helps mitigate the risk of injuries [21–23]. Team management and training tactics must be optimized to protect players equally, regardless of the first-team player status of athletes.

The absence of an association between injuries and the motivation for buying the footwear, the position on the field or the type of soccer shoe revealed how these variables do not significantly influence the risk of injury. This may suggest how intrinsic factors such as physical preparation, general health status and playing technique have a greater impact on injury prevention than the specific equipment used. These results have been described previously [15,24,25], indicating how individual characteristics and general preparation are more crucial for injury prevention than other extrinsic variables, such as the type of soccer shoe used or the position on the pitch. In addition, personal preferences and comfort with equipment can vary considerably between players, making it difficult to establish a direct relationship between the type of soccer shoe and the risk of injury. It is possible that other factors, such as individual biomechanics and adaptation to the type of shoe, play a more important role in the incidence of injuries [26–28]. In this way, coaches, trainers and health personnel of the teams should focus on evaluating and optimizing the physical and technical condition of each player, instead of focusing excessively on the type of equipment.

We have observed in our predictive model how the training load is a predictive factor of risk of injury. The more players train, the lower is their risk of injury. This relationship may indicate how better physical conditioning and progressive adaptation of the body to exertion prevents the development of injuries [29]. Therefore, a well-planned training load can allow a gradual progression in the intensity and volume of the sessions, increasing the effectiveness in muscle strengthening and endurance, thus reducing the susceptibility to injuries [30].

The predictive model also showed that younger players have a lower risk of injury. This protective effect may be due to the greater recovery capacity and the lower accumulated wear of younger athletes [31]. Younger age is associated with greater muscle plasticity and a faster ability to adapt to the physical demands of sport [32]. However, looking at the age range of the athletes included in the study, this variability could be because older players do less exercise due to their status on the team, where they may be more established due to their experience.

Finally, the use of multi-cleat boots was associated with a lower risk of injury. This can probably be due to offering a better pressure distribution and greater stability [33]. These types of boots can reduce the risk of sprains and other joint problems by providing a more solid and secure grounding during rapid movements and changes of direction. The inclusion of the type of soccer shoe in the predictive model of the risk of developing muscle injury is in agreement with previous studies where the importance of using specially designed equipment to reduce the risk of injuries is underlined [34,35].

The findings of this study may be relevant to sports professionals. The identification of the most relevant risk factors as well as the predictive model of injury in this population of football players may help in the implementation of more effective and personalized prevention strategies. In this way, it could contribute to reduce the incidence of injuries and improve the performance of these players. These results are also in line with the importance of conducting regular assessments and adjusting prevention strategies according to the individual needs of the players, which could include changes in equipment, modification of training regimes and incorporation of advanced recovery techniques.

Limitations of the Study

The collection of data through self-reported surveys can introduce a bias in the collection of information. The tendency of players to minimize or exaggerate their injury and training experiences can modify the analyzed data. The absence of a thorough control in the evaluation of variables such as intensity and the specific type of training can affect the results and the accuracy of the conclusions. Similarly, a relevant limitation of this study is the non-inclusion of variables such as the weekly competition load (in hours), muscle overload and fatigue, or the intensity of the training or competition (distance covered, heart rate, etc.). This limits the interpretation and generalization of the results of this study. It is possible that different training programs, with variations in intensity, duration, and type of exercise, may significantly affect the results, something that could not be controlled in this study. Therefore, future studies should collect data through direct monitoring of training. Similarly, as only male soccer players were included, these results cannot be generalized to female amateur soccer players. Although female professional soccer players show injury incidence rates and patterns comparable to those of male players [36], in non-professional female soccer players, these data need to be confirmed. Specific studies on female soccer players or comparing both sexes could help to identify risk factors more globally and whether sex influences the risk of muscle injury in these non-professional athletes.

5. Conclusions

The risk of injury is higher for non-professional players competing on artificial turf. This risk of muscle injury is also higher in players who are regular starters in their football teams than in substitutes. Field position, boot type and motivation to buy the boot are not related to an increased risk of muscle injury in these non-professional soccer players.

The best predictive model of risk of injury in non-professional soccer players includes age, training load and shoe type.

Author Contributions: Conceptualization, I.I.-R. and R.C.-B.; methodology, I.I.-R. and R.C.-B.; software, R.C.-B.; formal analysis, R.C.-B.; investigation, I.I.-R.; resources, R.C.-B.; data curation, R.C.-B.; writing—original draft preparation, I.I.-R. and R.C.-B.; writing—review and editing, I.I.-R. and R.C.-B.; visualization, I.I.-R. and R.C.-B.; supervision, I.I.-R. and R.C.-B.; project administration, I.I.-R. and R.C.-B. All authors have read and agreed to the published version of the manuscript.

Funding: This research received no external funding.

Institutional Review Board Statement: The study was conducted in accordance with the Declaration of Helsinki and approved by the Research Ethics Committee of the Principality of Asturias (protocol code CEImPA 2024.107; February 2024).

Informed Consent Statement: Informed consent was obtained from all subjects involved in the study.

Data Availability Statement: The data that support the findings of this study are available on request from the corresponding author. The data are not publicly available due to privacy or ethical restrictions.

Acknowledgments: We would like to thank the study participants for taking the time to take part in the assessments.

Conflicts of Interest: The authors declare no conflicts of interest.

References

1. Gurau, T.V.; Gurau, G.; Musat, C.L.; Voinescu, D.C.; Anghel, L.; Onose, G.; Munteanu, C.; Onu, I.; Iordan, D.A. Epidemiology of Injuries in Professional and Amateur Football Men (Part II). *J. Clin. Med.* **2023**, *12*, 6293. [CrossRef] [PubMed]
2. Jones, A.; Jones, G.; Greig, N.; Bower, P.; Brown, J.; Hind, K.; Francis, P. Epidemiology of Injury in English Professional Football Players: A Cohort Study. *Phys. Ther. Sport* **2019**, *35*, 18–22. [CrossRef] [PubMed]
3. Dekkers, T.; O'Sullivan, K.; Blake, C.; McVeigh, J.G.; Collins, K. Epidemiology and Moderators of Injury in Gaelic Football: A Systematic Review and Meta-Analysis. *J. Sci. Med. Sport* **2022**, *25*, 222–229. [CrossRef] [PubMed]
4. López-Valenciano, A.; Ruiz-Pérez, I.; Garcia-Gómez, A.; Vera-Garcia, F.J.; De Ste Croix, M.; Myer, G.D.; Ayala, F. Epidemiology of Injuries in Professional Football: A Systematic Review and Meta-Analysis. *Br. J. Sports Med.* **2020**, *54*, 711–718. [CrossRef]
5. Gurau, T.V.; Gurau, G.; Voinescu, D.C.; Anghel, L.; Onose, G.; Iordan, D.A.; Munteanu, C.; Onu, I.; Musat, C.L. Epidemiology of Injuries in Men's Professional and Amateur Football (Part I). *J. Clin. Med.* **2023**, *12*, 5569. [CrossRef]
6. Randers, M.B.; Hagman, M.; Christensen, J.F.; Póvoas, S.; Nielsen, J.J.; Krustrup, P. Health and Performance Effects of 12 Weeks of Small-Sided Street Football Training Compared to Grass Football Training in Habitually Active Young Men. *Eur. J. Appl. Physiol.* **2024**, *124*, 805–813. [CrossRef]
7. Ishøi, L.; Krommes, K.; Husted, R.S.; Juhl, C.B.; Thorborg, K. Diagnosis, Prevention and Treatment of Common Lower Extremity Muscle Injuries in Sport—Grading the Evidence: A Statement Paper Commissioned by the Danish Society of Sports Physical Therapy (DSSF). *Br. J. Sports Med.* **2020**, *54*, 528–537. [CrossRef]
8. Seif Barghi, T.; Khazaei, S.; Heydari, B.; Naderifar, H. The frequency of injuries of Iranian male professional soccer players: A cross-sectional study. *J. Inj. Violence Res.* **2024**, *16*. [PubMed]
9. Etzel, C.M.; Meghani, O.; Owens, B.D.; Kocher, M.S.; Field, A.E. Predictors of Anterior Cruciate Ligament Tears in Adolescents and Young Adults. *Orthop. J. Sports Med.* **2024**, *12*, 23259671241272699. [CrossRef]
10. Sánchez Hernández, N.; García-Fernández, A.; Alonso-Calvar, M. Propuesta de Protocolo de Prevención En El Uso de Calzado Según El Terreno de Juego Para Futbolistas Jóvenes. *Rev. Prep. Fís. Fútb.* **2021**, *37*, 30–43.
11. Smeets, K.; Jacobs, P.; Hertogs, R.; Luyckx, J.-P.; Innocenti, B.; Corten, K.; Ekstrand, J.; Bellemans, J. Torsional Injuries of the Lower Limb: An Analysis of the Frictional Torque between Different Types of Football Turf and the Shoe Outsole. *Br. J. Sports Med.* **2012**, *46*, 1078–1083. [CrossRef] [PubMed]
12. Almutawa, M.; Scott, M.; George, K.P.; Drust, B. The Incidence and Nature of Injuries Sustained on Grass and 3rd Generation Artificial Turf: A Pilot Study in Elite Saudi National Team Footballers. *Phys. Ther. Sport* **2014**, *15*, 47–52. [CrossRef] [PubMed]
13. Wik, E.H.; Lolli, L.; Chamari, K.; Materne, O.; Di Salvo, V.; Gregson, W.; Bahr, R. Injury Patterns Differ with Age in Male Youth Football: A Four-Season Prospective Study of 1111 Time-Loss Injuries in an Elite National Academy. *Br. J. Sports Med.* **2021**, *55*, 794–800. [CrossRef] [PubMed]
14. Gabbett, T.J. The Training-Injury Prevention Paradox: Should Athletes Be Training Smarter and Harder? *Br. J. Sports Med.* **2016**, *50*, 273–280. [CrossRef] [PubMed]
15. Hägglund, M.; Waldén, M.; Magnusson, H.; Kristenson, K.; Bengtsson, H.; Ekstrand, J. Injuries Affect Team Performance Negatively in Professional Football: An 11-Year Follow-Up of the UEFA Champions League Injury Study. *Br. J. Sports Med.* **2013**, *47*, 738–742. [CrossRef]
16. Ekstrand, J.; Timpka, T.; Hägglund, M. Risk of Injury in Elite Football Played on Artificial Turf versus Natural Grass: A Prospective Two-Cohort Study. *Br. J. Sports Med.* **2006**, *40*, 975–980. [CrossRef]

17. Miyamori, T.; Nagao, M.; Sawa, R.; Tumilty, S.; Yoshimura, M.; Saita, Y.; Ikeda, H.; Kaneko, K. Playing Football on Artificial Turf as a Risk Factor for Fifth Metatarsal Stress Fracture: A Retrospective Cohort Study. *BMJ Open* **2019**, *9*, e022864. [CrossRef]
18. Mears, A.C.; Osei-Owusu, P.; Harland, A.R.; Owen, A.; Roberts, J.R. Perceived Links Between Playing Surfaces and Injury: A Worldwide Study of Elite Association Football Players. *Sports Med. Open* **2018**, *4*, 40. [CrossRef]
19. Sousa, H.; Clemente, F.M.; Sarmento, H.; Gouveia, É.R.; Musa, R.M. Comparing Locomotor Intensity Indicators in Soccer Training and Competition across Contextual Factors: A Study of Replaced Coaches in a Portuguese Professional 1st League Team. *Front. Sports Act. Living* **2024**, *6*, 1391784. [CrossRef]
20. Freckleton, G.; Pizzari, T. Risk Factors for Hamstring Muscle Strain Injury in Sport: A Systematic Review and Meta-Analysis. *Br. J. Sports Med.* **2013**, *47*, 351–358. [CrossRef]
21. Querido, S.M.; Brito, J.; Figueiredo, P.; Carnide, F.; Vaz, J.R.; Freitas, S.R. Post-Match Recovery Practices in Professional Football: Design, Validity, and Reliability of a New Questionnaire. *Front. Sports Act. Living* **2021**, *3*, 680799. [CrossRef] [PubMed]
22. Marqués-Jiménez, D.; Calleja Gonzalez, J.; Arratibel, I.; Delextrat, A.; Terrados, N. Fatigue and Recovery in Soccer: Evidence and Challenges. *Open Sports Sci. J.* **2017**, *10*, 52–70. [CrossRef]
23. Dupont, W.G.; Nédélec, M.; McCall, A.; Berthoin, S.; Maffiuletti, N.A. Practical Aspects of Blending Science and Reality. *ASPETAR Sports Med. J.* **2015**, *4*, 20–27.
24. Gehring, D.; Rott, F.; Stapelfeldt, B.; Gollhofer, A. Effect of Soccer Shoe Cleats on Knee Joint Loads. *Int. J. Sports Med.* **2008**, *28*, 1030–1034. [CrossRef]
25. Mallo, J.; González, P.; Veiga, S.; Navarro, E. Injury Incidence in a Spanish Sub-Elite Professional Football Team: A Prospective Study during Four Consecutive Seasons. *J. Sports Sci. Med.* **2011**, *10*, 731–736.
26. Shan, G.; Zhang, X. From 2D Leg Kinematics to 3D Full-Body Biomechanics-the Past, Present and Future of Scientific Analysis of Maximal Instep Kick in Soccer. *Sports Med. Arthrosc. Rehabil. Ther. Technol.* **2011**, *3*, 23. [CrossRef]
27. Kolodziej, M.; Willwacher, S.; Nolte, K.; Schmidt, M.; Jaitner, T. Biomechanical Risk Factors of Injury-Related Single-Leg Movements in Male Elite Youth Soccer Players. *Biomechanics* **2022**, *2*, 281–300. [CrossRef]
28. Jiang, Z.; Hao, Y.; Jin, N.; Li, Y. A Systematic Review of the Relationship between Workload and Injury Risk of Professional Male Soccer Players. *Int. J. Environ. Res. Public Health* **2022**, *19*, 13237. [CrossRef]
29. Nyhus Hagum, C.; Tønnessen, E.; Hisdal, J.; Shalfawi, S.A.I. The Effect of Progressive and Individualised Sport-Specific Training on the Prevalence of Injury in Football and Handball Student Athletes: A Randomised Controlled Trial. *Front. Sports Act. Living* **2023**, *5*, 1106404. [CrossRef]
30. Stephenson, S.D.; Kocan, J.W.; Vinod, A.V.; Kluczynski, M.A.; Bisson, L.J. A Comprehensive Summary of Systematic Reviews on Sports Injury Prevention Strategies. *Orthop. J. Sports Med.* **2021**, *9*, 23259671211035776. [CrossRef]
31. Chena Sinovas, M.; Rodríguez Hernández, M.L.; Bores Cerezal, A. Epidemiology of Injuries in Young Spanish Soccer Players According to the Playing Positions (Epidemiología de Las Lesiones En Futbolistas Jóvenes Españoles Según La Demarcación). *Retos* **2020**, *38*, 459–464. [CrossRef]
32. Azzolino, D.; Spolidoro, G.C.I.; Saporiti, E.; Luchetti, C.; Agostoni, C.; Cesari, M. Musculoskeletal Changes Across the Lifespan: Nutrition and the Life-Course Approach to Prevention. *Front. Med.* **2021**, *8*, 697954. [CrossRef] [PubMed]
33. Hennig, E.M.; Sterzing, T. The Influence of Soccer Shoe Design on Playing Performance: A Series of Biomechanical Studies. *Footwear Sci.* **2010**, *2*, 3–11. [CrossRef]
34. Engebretsen, A.H.; Myklebust, G.; Holme, I.; Engebretsen, L.; Bahr, R. Prevention of Injuries among Male Soccer Players: A Prospective, Randomized Intervention Study Targeting Players with Previous Injuries or Reduced Function. *Am. J. Sports Med.* **2008**, *36*, 1052–1060. [CrossRef]
35. Thacker, S.B.; Stroup, D.F.; Branche, C.M.; Gilchrist, J.; Goodman, R.A.; Weitman, E.A. The Prevention of Ankle Sprains in Sports. A Systematic Review of the Literature. *Am. J. Sports Med.* **1999**, *27*, 753–760. [CrossRef]
36. Medina-Porqueres, I.; Sancho-Garcia, S.; Gomez-Caceres, A.; Mondragon-Cortes, R.; Ma-drid-Rodríguez, A.; Rosado-Velazquez, D. Injury surveillance in Spanish professional female soccer players: A three-season retrospective study. *Injury* **2024**, *55*, 111922. [CrossRef]

sports

MDPI

Article

Comparison of Inter-Rater and Intra-Rater Reliability of Raters with Different Levels of Experience When Using Landing Error Scoring System (LESS) in Field-Based Screening of Professional Football Players

Nikolaos I. Liveris, Charis Tsarbou, Sofia A. Xergia , Angelos Papadopoulos and Elias Tsepis *

Department of Physiotherapy, School of Health Rehabilitation Sciences, University of Patras, Rio, GR26504 Patras, Greece; n.liveris@upatras.gr (N.I.L.); ctsarmpou@upatras.gr (C.T.); sxergia@upatras.gr (S.A.X.); angpap1997@gmail.com (A.P.)

* Correspondence: tsepis@upatras.gr; Tel.: +30-2610962413

Abstract: It is essential for physical sports therapists to use reliable field-based tests to identify potential injury risk factors in athletes. The purpose of this study was to compare the inter- and intra-rater reliability of experienced and novice raters during use of the Landing Error Scoring System (LESS) in a field-based examination of professional football athletes. Thirty-seven male football athletes underwent pre-season LESS assessment. Two raters independently evaluated the recorded landing techniques at two separate intervals, two months apart, following the LESS standard protocol. Inter-and intra-rater values were calculated for the LESS total scores and individual scoring items. The overall LESS scores had excellent intra-rater reliability values for both the experienced (interclass correlation coefficient (ICC) = 0.95, 95% CI, 0.89–0.97; $p < 0.001$) and novice rater (ICC = 0.95, 95% CI, 0.90–0.97; $p < 0.001$), and very good to excellent inter-rater values for the first (ICC = 0.90, 95% CI, 0.77–0.95; $p < 0.001$) and second (ICC = 0.86, 95% CI, 0.71–0.93; $p < 0.001$) evaluation. Most of the individual scoring items ranged from moderate to perfect agreement. In conclusion, sports physical therapists, regardless of experience, can reliably use the LESS's total score, through video analysis of the regime. Individual scoring items can inform clinicians about impairments in the landing mechanism but data should be interpreted cautiously.

Keywords: pre-season screening; reliability; field-based examination; landing; risk factors

1. Introduction

Athletes' screening is considered an essential first step in order to identify potential risk factors that may increase the likelihood of injury. The information gained by the application of screening tests can guide sports physical therapists to apply targeted preventive interventions that may reduce the risk of injury [1,2]. Despite pre-season screening being a standard procedure for football teams, sports injuries remain a substantial problem for teams' performance and financial integrity [3]. The multifactorial and complex nature of injuries as well as the questionable validity of many screening tests make the prevention of injuries a challenging task [4,5]. Biomechanical predisposing factors, such as kinematic and kinetic parameters of landing and cutting movements, play a key role in the injury mechanism [6,7]. Laboratory-based examination using sophisticated motion analysis systems can identify kinematic and kinetic impairments during jumping or cutting tasks [6,8]. These systems are highly reliable; however, they are costly, time-consuming, and challenging to use in a field-based setting [9]. Therefore, the availability of reliable, low-cost, and time-efficient tools such as the Landing Error Scoring System (LESS) represents a crucial initial step [1]. In addition, the predictive value of separate tests is ambiguous, and the current trend is towards the use of test batteries, which approach athletes' functionality in a more holistic manner [4,10].

The LESS, consisting of 17 separate items, has been suggested to suit this purpose [9,10], as a tool that can be successfully applied during clinical or field-based examinations, with minimal and low-cost equipment [9]. It can also be applied frequently during the season to provide an updated assessment of athletes' functional status [10]. This is fundamental, because the latter is susceptible to fluctuations during the season, due to injury, illnesses, detraining, and various other factors [4]. In clinical practice, the consideration of the individual scoring items in addition to total scores can provide valuable information about specific deficiencies in landing mechanisms which are crucial for injury prevention [11–13]. In addition, combined with other evaluation measures such as strength asymmetries, ballistic function, previous injuries, and workload characteristics, LESS can contribute to the targeted formulation of injury prevention programs and re-evaluate the impact of prevention programs on athletes during the season [10,12].

The reliability of LESS depends heavily on examiners paying the appropriate attention to the guidelines while scoring each item. The results of previous studies [9,11,14,15] have indicated good to excellent reliability values of LESS total scores using standard LESS scoring instructions [9]. From these investigations, two reported the inter-rater reliability of the overall instrument, including specific scoring items. Regarding intra-rater reliability, only Everard et al. [15] reported reliability values of a single rater for the individual scoring items except for the total scores. According to these investigations [14,15], despite the range of reliability values of LESS's specific scoring items, these items provide acceptable reliability.

The need for additional investigation is dictated by methodological constraints. Earlier research has explored LESS's reliability in scoring either freshman military subjects or various sports athletes in controlled laboratory settings [14,15]. Expanding the analysis of its reliability in particular groups, such as professional football players or individuals with injuries, would enhance the generalizability of the outcomes [11]. Moreover, it is questionable whether the reliability is similar during in field-based testing, and this has not been tried before. In contrast to evaluations conducted in controlled indoor laboratory settings, outdoor field assessments may be subject to fluctuations in environmental factors and surface conditions, which could impact the assessment of LESS by evaluators. It is also vital to establish reliability among raters with different levels of experience, using solely baseline LESS instructions [9] without further training. In the study by Onate et al. [14], the novice rater had training by the founders of the instrument in the proper scoring technique before the examination of LESS reliability. In case of no requirement for additional training, its use would be expanded.

Therefore, the main aim of the present study was to examine the inter- and intra-rater reliability of LESS in comparing between experienced and novice raters using the standard scoring guidelines proposed by Padua et al. [9]. A secondary aim was to conduct the aforementioned examination on field, since it has been carried out indoors only so far. In this way, this study will provide valuable information for the medical and training staff of football teams for the reliable use of the LESS standard version as part of a team's injury risk screening protocol, regardless of the venue.

2. Materials and Methods

2.1. Participants

Thirty-seven male professional football players from two Greek second-division teams voluntarily participated in this study. The participants' characteristics are presented in Table 1. The sample of this study was involved in a more extensive prospective cohort investigation examining the risk factors for lower-limb injuries. To assess LESS reliability, participants were chosen randomly from a larger sample. The football athletes involved in this study were free of injury or fully rehabilitated from a previous one, and they participated in their teams' activities without restrictions. All volunteers were informed of the study's aim and signed a consent form. Ethical approval was obtained from the Committee of the University of Patras (ID: 12126).

Table 1. Samples' demographic characteristics.

	Minimum	Maximum	Mean ± SD
Age	17	32	21.49 ± 4.06
Weight (kg)	63.68	93.13	74.92 ± 7.25
Height (m)	1.66	1.92	1.81 ± 0.07
BMI	20.47	25.77	22.92 ± 1.37

2.2. Procedure

During the pre-season period, 37 athletes participated in a field-based drop jump assessment to identify potential risk factors for lower limb injuries. Initially, they were informed of the purpose of the evaluation and signed a consent form. Demographic characteristics, previous season's training exposure, and injury history were also recorded using a structured questionnaire. Subsequently, after a ten-minute sports-specific warm-up, including running and stretching, athletes performed a bilateral drop-jump task assessment using the LESS guidelines [9].

LESS assessment was conducted in accordance with the instructions provided by Padua et al. [9]. Following the instructions for the appropriate test setup [9], the participants jumped from a 30 cm box at a distance equal to 50% of their height and immediately performed a vertical jump (Figure 1). The athletes were instructed on the proper execution of the task and performed two familiarization trials. Three successful attempts were recorded for analysis. Each athlete spent two to three minutes to complete the test. No instructions regarding the proper landing technique were provided. Two conventional cameras (Sony HDR-CX625 and Panasonic HC-V770) recorded the landing tasks in the sagittal and frontal planes. The recorded videos were stored on the personal computers of two raters for analysis.

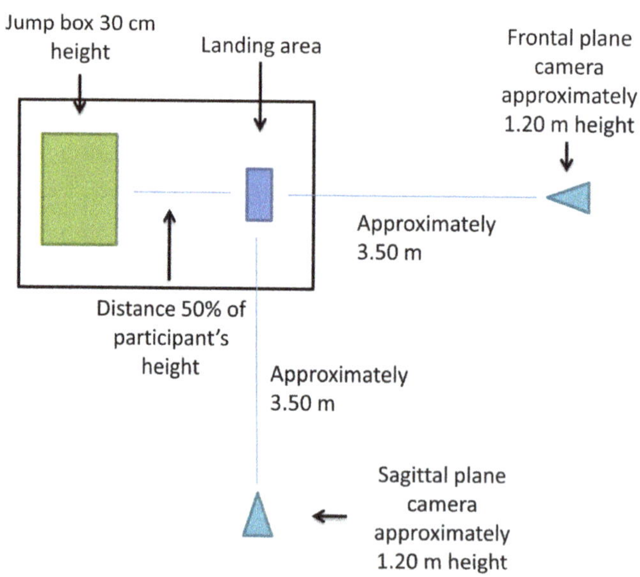

Figure 1. Test setup. Landing area and camera placement.

2.3. Data Collection

Two raters evaluated the recorded videos of the landings based on published guidelines [9]. To calculate the intra-rater reliability, both raters performed two evaluations of the videos, separated by approximately two months. The videos were evaluated randomly during the second assessment to prevent recall bias. The two raters had different experience levels. The first one had previously used the instructions of Padua et al. [9] when performing approximately 150 LESS evaluations for the purpose of other studies [10,16,17]. The novice rater used the LESS for the first time. Both raters applied the recommended guidelines [9] without further education regarding proper LESS evaluation. The reliability results of the experienced and a novice rater were compared to cover a broad spectrum of raters' familiarization, since clinical or sports physical therapists usually have little or no respective experience. It is essential to identify the degree to which novice examiners can be trusted when they report LESS values. The experienced rater was a Ph.D. student in sports physical therapy with 10 years of experience in clinical practice, and the novice rater was an M.Sc. student in physical therapy and therapeutic exercise without previous experience in LESS use but with 6 years of experience in clinical practice.

The investigators analyzed the recorded videos of the three bilateral drop-jumps using the scoring sheet that included 17 scoring items [9]. This scoring form focused on the assessment of trunk position, knee (flexion angles, valgus), and hip flexion angle at the initial contact (IC) and the maximum knee flexion during landing (Figure 2). In addition, foot rotation, symmetrical foot initial contact, and base of support width were also considered. Finally, items 16 and 17 reflected the rater's subjective view of the sagittal plane joint displacement during landing and the overall impression of the landing. For items 1–15, if an error in the landing mechanism existed, the rater scored "1". For items 16 and 17, the rater scored "0" for soft or excellent landing, "1" for average, and "2" for stiff or poor landing mechanisms. The total LESS score was calculated as the average of the LESS scores of the three trials [12]. Specific errors were recorded if an error existed in at least two of the three trials for items 1–15. For items 16–17, average scoring of "1" is considered when it has been recorded in at least two of the three trials, and for poor/stiff landing scoring, "2" is recorded when it has been recorded in at least in one of three trials. Higher total LESS scores indicate more landing errors. To increase the objectivity of the landing assessment, the videos were evaluated using the two-dimensional video analysis software of Kinovea (Version 0.9.5).

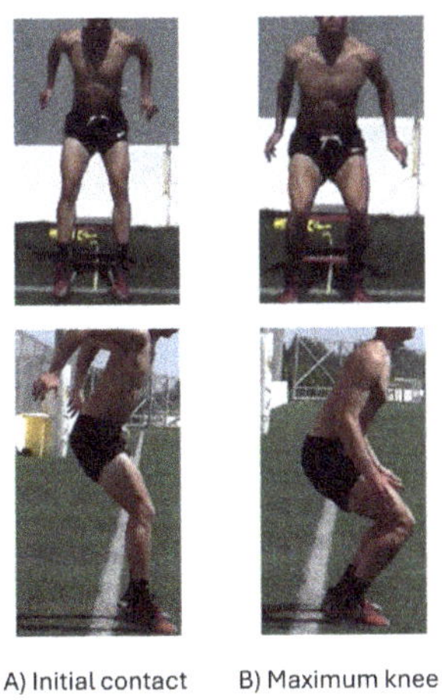

Figure 2. Evaluation of landing mechanism during initial contact (**A**) and maximum knee flexion (**B**) from sagittal and frontal view.

2.4. Statistical Analysis

The SPSS software, version 28, was used for the statistical analysis. The inter- and intra-rater reliability of the total LESS scores were assessed using the average interclass correlation coefficient (ICC) measures for 2-way mixed modes with 95% confidence intervals (CIs). The type of absolute agreement for ICC was used. The kappa statistic was used to evaluate the reliability of the individual scoring items of the LESS, which were categorical/dichotomous (0–1) variables. The kappa statistic has proven to be a more suitable measurement than the percentage agreement [14]. The inter-rater reliability values for the total LESS scores and individual scoring items were calculated for the first and second LESS assessments. For the interpretation of kappa statistics, values of 0 represent poor agreement, 0.01–0.20 represents a slight agreement, 0.21–0.40 represents a fair agreement, 0.41–0.60 moderate agreement, 0.61–0.80 represents substantial agreement, and 0.81–1 almost perfect agreement [18]. Regarding the ICC values, agreement between raters of less than 0.5 indicates weak reliability, 0.5 to 0.75 indicates moderate reliability, 0.75 to 0.90 indicates good reliability, and greater than 0.90 indicates excellent reliability [19]. According to the recommendations of Koo and Li [19], the range of 95% CIs was also considered to provide a more thorough analysis of ICC outcomes.

3. Results

The intra-rater reliability of the LESS total scores was excellent for both the experienced and novice raters, with average ICC values of 0.95 (95% CI, 0.89–0.97; $p < 0.001$) and 0.95 (95% CI, 0.90–0.97; $p < 0.001$), respectively. Regarding the inter-rater reliability, the results indicated a good to excellent agreement among raters in the first and second LESS evaluations, with average ICC values of 0.90 (95% CI, 0.77–0.95; $p < 0.001$) and 0.86 (95% CI, 0.71–0.93; $p < 0.001$), respectively. The findings demonstrated a slight variation when examining the range of the 95% confidence intervals. According to the 95% CIs, the results indicated good to excellent intra-rater reliability for both experienced and novice raters. The findings from the inter-rater assessments demonstrated an acceptable level of agreement, with values indicating good to excellent reliability in the initial evaluation and moderate to excellent reliability in the subsequent evaluation. A comprehensive analysis of the descriptive statistics for the raters' total scores on the LESS scale is provided in Table 2.

Table 2. Descriptive statistics of LESS total scores.

	Minimum	Maximum	Mean ± SD
Experience 1	1.67	11	5.65 ± 1.88
Experience 2	2.67	10	5.95 ± 1.69
Novice 1	1.67	10.67	5.12 ± 1.89
Novice 2	2.33	11	5.4 ± 2.1

The inter-rater agreement of the specific scoring items of the LESS ranged from moderate to almost perfect for most individual scoring items in the first evaluation, and for all scoring items in the second LESS evaluation (Table 3). Low inter-rater agreement was observed in the assessment of the first evaluation for 13 (hip flexion displacement) and 17 (overall impression). However, these specific scoring items reached moderate kappa values when the inter-rater reliability of the second LESS evaluation was assessed. In addition, perfect agreement in both assessments was observed only for items 2 (hip flexion at IC) and 9 (internal foot position). These scoring items presented constant values for all observations. At the same time, we observed a range between substantial and almost perfect agreement when comparing the two evaluations for items 1 (knee flexion at IC), 4 (ankle plantar flexion at IC), 7 (wide stance), 8 (narrow stance), 10 (external foot position), and 12 (knee flexion displacement). Further, there was a moderate inter-rater agreement for item 11 (symmetric foot contact at IC) and a substantial agreement for items 3 (trunk flexion at IC) and 15 (knee valgus displacement) in both evaluations. Finally, we observed moderate to substantial agreement for items 5 (knee valgus at IC), 6 (lateral trunk flexion at IC), 14 (trunk flexion displacement), and 16 (overall joint displacement) when we compared the two evaluations.

Table 3. Inter- and intra-rater agreement of specific scoring items of the experienced and novice raters.

	Scoring Items	Inter-Rater Cohen's Kappa First Evaluation *	Inter-Rater Cohen's Kappa Second Evaluation *	Intra-Rater Cohen's Kappa Experienced Rater *	Intra-Rater Cohen's Kappa Novice Rater *
1	Knee flexion at IC	0.92	0.62	0.71	1.00
2	Hip flexion at IC	1.00 (constant)	1.00 (constant)	1.00 (constant)	1.00 (constant)
3	Trunk flexion at IC	0.65	0.64	1.00	1.00
4	Ankle plantar flexion at IC	0.80	0.87	0.93	1.00
5	Knee valgus at IC	0.59	0.68	0.80	0.65
6	Lateral trunk flexion at IC	0.72	0.53	0.65	0.80
7	Wide stance	0.65	1.00	0.65	1.00
8	Narrow stance	0.89	0.74	0.79	0.95
9	Internal foot position	1.00 (constant)	1.00 (constant)	1.00 (constant)	1.00 (constant)
10	External foot position	0.92	0.71	0.77	0.85
11	Symmetric foot contact at IC	0.60	0.60	0.80	0.80
12	Knee flexion displacement	1.00	0.68	0.68	1.00
13	Hip flexion displacement	0.36	0.53	0.64	0.64
14	Trunk flexion displacement	0.54	0.63	0.94	0.83
15	Knee valgus displacement	0.63	0.72	0.68	0.89
16	Overall joint displacement	0.66	0.62	0.71	0.83
17	Overall impression	0.20 **	0.44	0.51	0.43

* Statistically significant < 0.05; ** not statistically significant = 0.12; constant—all rates have the same value.

The intra-rater values of the experienced and novice raters ranged from moderate to almost perfect agreement (Table 3). Almost perfect intra-rater reliability for both raters was observed for items 2 (hip flexion at IC), 3 (trunk flexion at IC), 4 (ankle plantar flexion at IC), 9 (internal foot position), and 14 (trunk flexion displacement). In addition, raters achieved substantial intra-rater kappa values for items 11 (symmetric foot contact at the IC) and 13 (hip flexion displacement). The remaining items had substantial and almost perfect intra-rater agreement for both raters. Finally, there was moderate intra-rater agreement for both raters on item 17 regarding the overall impression of the landing technique, representing the lowest intra-rater values for both raters.

A final outcome revealed that determining an athlete's performance using the LESS necessitates diverse scoring durations among evaluators. A novice rater typically takes up to 20 min, while experienced rater spends an average of 10 min.

4. Discussion

The current research examined the reliability of LESS in and between raters with varying levels of experience in its application. Further, this study was conducted on field during pre-season screening of professional football players. The outcomes of our research showed that raters with varying backgrounds in LESS evaluation and without further training achieved excellent intra-rater reliability and very good to excellent inter-rater agreement in LESS total scores. These findings align with previous studies [14,15], which reported similar ICC values for LESS total scores. In addition, our study provides inter- and intra-rater reliability values for the individual scoring items. To the best of our knowledge, this is the first study to examine the reliability of LESS among professional football players in field-based situations. We chose to investigate the intra- and inter-rater reliability among raters with no previous training in adequately using the LESS instrument and following only the standard instruction and scoring sheets of Padua et al. [9]. Our purpose was to assess whether the LESS has the appropriate reliability to be adequately used by the football team's medical staff, using only the instructions given by the founders of the instrument as a guide [9].

According to the results, the LESS total scores had excellent intra-rater and very good to excellent inter-rater reliability values. These results agree with previous studies that examined the reliability of the LESS total scores in various sports athletes under laboratory conditions [11,14,15]. The total scores provide an overall impression of the landing technique, with lower values indicating a safer landing mechanism, with a lower risk of injury [9,12]. Athletes who score over five [12] or six [13] are categorized as having high-risk landing performance. Using these cutoff points, the team's medical and coaching staff can classify athletes as high- or low-risk for injury in combination with holistic field-based screening measurements, including isometric strength parameters, triple-hop landing, flexibility, and core stability measurements [10]. Subsequently, the team's staff can implement appropriate injury-prevention exercise programs for at-risk athletes [2,10, 11]. However, the total LESS score results may be similar on different occasions despite differences in the scores of individual scoring items [15].

The individual scoring items can provide insight into specific deficits of landing. In contrast to the good to excellent reliability values of the LESS total scores, the reliability values of individual scoring items should be considered more cautiously. Our findings indicate a degree of inconsistency in the reliability scores of the individual scoring items. Specifically, the results of some individual items, such as knee flexion at IC, hip flexion displacement, and wide stance, revealed a certain degree of variability in the inter-rater reliability values across the first and second evaluations. Furthermore, the overall impression (item 17) demonstrated low reliability values. Consequently, sports physical therapists must thoughtfully assess the outcomes of these specific items when assessing for possible risk factors or the efficacy of preventive measures based on individual LESS items. However, in agreement with previous studies [14,15], the inter- and intra-rater reliability for most of the scoring items in our research ranged from moderate to almost perfect agreement.

It is important to mention differences between our study and previous investigations, because these may affect the comparison of the results. Particularly, the study of Onate et al. [14] used only the first trial to calculate inter-rater reliability values and not the average results of the three trials proposed by Padua et al. [9]. On the other hand, the study of Everard et al. [15] reported that while raters had no experience using the LESS, they had significant experience with the Functional Movement Screen (FMS), which may have affected the results, as the authors mentioned in their paper. Finally, as Everard et al. [15] noted, the influence of rater background on LESS results requires further examination.

Specifically, regarding the inter-rater reliability values of individual scoring items, substantial and moderate agreement in the repeated evaluation of the videos was observed for most scoring items, which agrees with previous studies [14,15]. Nevertheless, in contrast with the relevant literature [14,15], low inter-rater kappa values (<0.40) were observed in the first evaluation of the videos regarding the hip flexion displacement between the IC and peak knee flexion (item 13). However, Everard et al. [15] reported an inter-rater agreement of 0.53, which was slightly different from the inter-rater agreement of item 13 (0.36) in this study. At the same time, lower inter-rater values than those reported in the literature [15] were observed in the evaluation of item 17 and, more precisely, in the first assessment. This can be attributed to the scoring of the overall impression of the landing technique (item 17), which is strongly subjective, despite instructions, and it is influenced by the level of the rater's experience as well as their specific training on the LESS or other relative tests such as the FMS [14,15]. However, we observed moderate kappa values for the 13 and 17 scoring items in the second inter-rater evaluation. As previously mentioned, our study raters had different experiences using LESS, but neither had received education about the proper technique of rating, which may have influenced the low inter-rater reliability values of items 13 and, more importantly, item 17.

In clinical practice, different clinicians may assess the landing technique of an individual before and after the implementation of injury prevention programs. Considering the subjective nature of individual scoring of some items, we calculated the inter-rater reliability of scoring items at two different time points to evaluate the stability of the reliability results. The results indicated that the inter-rater reliability values of most scoring items ranged between the two video assessments. A possible explanation for this phenomenon is that, because the scoring follows a dichotomous strategy (score 0 or 1) when a landing impairment is near the cutoff point, the score given by a rater may change at different scoring times. For instance, this may explain the low inter-rater reliability values for hip flexion displacement (item 13). Despite these variations in values, the scoring form seems to have an acceptable inter-rater agreement, and clinicians can be informed about the possible specific landing impairments of their athletes. In addition, clinicians should be aware that because of the dichotomous process of scoring each impairment, observation is not very sensitive. For instance, whereas we rated the existence of valgus during landing, the instrument does not inform us about the magnitude of the valgus presented in a participant. These observations can be added to the total score only when the rater scores item 17 regarding the overall impression of landing, which is clearly a subjective scoring criterion, as we have already mentioned.

To our knowledge, there is limited evidence in the literature regarding the intra-rater reliability of two raters with different experiences using the LESS instrument. Onate et al. [14] examined only the inter-rater agreement among an expert and novice rater, whereas the study of Everard et al. [15] provides intra-rater values only from the one rater. Similar to Everard et al. [15], our results indicate that the kappa values showed substantial and almost perfect agreement for most scoring items. Furthermore, both raters showed moderate agreement in overall landing impressions and substantial agreement in general joint displacement.

In addition, a side finding of the study revealed that the two raters differed in the time required to complete the scoring. Specifically, the novice rater spent up to 20 min rating each participant's three attempts, whereas the experienced rater spent 10 min on average. This may be because the novice rater usually spent more time scrutinizing and reading the scoring instructions. The control of scoring time, in future studies, will provide valuable information about the aforementioned observation. Finally, future attempts could add a specifically trained rater in LESS.

In conclusion, sports physical therapists can reliably use the LESS total scores to assess the landing technique of football players, following only the published instructions of the standard version of the instrument [9]. LESS is a valuable tool for medical teams, regardless of the examiners' level of experience, for field-based screening of football players. However, the individual scoring items should be viewed with caution since there was a considerable range in reliability. In any case, information of this assessment tool can draw attention to specific landing impairments of each individual, and along with additional testing, an individualized exercise prevention program can be planned. However, its direct connection to injuries remains to be further investigated.

Author Contributions: Conceptualization, N.I.L., C.T., E.T. and. S.A.X.; methodology, N.I.L., C.T., S.A.X. and E.T.; validation, N.I.L. and C.T.; formal analysis, E.T., A.P. and N.I.L.; investigation, N.I.L., C.T. and A.P.; data curation, N.I.L., C.T. and A.P; writing—original draft preparation, N.I.L. and C.T.; writing—review and editing, E.T. and S.A.X.; visualization, N.I.L., C.T., E.T. and S.A.X.; supervision, S.A.X. and E.T.; project administration, S.A.X. and E.T. All authors have read and agreed to the published version of the manuscript.

Funding: This research received no external funding.

Institutional Review Board Statement: This study was conducted in accordance with the Declaration of Helsinki and approved by the Institutional Ethics Committee of the University of Patras, Greece (ID 12126; date: 6 June 2023).

Informed Consent Statement: Written informed consent was obtained from all subjects involved in the study.

Data Availability Statement: The data presented in this study are available on request from the corresponding author. The data are not publicly available due to privacy and ethical restrictions.

Acknowledgments: We thank the team's medical and coaching staffs and players for their cooperation to execute the study's measurements.

Conflicts of Interest: The authors declare no conflicts of interest.

References

1. Read, P.J.; Oliver, J.L.; De Ste Croix, M.B.A.; Myer, G.D.; Lloyd, R.S. A Review of Field-Based Assessments of Neuromuscular Control and Their Utility in Male Youth Soccer Players. *J. Strength Cond. Res.* **2019**, *33*, 283–299. [CrossRef] [PubMed]
2. Mendonça, L.D.M. To Do or Not to Do?—The Value of the Preseason Assessment in Sport Injury Prevention. *Int. J. Sports Phys. Ther.* **2022**, *17*, 111–113. [CrossRef]
3. Eliakim, E.; Morgulev, E.; Lidor, R.; Meckel, Y. Estimation of Injury Costs: Financial Damage of English Premier League Teams' Underachievement Due to Injuries. *BMJ Open Sport Exerc. Med.* **2020**, *6*, e000675. [CrossRef] [PubMed]
4. Fonseca, S.T.; Souza, T.R.; Verhagen, E.; van Emmerik, R.; Bittencourt, N.F.N.; Mendonça, L.D.M.; Andrade, A.G.P.; Resende, R.A.; Ocarino, J.M. Sports Injury Forecasting and Complexity: A Synergetic Approach. *Sports Med.* **2020**, *50*, 1757–1770. [CrossRef] [PubMed]
5. Bahr, R. Why Screening Tests to Predict Injury Do Not Work—And Probably Never Will...: A Critical Review. *Br. J. Sports Med.* **2016**, *50*, 776–780. [CrossRef] [PubMed]
6. Aerts, I.; Cumps, E.; Verhagen, E.; Verschueren, J.; Meeusen, R. A Systematic Review of Different Jump-Landing Variables in Relation to Injuries. *J. Sports Med. Phys. Fit.* **2013**, *53*, 509–519.
7. Bates, N.A.; Ford, K.R.; Myer, G.D.; Hewett, T.E. Kinetic and Kinematic Differences between First and Second Landings of a Drop Vertical Jump Task: Implications for Injury Risk Assessments? *Clin. Biomech.* **2013**, *28*, 459–466. [CrossRef] [PubMed]
8. Boling, M.C.; Padua, D.A.; Marshall, S.W.; Guskiewicz, K.; Pyne, S.; Beutler, A. A Prospective Investigation of Biomechanical Risk Factors for Patellofemoral Pain Syndrome: The Joint Undertaking to Monitor and Prevent ACL Injury (JUMP-ACL) Cohort. *Am. J. Sports Med.* **2009**, *37*, 2108–2116. [CrossRef] [PubMed]
9. Padua, D.A.; Marshall, S.W.; Boling, M.C.; Thigpen, C.A.; Garrett, W.E.; Beutler, A.I. The Landing Error Scoring System (LESS) Is a Valid and Reliable Clinical Assessment Tool of Jump-Landing Biomechanics: The Jump-ACL Study. *Am. J. Sports Med.* **2009**, *37*, 1996–2002. [CrossRef] [PubMed]
10. Tsarbou, C.; Liveris, N.I.; Xergia, S.A.; Tsekoura, M.; Fousekis, K.; Tsepis, E. Pre-Season ACL Risk Classification of Professional and Semi-Professional Football Players, via a Proof-of-Concept Test Battery. *Appl. Sci.* **2023**, *13*, 7780. [CrossRef]
11. Hanzlíková, I.; Hébert-Losier, K. Is the Landing Error Scoring System Reliable and Valid? A Systematic Review. *Sports Health* **2020**, *12*, 181–188. [CrossRef] [PubMed]
12. Padua, D.A.; DiStefano, L.J.; Beutler, A.I.; De La Motte, S.J.; DiStefano, M.J.; Marshall, S.W. The Landing Error Scoring System as a Screening Tool for an Anterior Cruciate Ligament Injury—Prevention Program in Elite-Youth Soccer Athletes. *J. Athl. Train.* **2015**, *50*, 589–595. [CrossRef] [PubMed]
13. Smith, H.C.; Johnson, R.J.; Shultz, S.J.; Tourville, T.; Holterman, L.A.; Slauterbeck, J.; Vacek, P.M.; Beynnon, B.D. A Prospective Evaluation of the Landing Error Scoring System (LESS) as a Screening Tool for Anterior Cruciate Ligament Injury Risk. *Am. J. Sports Med.* **2011**, *40*, 521–526. [CrossRef] [PubMed]
14. Onate, J.; Cortes, N.; Welch, C.; Van Lunen, B. Expert versus Novice Interrater Reliability and Criterion Validity of the Landing Error Scoring System. *J. Sport Rehabil.* **2010**, *19*, 41–56. [CrossRef] [PubMed]
15. Everard, E.; Lyons, M.; Harrison, A.J. Examining the Reliability of the Landing Error Scoring System with Raters Using the Standardized Instructions and Scoring Sheet. *J. Sport Rehabil.* **2020**, *29*, 519–525. [CrossRef] [PubMed]
16. Liveris, N.I.; Tsarbou, C.; Tsimeas, P.D.; Papageorgiou, G.; Xergia, S.A.; Tsiokanos, A. Evaluating the Effects of Match-Induced Fatigue on Landing Ability; the Case of the Basketball Game. *Int. J. Exerc. Sci.* **2021**, *14*, 768–778. [PubMed]
17. Tsarbou, C.; Liveris, N.I.; Tsimeas, P.D.; Papageorgiou, G.; Xergia, S.A.; Tsiokanos, A. The Effect of Fatigue on Jump Height and the Risk of Knee Injury after a Volleyball Training Game: A Pilot Study. *Biomed. Hum. Kinet.* **2021**, *13*, 197–204. [CrossRef]
18. Sim, J.; Wright, C.C. The Kappa Statistic in Reliability Studies: Use, Interpretation, and Sample Size Requirements. *Phys. Ther.* **2005**, *85*, 257–268. [CrossRef] [PubMed]
19. Koo, T.K.; Li, M.Y. A Guideline of Selecting and Reporting Intraclass Correlation Coefficients for Reliability Research. *J. Chiropr. Med.* **2016**, *15*, 155–163. [CrossRef] [PubMed]

sports

MDPI

Article

The Relationship between Functional Movement Quality and Speed, Agility, and Jump Performance in Elite Female Youth Football Players

Dan Iulian Alexe [1], Denis Čaušević [2], Nedim Čović [2], Babina Rani [3], Dragoș Ioan Tohănean [4,*], Ensar Abazović [2], Edi Setiawan [5] and Cristina Ioana Alexe [6,*]

1 Department of Physical and Occupational Therapy, "Vasile Alecsandri" University of Bacău, 600115 Bacău, Romania; alexedaniulian@ub.ro
2 Faculty of Sport and Physical Education, University of Sarajevo, 71000 Sarajevo, Bosnia and Herzegovina; denis.causevic@fasto.unsa.ba (D.Č.); nedim.covic@fasto.unsa.ba (N.Č.); ensar.abazovic@fasto.unsa.ba (E.A.)
3 Department of Physical Rehabilitation & Medicine (Physiotherapy), Post Graduate Institute of Medical Education and Research, Chandigarh 160012, India; says2babina@gmail.com
4 Department of Motric Performance, Transilvania University of Brașov, 500036 Brașov, Romania
5 Faculty of Teacher Training and Education, Suryakancana University, Cianjur Kidul 43216, Indonesia; edi_setiawan@unsur.ac.id
6 Department of Physical Education and Sports Performance, "Vasile Alecsandri" University of Bacău, 600115 Bacău, Romania
* Correspondence: dragos.tohanean@unitbv.ro (D.I.T.); alexe.cristina@ub.ro (C.I.A.)

Abstract: The association between movement screening and physical fitness testing in athletes is conflicting, and therefore, this study aimed to examine the relationship between Functional Movement Screen (FMS) performance and physical performance in elite female youth football players. Twenty-two players from the national U16 team of Bosnia and Herzegovina underwent FMS and physical performance tests, including speed, agility, and jump assessments. Jump and speed performance score correlated well with ASLR, while the overall FMS score was not associated with any of the performance variables. These findings suggest that while certain movement patterns may impact athletic performance, the relationship between movement screening and physical performance is delicate. Coaches and practitioners should consider individual variations and sport-specific demands when interpreting FMS results in order to optimize and maximize athlete performance and reduce injury risks.

Keywords: FMS; mobility; stability; athletic performance; female football; soccer

1. Introduction

Football is an immensely popular and an intense sport that involves high-demand tasks such as landing, cutting, and rapid change of direction. Players are also expected to have higher performance in strength, speed, endurance, and power [1]. This necessitates a holistic approach to training and assessment.

The screening tests that can detect modifiable intrinsic risk factors for musculoskeletal injury have always been of interest to the practitioners of sport and exercise medicine. It has been documented previously that football players' performance is affected by their ability to execute movements correctly, which is emphasized in the literature as crucial for long-term safety and effectiveness [2,3].

The variety of tests used to evaluate different sport-specific parameters do not directly implicate any information on the efficient movement proficiency of the player. For resolving this, a battery of assessment tools was developed with Functional Movement Screening (FMS). Pre-participation screening and sports performance can be linked together with the use of FMS, the most popular movement screening technique used by specialists to evaluate an individual's fundamental movement patterns [4]. By assessing any asymmetries, the dysfunctional patterns and higher musculoskeletal injury risks can be identified with FMS. A score of <14 on FMS has been linked to greater chances of injury [5,6]. However, this cutoff score can be influenced by multiple factors, like gender, age, body composition, type of sport, training state, and diet, among others. Through such stratification, targeted interventions can be delivered to groups considered "at-risk" in order to reduce the likelihood of injury, thereby enhancing the performance.

FMS has gained popularity as a comprehensive assessment tool in sports science [4]. However, its relationship to sport-specific performance metrics remains a subject of debate among researchers and practitioners [7,8]. While FMS aims to evaluate fundamental movement patterns, it is essential to consider how these patterns translate into actual athletic performance. The correlation between FMS scores and various sport-specific parameters, such as speed, agility, and power, has yielded inconsistent results across different studies and sports disciplines [9,10]. This variability in findings highlights the need for sport-specific investigations to determine the true value of FMS in predicting and enhancing athletic performance.

The relationship of movement screening with physical fitness testing in athletes is conflicting in the available literature for different sports. Zhang et al. [11] have reported the inaccuracy of FMS in predicting jump and sprint performance, while few studies found FMS to correlate significantly with vertical jump [10], agility [2,10], and lower limb strength [9]. However, such an association in young female football players, per se, is so far under-explored.

This study is therefore an effort to provide a clear picture of the strength and conditioning coaches and the treating physical therapists of whether any association exists between physical performance and efficient movement (FMS) in young female football players. Therefore, the present study aimed to investigate the correlations between functional movement quality (FMS) and speed, agility, and jump performance in elite female youth football players.

2. Materials and Methods

2.1. Experimental Approach to the Problem

This was a transversal observational and descriptive study. This study obtained preseason measures of physical performance (speed, planned agility, and vertical jump) and movement quality (FMS) in elite junior football athletes in Bosnia and Herzegovina. A cross-sectional analysis was conducted on each participant to examine the relationship between their movement quality and physical performance metrics. To address the research questions, this study employed a multivariate correlation analysis approach.

2.2. Participants

Twenty-two elite female youth football players (age: 15.59 ± 0.57) from the national U16 team of Bosnia and Herzegovina participated in this study. All participants had a minimum of 5 years training experience. Before this study, all athletes were provided information about the procedures and study objectives. Subjects with a history of recent (previous 30 days) injury or surgery prohibiting full participation in the regular training schedule were excluded. Participants were excluded if they were in their menstrual cycle. The study was approved by the Ethics Committee of the Faculty of Sports and Physical Education, University of Sarajevo (No: 01−2603/22; 1 July 2022) and was carried out in accordance with the Declaration of Helsinki. After the procedures were fully explained, parents provided written consent for their minor children to participate in the study, ensuring complete ethical compliance and explicitly stating that participants could withdraw from the study at any time without consequence.

2.3. Measurement Procedure

All the tests/measurements were performed at the Institute of Sport at the Faculty of Sports and Physical Education, University of Sarajevo. For this study, an appropriate training/testing cycle was developed, consisting of a single day of testing. The testing session was performed on the last day of 5 days of national training camp in the morning between 09:00 and 12:00. The research procedure started with the evaluation of body composition (body height, body mass, percentage of body fat (PBF), body mass index (BMI), and fat free mass (FFM)) by digital stadiometer (InBody BSM 370; Biospace Co., Ltd., Seoul, Republic of Korea) [12], and a direct segmental high-frequency bioelectrical impedance scale (InBody 720; Biospace Co., Ltd., Seoul, Republic of Korea). A general independent warm-up was provided by the national selection strength and conditioning coach. After warming up, subjects completed the FMS movement assessment and a battery of physical performance tests. The physical performance tests included a 5, 10, 20, and 30 m sprint, countermovement jump—free arms (CMJ free arms) height, zig-zag agility test, and *t*-test. All physical performance testing was conducted by trained staff with previous experience in physical performance assessment.

2.4. Functional Movement Screen (FMS)

Participants were screened using the functional movement screen protocol (FMS) that used 7 movement patterns [4,13]. FMS reliability has been previously established [14]. Each participant performed three trials of every movement pattern. An experienced rater, with two years of screening experience, evaluated these trials in real time using a 4-point scale (Table 1), adhering to the FMS rater manual and established research protocols [4]. The testing procedure incorporated rest periods of approximately 5 s between trials, 1 min between different tests, and participants returned to the starting position after each trial. In line with FMS criteria, the highest score from the three trials was recorded for subsequent analysis. For bilateral tests, the lower of the two scores was documented.

Table 1. FMS criteria.

Score	Criteria
0	The participant experiences pain in any part of the body at any point during the test.
1	The participant either fails to finish the movement pattern or is unable to acquire the position required to conduct the movement.
2	The participant may finish the exercise but does so with compensation(s).
3	The participant can complete the activity accurately without any assistance.

2.5. Speed

The assessment of running speed involved participants performing 30 m maximal sprints. Each sprint began from a stationary standing position, with the athlete's lead foot positioned 20 cm behind the initial photocell. Four photocells (Witty, Microgate, Bolzano, Italy) were used to measure 5 m, 10 m, 20 m, and 30 m maximal sprint times (in seconds) [15,16]. Each player performed two trials (ICC > 0.81) with a 3 min rest in between, and the best of the two was analyzed. Photocells were placed at a height of 120 cm [17].

2.6. Agility

Agility was evaluated using the same photocells (Microgate, Bolzano, Italy) through the zig-zag and *t*-test, as recommended by previous studies [18–20].

The zig-zag agility test was selected for its ability to assess multiple facets of agility, including short acceleration, deceleration, and balance control. Conducted on an outdoor football field, the test comprised four 5 m sections totaling 20 m of linear sprinting. Cones were positioned at 100° angles to mark the course, following established protocols from previous research [20]. Each participant completed the test twice (ICC > 0.84), with the best score being recorded for analysis.

The T-test assessed athletes' agility through a series of movements. Participants began with their lead foot 20 cm behind the initial photocell, then sprinted 9.14 m forward to touch a center cone with their right hand. They then shuffled 4.57 m left to touch a second cone, followed by a 9.50 m right shuffle to a third cone, before shuffling back 4.75 m to touch the center cone with their left hand. Finally, they ran backward to the starting point [20]. The timing was recorded in seconds using photocells (Microgate, Bolzano, Italy) at the starting line. Each athlete completed two trials (ICC > 0.79) with a 3 min rest between attempts, and the best time was recorded.

2.7. Jumping Performance

For assessment of the jumping performance, the countermovement jump with free arms (CMJ free arms), which was found to be reliable previously [21], was performed [15]. Protocols included two data collection trials and were performed using Optojump Next system (Microgate, Bolzano, Italy). At the beginning, players started from an upright standing position with feet shoulder-width apart and hands next to the body for arm swing. They performed a preliminary downward countermovement to a self-selected depth by flexing the hips and knees. Players then immediately extended their hips and knees to execute a vertical jump. After the jump, the player returned to the starting position. This procedure was repeated twice (ICC > 0.91), and the best of the two attempts was used for analysis. The trial was considered invalid if knee flexion occurred upon landing.

2.8. Statistics

The results were presented as mean ± standard deviation (SD). Spearman's rank correlation analysis was used to quantify associations between FMS—tests and sprint, agility, and jump performance variables. The strength of correlation was determined as small (<0.29), moderate (0.3–0.49), large (0.5–0.69), or very large (>0.7) [22]. The statistical analysis was performed using SPSS (Version 22. For Windows, Armonk, NY, USA. IBM Corp.). Statistical significance was set at $p < 0.05$.

3. Results

Twenty-two players (four strikers, nine midfielders, seven fullbacks, and two goalkeepers) completed the testing procedure and were included in a final analysis. Table 2 shows the descriptive statistics for the morphological, performance, and FMS variables.

Table 3 shows all the correlation coefficients between morphological, performance, and FMS variables. Significant correlation was found between shoulder mobility and two agility (−0.39 and −0.42) and two sprint (−0.42 and −0.38) tests and variables, respectively. Furthermore, the active straight leg raise test correlated significantly to jump (0.45) and speed (ranging −0.41 to −0.47) performance and the in-line lounge test correlated significantly to the zig-zag test (−0.44). It is interesting to note that no correlation was found between the overall FMS score and any performance variable.

Table 2. Descriptive statistics and post hoc comparisons for body composition and physical fitness tests.

Variables	Total (n = 22)		Striker (n = 4)		Midfielder (n = 9)		Fullback (n = 7)		Goalkeeper (n = 2)	
	Mean	SD	Mean	SD	Mean	SD	Mean	SD	Mean	SD
Age (years)	15.59	0.57	15.90	0.27	15.42	0.66	15.55	0.51	15.90	0.84
Body height (cm)	168.30	6.43	167.05	9.98	167.64	6.79	169.24	4.30	170.45	7.99
Body mass (kg)	59.83	7.25	60.52	12.02	57.46	7.00	62.17	3.26	60.90	11.03
BMI (kg/m^2)	21.06	1.57	21.52	2.14	20.38	1.46	21.71	1.26	20.90	1.83
PBF (%)	20.49	3.49	21.00	4.41	19.15	2.98	21.85	3.14	20.75	6.15
FFM (kg)	47.42	4.87	47.62	8.30	46.38	5.42	48.51	1.45	47.90	4.94
FMS score	16.50	2.22	17.25	1.50	15.88	3.05	17.28	1.11	15.00	0.00

Table 2. *Cont.*

Variables	Total (n = 22)		Striker (n = 4)		Midfielder (n = 9)		Fullback (n = 7)		Goalkeeper (n = 2)	
	Mean	SD	Mean	SD	Mean	SD	Mean	SD	Mean	SD
Deep squat	2.45	0.59	2.50	0.58	2.33	0.70	2.71	0.48	2.00	0.00
Hurdle step	2.36	0.66	2.75	0.50	2.33	0.70	2.28	0.75	2.00	0.00
In-line lunge	2.59	0.59	3.00	0.00	2.44	0.72	2.71	0.48	2.00	0.00
Shoulder mobility	2.59	0.66	2.50	1.00	2.33	0.70	2.85	0.37	3.00	0.00
ASLR	2.59	0.50	2.25	0.50	2.55	0.52	2.71	0.48	3.00	0.00
TSPU	1.86	0.83	2.00	0.52	1.88	0.93	2.00	0.81	1.00	0.00
Rotary stability	2.04	0.21	2.25	0.50	2.00	0.00	2.00	0.00	2.00	0.00
CMJ free arms (cm)	28.88	4.01	28.47	2.80	29.95	3.86	27.70	5.19	29.00	3.39
Zig-zag (s)	6.29	0.29	6.41	0.26	6.24	0.24	6.22	0.39	6.49	0.91
T-test (s)	11.37	0.54	11.91	0.54	11.12	0.38	11.31	0.56	11.61	0.53
5 m sprint (s)	1.12	0.06	1.17	0.09	1.12	0.06	1.08	0.05	1.13	0.14
10 m sprint (s)	1.94	0.08	2.00	0.10	1.95	0.07	1.90	0.09	1.93	0.14
20 m sprint (s)	3.38	0.15	3.48	0.16	3.40	0.13	3.31	0.16	3.36	0.03
30 m sprint (s)	4.78	0.22	4.92	0.23	4.80	0.20	4.67	0.24	4.79	0.04

BMI: Body mass index; PBF: Percentage of body fat; FFM: Fat-free mass; FMS: Functional movement screen; ASLR: Active straight leg raise; TSPU: Trunk stability push-up; CMJ: Countermovement jump.

Table 3. Correlation between FMS tests and sprint, agility, and jump performance variables.

Variables	CMJ Free Arms	Zig-Zag	T-Test	5 m	10 m	20 m	30 m
FMS score	0.17 (−0.27, 0.55)	−0.13 (−0.52, 0.31)	−0.18 (−0.56, 0.26)	−0.27 (−0.62, 0.17)	−0.14 (−0.53, 0.30)	−0.18 (−0.56, 0.26)	−0.21 (−0.58, 0.23)
Deep squat	0.22 (−0.22, 0.59)	−0.17 (−0.55, 0.27)	−0.15 (−0.54, 0.29)	−0.11 (−0.51, 0.33)	0.17 (−0.27, 0.55)	−0.17 (−0.55, 0.27)	0.09 (−0.34, 0.49)
Hurdle step	0.13 (−0.31, 0.52)	−0.15 (−0.54, 0.29)	−0.14 (−0.53, 0.29)	−0.19 (−0.57, 0.25)	−0.08 (−0.49, 0.35)	−0.11 (−0.51, 0.33)	−0.17 (−0.55, 0.27)
In-line lunge	0.28 (−0.16, 0.62)	−0.44 * (−0.72, −0.02)	−0.19 (−0.57, 0.25)	−0.10 (−0.50, 0.34)	−0.06 (−0.47, 0.37)	−0.10 (−0.50, 0.34)	−0.09 (−0.49, 0.34)
Shoulder mobility	0.20 (−0.24, 0.57)	−0.39 * (−0.70, 0.03)	−0.39 * (−0.70, 0.04)	−0.42 * (−0.72, 0.00)	−0.38 * (−0.69,0.05)	−0.29 (−0.63, 0.15)	−0.28 (−0.63, 0.16)
ASLR	0.45 * (0.03, 0.73)	−0.30 (−0.64, 0.14)	−0.30 (−0.64, 0.14)	−0.35 (−0.67, 0.08)	−0.41 * (−0.71, 0.01)	−0.47 * (−0.74, −0.06)	−0.46 * (−0.73, −0.05)
TSPU	0.06 (−0.38, 0.47)	−0.24 (−0.60, 0.20)	−0.17 (−0.55, 0.27)	−0.22 (−0.59, 0.22)	−0.16 (−0.54, 0.28)	−0.05 (−0.46, 0.38)	−0.07 (−0.48, 0.36)
Rotary stability	0.25 (−0.19, 0.61)	−0.02 (−0.44, 0.40)	−0.13 (−0.52, 0.31)	−0.18 (−0.56, 0.26)	−0.27 (−0.62, 0.17)	−0.23 (−0.59, 0.21)	−0.25 (−0.61, 0.19)

FMS: Functional movement screen; ASLR: Active straight leg raise; TSPU: Trunk stability push-up; CMJ: Countermovement jump. * Correlation is significant at the $p < 0.05$ level.

4. Discussion

This study aimed to elucidate whether a relationship exists between physical performance and efficient movement (FMS) in young female football players. Results suggested that the FMS score, surpassing the cutoff of 14.5 as proposed by Zhang et al. [11], was sufficient to indicate good sensitivity and a lower false-positive rate of FMS in female football players.

Overall, the FMS score had a very weak positive influence on zig-zag and T-test agility and 5 m, 10 m, 20 m, and 30 m sprint times along with CMJ free arms performance. These findings contrast with those of Zhang et al. [11] for elite young female players, who reported a moderate correlation between FMS score and 10 m and 20 m sprint times. Prior studies examining this association have yielded ambiguous outcomes. Several investigations have identified slight to moderate correlations between FMS scores and diverse physical performance metrics, such as jumping, agility, or speed assessments, specifically in female populations [2,8,11,23,24]. The inconclusive results could likely be attributed to the participants' level of maturity, as it is widely acknowledged that rapid growth during adolescence can impact performance in young athletes. Despite the lack of significant difference in the total FMS score between playing position groups, this factor could still provide a plausible explanation for the variability in results. Moreover, in our study, participants exhibited notably higher body size (21 vs. 19 kg/m^2) and had better sprint and

FMS scores but lower jump performance when compared to the participants in a previous study [11]. This difference in performance could potentially be attributed to higher muscle mass among our study participants, who were approximately 9 months older and had more training experience. Our findings suggest that in young athletes, functional movements may play a more significant role in performance, whereas in more mature players, performance may rely more on power and strength. Moreover, Bennett et al. [25] demonstrated the potential of FMS during athletic performance optimization since FMS can determine acceptable movement capabilities. They found a significant, albeit slight, association of FMS score to the 5 m sprint time as well as the agility performance. Additionally, they observed a significant increase in both FMS score and speed performance after one year, although no significant relationships were found between these improvements, supporting the importance of our assumption previously explained. These findings underscore the significance of adequate movement ability to enhance physical performance, but it should not be underestimated since this potentially can reduce the risk of injuries [26]. As stated by Bennet et al. [25] "If movement quality does play a role in physical performance capacity, it is likely to be only one small part of the puzzle".

Observing relations between each test, it was evident that a higher in-line lunge score was associated with better zig-zag results, higher shoulder mobility with better agility (zig-zag and T-test), and acceleration capabilities (5 and 10 m), with small but significant correlations, respectfully. These results align with those presented by Zhang et al. [11]. Higher active straight leg raise score contributed to better CMJ and maximal speed (10 m, 20 m, and 30 m) test performance. As far as athletic performance goes, movement quality has a limited impact. Although the FMS evaluates specific isolated fundamental movement patterns, it cannot predict abilities like agility and execution speed [27]. Moreover, the precise technical skill of force application significantly impacts sprint performance, highlighting the inadequacy of fundamental movement alone.

Moreover, the present study further demonstrated that increased range of motion (ROM) in shoulders and dorsal lower body did correlate with enhanced agility and acceleration physical performance. Such findings could be the result of increased ROM ability to facilitate a more extensive arm swing during sprinting, leading to increased propulsion and higher speed, and enabling better coordination between upper and lower body movements, enhancing the transfer of force and thus improving power production. Additionally, increased shoulder mobility contributes to better balance and stability, crucial for maintaining proper body position [28]. Optimal shoulder and lower limb ROM are essential for proper body mechanics and posture, which can enhance movement efficiency. However, individual responses may vary, highlighting the importance of tailored training programs focusing on flexibility, mobility, and strength to maximize the benefits of increased shoulder ROM on athletic performance. Consequently, strength and conditioning coaches should recognize that ROM assessments may offer good insights into the possible issues regarding low basic performance of female athletes [29].

As observed in a study by Alicea-Kulian et al. [30] using stepwise multiple regression analysis, deep squats predicted vertical jump height (in centimeters) most effectively ($r = 0.416$). Our results indicate that active straight leg raises correlate to vertical jump performance. These findings emphasize the significance of hamstring flexibility and hip functionality as potential predictors of performance variables, especially for power movements such as the vertical jump.

These results suggest that there are associations between FMS scores and certain physical performance measures in elite female youth football players, indicating the importance of functional movement quality in athletic performance.

The investigations of Functional Movement Screening (FMS) and its relationship with physical performance in young female football players have several potential reasons for variations in correlations between FMS and tests of strength, speed, and agility. Objective limitations arise when comparing outcomes across different studies in this population.

While football is played similarly worldwide, variations in training approaches and regimes can influence the development of diverse movement patterns and aspects of strength, speed, and agility. Moreover, identical, or similar movements may be cultivated using different training methods, impacting test results. Even slight differences in testing methodologies can lead to varying outcomes and levels of correlation. Our results align well with a series of studies that focused on the interrelationship between the components of agility, strength, explosive power, reaction time, and balance which highlighted that sports performance in team sports is conditioned by the level of development of all components of motor capacity [22,31].

Furthermore, young athletes with differing levels of experience may demonstrate varying correlation levels between functional movement tests and assessments of strength, speed, and agility. Those with greater experience may exhibit superior movement techniques, resulting in heightened correlations between tests. Genetic factors, body morphology, and anthropometric measures can also influence the levels of strength, speed, and agility, consequently affecting correlations with functional movement tests.

The current physical condition of players, including factors such as injuries or fatigue, can also significantly influence test outcomes and correlations between tests. Variations in measurement error or uncertainty can further impact correlations between tests. Therefore, for future studies, it is imperative to clearly state measurement errors to allow for comparison and interpretation of results.

This study has a few limitations. The study's conclusions and statistical strength may be constrained by its limited participant pool of only 22 subjects. Larger sample sizes in future studies could provide more generalizable results. Additionally, the study employed a single day of testing, which might not capture the variability in performance that could occur over multiple testing sessions. Furthermore, the young athletes with differing levels of training experience may demonstrate varying correlation levels between functional movement tests and assessments of strength, speed, and agility. Those with greater experience might exhibit superior movement techniques, leading to heightened correlations between tests.

5. Conclusions

The findings of this study underline the importance and significance of a holistic approach. Furthermore, FMS assessment can be a valuable tool in injury prevention and its results do not influence physical performance since the correlation coefficients we found were, at most, moderate in elite female youth football players. Additionally, individual variations and factors such as training background, fitness level, and sport-specific demands should always be considered. A clear limitation of this study arose, namely, in the population studied. Considering that this is the national team, which has already undergone a detailed selection process, future studies should focus on lower-league female footballers.

Author Contributions: Conceptualization, D.I.A., D.Č. and N.Č.; methodology, D.I.A., D.Č. and C.I.A.; software, N.Č., B.R., E.A., D.I.T. and E.S.; validation, D.I.A., C.I.A. and D.Č.; formal analysis, D.I.A., C.I.A. and N.Č.; investigation, D.I.A., D.Č. and N.Č.; resources, D.I.T., B.R., D.Č., E.A. and E.S.; data curation, D.I.A., E.A. and N.Č.; writing—original draft preparation, D.I.A., D.Č. and N.Č.; writing—review and editing, D.I.A., D.Č., B.R., E.S., E.A., C.I.A., D.I.T. and N.Č.; visualization, B.R., E.S., C.I.A. and D.I.T.; supervision, D.I.A., C.I.A. and D.Č.; project administration, D.I.A. and D.Č.; funding acquisition, D.I.A., D.I.T. and C.I.A.; All authors have read and agreed to the published version of the manuscript.

Funding: This research received no external funding.

Institutional Review Board Statement: The study was conducted in accordance with the Declaration of Helsinki, and approved by the Ethics Committee of the Faculty of Sports and Physical Education, University of Sarajevo (No: 01−2603/22; 1 July 2022).

Informed Consent Statement: The parents provided informed consent by signing a written document that allowed the minor subjects to participate in the study.

Data Availability Statement: The data presented in this study are available upon reasonable request from the corresponding author.

Acknowledgments: A great thank you to all collaborators and volunteers for their availability and contribution to this study. Cristina Ioana Alexe and Dan Iulian Alexe thank the "Vasile Alecsandri" University in Bacău, Romania, for the support and assistance provided.

Conflicts of Interest: The authors declare no conflicts of interest.

References

1. Mustafovic, E.; Causevic, D.; Covic, N.; Ibrahimovic, M.; Alic, H.; Abazovic, E.; Masic, S. Talent Identification in Youth Football: A Systematic Review. *J. Anthropol. Sport Phys. Educ.* **2020**, *4*, 37–43.
2. Kramer, T.A.; Sacko, R.S.; Pfeifer, C.E.; Gatens, D.R.; Goins, J.M.; Stodden, D.F. The association between the functional movement screentm, Y-balance test, and physical performance tests in male and female high school athletes. *Int. J. Sports Phys. Ther.* **2019**, *14*, 911. [CrossRef] [PubMed]
3. Lim, K.H.; Seo, T.B.; Kim, Y.P. Relationship between movement dysfunctions and sports injuries according to gender of youth soccer player. *J. Exerc. Rehabil.* **2020**, *16*, 427. [CrossRef]
4. Cook, G.; Burton, L.; Hoogenboom, B. Pre-participation screening: The use of fundamental movements as an assessment of function—Part 1. *N. Am. J. Sports Phys. Ther.* **2006**, *1*, 62–72. [PubMed]
5. Smith, L.J.; Creps, J.R.; Bean, R.; Rodda, B.; Alsalaheen, B. Performance of high school male athletes on the Functional Movement Screen™. *Phys. Ther. Sport* **2017**, *27*, 17–23. [CrossRef] [PubMed]
6. Scudamore, E.M.; Stevens, S.L.; Fuller, D.K.; Coons, J.M.; Morgan, D.W. Functional movement screen items predict dynamic balance under military torso load. *Mil. Med.* **2020**, *185*, 493–498. [CrossRef] [PubMed]
7. Parchmann, C.J.; McBride, J.M. Relationship between functional movement screen and athletic performance. *J. Strength Cond. Res.* **2011**, *25*, 3378–3384. [CrossRef] [PubMed]
8. Lockie, R.G.; Schultz, A.B.; Callaghan, S.J.; Jordan, C.A.; Luczo, T.M.; Jeffriess, M.D. A preliminary investigation into the relationship between functional movement screen scores and athletic physical performance in female team sport athletes. *Biol. Sport* **2015**, *32*, 41–51. [CrossRef] [PubMed]
9. Okada, T.; Huxel, K.C.; Nesser, T.W. Relationship between core stability, functional movement, and performance. *J. Strength Cond. Res.* **2011**, *25*, 252–261. [CrossRef] [PubMed]
10. Lloyd, R.S.; Oliver, J.L.; Radnor, J.M.; Rhodes, B.C.; Faigenbaum, A.D.; Myer, G.D. Relationships between functional movement screen scores, maturation and physical performance in young soccer players. *J. Sports Sci.* **2015**, *33*, 11–19. [CrossRef]
11. Zhang, J.; Lin, J.; Wei, H.; Liu, H. Relationships between Functional Movement Quality and Sprint and Jump Performance in Female Youth Soccer Athletes of Team China. *Children* **2022**, *9*, 1312. [CrossRef] [PubMed]
12. Ćović, N.; Čaušević, D.; Alexe, C.I.; Rani, B.; Dulceanu, C.R.; Abazović, E.; Lupu, G.S.; Alexe, D.I. Relations between specific athleticism and morphology in young basketball players. *Front. Sports Act. Living* **2023**, *5*, 1276953. [CrossRef] [PubMed]
13. Cook, G.; Burton, L.; Hoogenboom, B. Pre-participation screening: The use of fundamental movements as an assessment of function—Part 2. *N. Am. J. Sports Phys. Ther.* **2006**, *1*, 132–139.
14. McCunn, R.; aus der Fünten, K.; Fullagar, H.H.; McKeown, I.; Meyer, T. Reliability and association with injury of movement screens: A critical review. *Sports Med.* **2016**, *46*, 763–781. [CrossRef]
15. Zelenović, M.; Kontro, T.; Čaušević, D.; Bjelica, B.; Aksović, N.; Milanović, Z. Warm-up is an efficient strategy to prevent diur-nal variation of short-term maximal performance in young basketball players. *Chronobiol. Int.* **2024**, *41*, 439–446. [CrossRef]
16. Krolo, A.; Gilic, B.; Foretic, N.; Pojskic, H.; Hammami, R.; Spasic, M.; Uljevic, O.; Versic, S.; Sekulic, D. Agility testing in youth football (soccer) players; evaluating reliability, validity, and correlates of newly developed testing protocols. *Int. J. Environ. Res. Public Health* **2020**, *17*, 294. [CrossRef]
17. Čaušević, D.; Ćović, N.; Abazović, E.; Rani, B.; Manolache, G.M.; Ciocan, C.V.; Zaharia, G.; Alexe, D.I. Predictors of speed and agility in youth male basketball players. *Appl. Sci.* **2023**, *13*, 7796. [CrossRef]
18. Yapici, H.; Soylu, Y.; Gulu, M.; Kutlu, M.; Ayan, S.; Muluk, N.B.; Aldhahi, M.I.; AL-Mhanna, S.B. Agility Skills, Speed, Balance and CMJ Performance in Soccer: A Comparison of Players with and without a Hearing Impairment. *Healthcare* **2023**, *11*, 247. [CrossRef] [PubMed]
19. Matsentides, D.; Christou, M.; Zaras, N. The Effects of Different Re-Warm-Up Strategies on Power, Changing of Direction and Ball Shooting Velocity in Well-Trained Soccer Players. *Sports* **2023**, *11*, 169. [CrossRef]
20. Čaušević, D.; Mašić, S.; Doder, I.; Matulaitis, K.; Spicer, S. Speed, agility and power potential of young basketball players. *Balt. J. Sport Health Sci.* **2022**, *4*, 29–34. [CrossRef]
21. Heishman, A.D.; Daub, B.D.; Miller, R.M.; Freitas, E.D.; Frantz, B.A.; Bemben, M.G. Countermovement jump reliability performed with and without an arm swing in NCAA division 1 intercollegiate basketball players. *J. Strength Cond. Res.* **2020**, *34*, 546–558. [CrossRef] [PubMed]

22. Gidu, D.V.; Badau, D.; Stoica, M.; Aron, A.; Focan, G.; Monea, D.; Stoica, A.M.; Calota, N.D. The Effects of Proprioceptive Training on Balance, Strength, Agility and Dribbling in Adolescent Male Soccer Players. *Int. J. Environ. Res. Public Health* **2022**, *19*, 2028. [CrossRef]
23. Martín-Moya, R.; Rodríguez-García, L.; Moreno-Vecino, B.; Clemente, F.M.; González, A.L.; González-Fernández, F.T. Differences and relationship in functional movement screen (FMS™) scores and physical fitness in males and female semi-professional soccer players. *PeerJ* **2023**, *11*, e16649. [CrossRef] [PubMed]
24. Fitton Davies, K.; Sacko, R.S.; Lyons, M.A.; Duncan, M.J. Association between Functional Movement Screen scores and athletic performance in adolescents: A systematic review. *Sports* **2022**, *10*, 28. [CrossRef]
25. Bennett, H.; Fuller, J.; Milanese, S.; Jones, S.; Moore, E.; Chalmers, S. Relationship between movement quality and physical performance in elite adolescent Australian football players. *J. Strength Cond. Res.* **2022**, *36*, 2824–2829. [CrossRef] [PubMed]
26. Moore, E.; Chalmers, S.; Milanese, S.; Fuller, J.T. Factors influencing the relationship between the functional movement screen and injury risk in sporting populations: A systematic review and meta-analysis. *Sports Med.* **2019**, *49*, 1449–1463. [CrossRef]
27. Delecluse, C. Influence of strength training on sprint running performance: Current findings and implications for training. *Sports Med.* **1997**, *24*, 147–156. [CrossRef]
28. Mašić, S.; Čaušević, D.; Čović, N.; Spicer, S.; Doder, I. The benefits of static stretching on health: A systematic review. *J. Kinesiol. Exerc. Sci.* **2024**, *34*, 1–7. [CrossRef]
29. Kritz, M.; Cronin, J.; Hume, P. The bodyweight squat: A movement screen for the squat pattern. *Strength Cond. J.* **2009**, *31*, 76–85. [CrossRef]
30. Alicea-Kulian, K.; Thomas, K.; Wolf, D.; Cuestas, R.V.; Wall, J.; Avery, A.; Batchelor, V.; Crowley, S.; Magal, M. Does Lower Extremity Fms Performance Predict Vertical Jump Height In Female Ncaa Division Iii Footballers. In Proceedings of the Medicine and Science in Sports and Exercise, Virtual, 27 May 2020; p. 50.
31. Gherghel, A.; Badau, D.; Badau, A.; Moraru, L.; Manolache, G.M.; Oancea, B.M.; Tifrea, C.; Tudor, V.; Costache, R.M. Optimizing the Explosive Force of the Elite Level Football-Tennis Players through Plyometric and Specific Exercises. *Int. J. Environ. Res. Public Health* **2021**, *18*, 8228. [CrossRef]

sports

MDPI

Article

Factors Affecting the Running Performance of Soccer Teams in the Turkish Super League

Spyridon Plakias [1] and Yiannis Michailidis [2,*]

[1] Department of Physical Education and Sport Science, University of Thessaly, 38221 Trikala, Greece; spyros_plakias@yahoo.gr
[2] Laboratory of Evaluation of Human Biological Performance, New Buildings of Laboratories, Department of Physical Education and Sports Sciences, Aristotle University of Thessaloniki, 57001 Thessaloniki, Greece
* Correspondence: ioannimd@phed.auth.gr; Tel.: +30-2310992248

Abstract: Performance analysis in sports is a rapidly evolving field, where academics and applied performance analysts work together to improve coaches' decision making through the use of performance indicators (PIs). This study aimed to provide a comprehensive analysis of factors affecting running performance (RP) in soccer teams, focusing on low (LI), medium (MI), and high-speed distances (HI) and the number of high-speed runs (NHI). Data were collected from 185 matches in the Turkish first division's 2021–2022 season using InStat Fitness's optical tracking technology. Four linear mixed-model analyses were conducted on the RP metrics with fixed factors, including location, team quality, opponent quality, ball possession, high-press, counterattacks, number of central defenders, and number of central forwards. The findings indicate that high-press and opponent team quality affect MI ($d = 0.311$, $d = 0.214$) and HI ($d = 0.303$, $d = 0.207$); team quality influences MI ($d = 0.632$); location and counterattacks impact HI ($d = 0.228$, $d = 0.450$); high-press and the number of central defenders affects NHI ($d = 0.404$, $d = 0.319$); and ball possession affects LI ($d = 0.287$). The number of central forwards did not influence any RP metrics. This study provides valuable insights into the factors influencing RP in soccer, highlighting the complex interactions between formations and physical, technical–tactical, and contextual variables. Understanding these dynamics can help coaches and analysts optimize team performance and strategic decision making.

Keywords: football; performance analysis; tactics; formations; running performance metrics; contextual variables

1. Introduction

Performance analysis in sports is a great and rapidly evolving field [1]. On one hand, academics continually provide new research data, while on the other, applied performance analysts (PAs) join the coaching staff of teams, assisting in improving coaches' decision making [2–4]. PAs use performance indicators (PIs) to draw conclusions [5]. PIs can be categorized based on whether their data originate from event or positional-tracking data [6], while to strengthen the meaningfulness of these, the importance of contextual variables has been highlighted [7]. Event data provide information on technical and tactical issues [8], tracking data are useful for analyzing running performance (RP) and tactics [9], while contextual variables enhance the quality of both [10]. Running performance (RP) is a crucial element of the overall performance of soccer players, contributing along with technical, tactical, and mental components [11]. However, on its own, it is not sufficient to interpret match outcomes [12,13], and it can be influenced by many factors [14]. Therefore, when interpreting RP in soccer, one should include contextual variables that may also explain part of the mental components [15,16], as well as technical–tactical variables. Such a holistic approach can provide genuinely useful information to team coaches.

The role of contextual variables in the RP of teams has been documented by research for many years, as Lago-Peñas [17] states in his review article. Regarding the most recent research, several contradictory findings have emerged. Modric et al. [18] found that away matches were associated with increased total distance (TD) and low-intensity (<4 m/s) running. Jerkovic et al. [19] found a greater amount of distance covered in the running zone (4–5.48 m/s) for away matches, while Gonçalves et al. [20] observed higher values of high-intensity running (60–100% of the individual maximum running speed) in home matches compared to away matches. Additionally, Modric et al. [18] found that team quality was not associated with RP, whereas Aquino et al. [21] reported that the top-ranked team covered greater total distance with high acceleration compared to the bottom-ranked team. Finally, regarding opponent quality, Modric et al. [18] and Jerkovic et al. [19] concluded that the quality of the opponent team was not associated with RP. Conversely, Gonçalves et al. [22] found that starters playing against strong opponents exhibited higher values of distance in high-speed running (5.5–7 m/s), and Gonçalves et al. [20] found that matches against strong opponents resulted in greater total distance covered.

However, analyzing situational variables in isolation seems to offer only a limited understanding of the complicated nature of team sports performance, since research has shown that ball possession, as well as other technical and tactical actions, is also affected by the location of the match and the opponents' strength [17]. In examining the effects of tactical behavior, several researchers have studied the impact of ball possession on RP. For example, Modric et al. [23] found that in the UEFA Champions League 2020–2021, teams with high ball possession covered more distance in high-speed running (5.5–7 m/s) and sprinting (>7 m/s) than teams with low ball possession. In contrast, da Mota et al. [24] found that in the 2014 FIFA World Cup, teams with high ball possession covered similar distances at medium (3–3.9 m/s) and high speeds (>3.9 m/s) but covered greater distances in total and at low speed ($\leq$3 m/s) compared to teams with low ball possession. Additionally, Modric et al. [23] found no differences in counterattacks and high-pressing regardless of whether teams covered greater or smaller distances both overall and at high intensities. Conversely, Forcher et al. [25] identified differences in RP between teams that adopt a counterattacking style compared to those that favor a ball possession style, and Low et al. [26] found differences in RP between teams employing deep-defending and high-press strategies. These studies highlight the complex and varied effects of tactical behaviors on RP in soccer, indicating that different styles of play can significantly influence physical demands on players, something that also emerged in the research of Plakias et al. [27], who made a direct comparison between two opposite styles in 19 tactical situations.

Finally, regarding formations, which constitute another tactical aspect of soccer [28], Modric et al. [29] demonstrated that the values for almost all of the RP metrics are greater with three central defenders than with two central defenders. This conclusion was also reached by Tierney et al. [30], who found greater distances covered at high speeds ($\geq$5.5 m/s) with three central defenders. Additionally, Borghi et al. [31] found that formations with two central forwards cover greater distances at high intensities (>5.5 m/s) than those with one central forward (3-5-2 > 4-4-2 > 4-3-3). This finding aligns with the results of Bradley et al. [32] (4-4-2 > 4-3-3 > 4-5-1) and Arjol-Serrano et al. [33] (4-4-2 > 4-2-3-1), but not with those of Aquino et al. [34] and Vieira et al. [35], who found that mean speed and high-intensity activities are greater in the 4-3-3 formation compared to the 4-4-2. It is worth noting that all the aforementioned studies on formations had sample sizes ranging from 20 to 59 matches, limiting the generalizability of the conclusions regarding formations. For this reason, the authors focused more on the differences between player positions.

All the aforementioned conflicting findings indicate that RP may be influenced differently in each competition, depending on the level and type of competition. Additionally, examining factors in isolation may yield some results, but it cannot explain the complex nature of soccer, where physical, technical–tactical, and contextual factors interact with each other. Building on the existing literature, we hypothesized that a combination of eight factors, including location, team quality, opponent team quality, ball possession, high-press, counterattacks, number of central defenders, and number of central forwards, significantly affect various aspects of running performance. Specifically, we anticipate that these factors will differentially impact low-speed distance (LI), medium-speed distance (MI), high-speed distance (HI), and the number of high-speed runs (NHI).

Using a large sample of matches that included all teams from the first Turkish league in the 2021–2022 season, we aimed to address an additional gap in the existing literature. Specifically, most studies examining factors affecting team RP often rely on samples from a single team with GPS data access or a limited number of matches from international competitions like the UEFA Champions League or the FIFA World Cup. Therefore, the purpose of this study is to provide a comprehensive analysis of the factors (including formations, technical–tactical variables, and contextual factors) that affect the RP of soccer teams, focusing on LI, MI, HI, and NHI. This holistic approach aims to enhance the understanding of how different elements interact to affect RP in soccer. By doing so, it seeks to fill the existing gaps in the literature and offer practical insights for optimizing team performance at a competitive level. Understanding these dynamics can help coaches and analysts design better training and game strategies, ultimately improving team performance and success in matches.

2. Material and Methods

2.1. Sample

This study analyzed data from the Turkish first division's 2021–2022 season, encompassing 20 teams over 38 matchdays, with each matchday featuring 10 games. Instatscout supplied data for the first 24 matchdays, covering 240 matches. Due to missing data for two matches and the exclusion of 53 matches because of red card incidents, the final sample included 185 matches, resulting in 370 (i.e., 2 × 185) observations, with each team in a match providing one observation.

2.2. Procedure

Data collection of the running variables was performed using InStat Fitness's optical tracking technology (https://football.instatscout.com/, accessed on 1 May 2024), a FIFA-certified system known for its high precision and reliability, as confirmed on the FIFA website [36] and referenced in previous studies [37,38]. For the 2021–2022 season, InStat's system was designated as the official Electronic Performance and Tracking System (EPTS) for the league [27]. For the technical–tactical variables the data were obtained from the Instatscout platform. As reported in previous studies, the reliability of Instatscout data is very high (K values 0.90 to 0.98) [39–41].

2.3. Ethics

Ethics committee approval of the current study was gained from the University of Thessaly (No. 1973, 12 October 2022). Additionally, InStat Ltd. granted written consent on 8 November 2022, for the utilization of the data in this research, ensuring adherence to all ethical standards for research and publication.

2.4. Statistical Analyses

Initially, cluster analysis was applied to create categorical variables concerning: (a) the quality of the teams and the opponents as strong or weak (based on the number of points each team collected in the final championship standings), (b) ball possession as high or low (based on the team's possession percentage in each observation), (c) the counterattacks of the match as many or few (based on the total number of counterattacks for both teams in the match for each observation), and (d) the high-pressing actions as many or few (based on the number of high-pressing actions of the team in each observation).

Next, after checking the normality of the distribution of the four dependent variables shown in Table 1, a linear mixed-model analysis was performed four times, correspondingly. In all cases, the eight independent variables shown in Table 1 were used as fixed factors, and the variable TEAM was used as a random factor. The definitions in Table 1 for high press, counterattacks, and ball possession are derived from the glossary of Instatscout, the platform from which the data for the respective variables were obtained. The variable TEAM represented the 20 different teams participating in the Turkish league in the 2021–2022 season. The thresholds for creating the running variables are those used in previous research [27,29,42]. However, in this study, the intensities of standing (<0.2 m/s), walking (0.21–2 m/s), and jogging (2.01–4 m/s) were combined as low-intensity, the intensity of running (4.01–5.5 m/s) was named medium-intensity, and the intensities of high speed (5.51–7 m/s) and sprint (>7 m/s) were combined as high-intensity. All statistical analyses were conducted using the IBM SPSS statistical package (version 29.00, IBM Corporation, Armonk, NY, USA), with a significance level set at $p < 0.05$. Cohen's d was utilized to measure the effect size. The effect sizes were defined as follows: trivial (d = 0.0 to 0.19), small (d = 0.2 to 0.49), medium (d = 0.5 to 0.79), and large (d ≥ 0.8) [43].

Table 1. The variables used when performing the four linear mixed-model analyses.

Type	Abbreviation	Definition
Dependent variables	LI	Low-intensity (0–4 m/s) distance
	MI	Medium-intensity (4.01–5.5 m/s) distance
	HI	High-intensity (>5.51 m/s) distance
	NHI	Number of high-intensity runs (>5.51 m/s)
Independent variables (fixed factors)	LC	Location (home/away)
	TQ	Team's quality (strong/weak)
	OQ	Opponent's quality (strong/weak)
	CD	Number of central defenders (two/three)
	CF	Number of central forwards (one/two)
	HP	High-press (many/few): Pressing until 30 m from the opponent's goal. Pressing, in its turn, is counted for the opponents of a team that is building its attack when players are actively trying to get the ball back.
	BP	Ball possession (high/low): Percentage share of one team's ball possession in the total ball-in-play time. Ball possession is the sum of all time periods between the start of possession to the moment of transition or to the moment the ball went out.
	CA	Counterattacks (many/few): Attack from the open play that starts with winning the ball from a defensive position and then quickly transitioning to offense while the prior attacking team is caught in an offensive formation; the length of possession during the attack cannot exceed 8 s before the possession transitions or ends; alternatively, the length of possession can last between 8 and 30 s, but the speed of attack cannot be less than 2.6 m/s. A counterattack cannot begin with a pass from a goalkeeper if he controlled the ball for more than 4 s before the action.
Independent variable (random factor)	TEAM	The 20 teams that participated in the Turkish first division 2021–2022 season.

3. Results

3.1. Cluster Analyses

Based on the number of points they accumulated in the championship, the teams were classified into two categories (strong/weak). The strong category included teams that ranked 1st–13th with points ranging from 52 to 81 (cluster center 61.00), while the weak category included teams that ranked 14th–20th with points ranging from 20 to 47 (cluster center 36.57).

Based on the number of high-pressing actions performed by the teams in each match, the observations were classified into two categories (many/few). The many category included observations where the team had 10 to 21 high-pressing actions (cluster center 12.50), while the few category included observations where the team had 0 to 9 high-pressing actions (cluster center 5.96).

Based on ball possession percentage, the observations were classified into two categories (high/low). The high category included observations where the team had 50.01% to 80% possession (cluster center 56.54), while the low category included observations where the team had 20% to 49.99% possession (cluster center 42.67).

Finally, based on the number of counterattacks performed by both teams combined in each match, the observations were classified into two categories (many/few). The many category included observations where the match had 30 to 53 counterattacks (cluster center 34.76), while the few category included observations where the match had 13 to 29 counterattacks (cluster center 23.74).

3.2. Linear Mixed Models

Table 2 shows the means of the dependent variables across the categories of the independent variables. Table 3 shows F and p values of the type III tests of fixed effects for the four models that were generated for the corresponding four dependent variables.

Table 2. The mean of the dependent variables across the categories of the independent variables.

Independent Variables	Independent Variables' Categories	Dependent Variables			
		LI	MI	HI	NHI
CD	Two CDs	85,192.247	18,740.194	9780.509	632.877
	Three CDs	85,224.288	19,181.388	10,078.614	652.853
CF	One CF	85,132.495	18,919.433	9969.323	645.492
	Two CFs	85,284.040	19,002.149	9889.800	640.238
TQ	Strong	85,489.889	19,456.661	10,089.752	650.853
	Weak	84,926.646	18,464.921	9769.370	634.877
OQ	Strong	85,239.146	19,129.081	10,043.755	648.218
	Weak	85,177.389	18,792.501	9815.367	637.512
HP	Many	85,117.847	19,205.067	10,096.827	655.501
	Few	85,298.688	18,716.515	9762.295	630.228
BP	High	84,801.273	18,967.825	9991.655	644.705
	Low	85,615.262	18,953.757	9867.467	641.024
CA	Few	85,304.201	18,946.646	9680.661	640.152
	Many	85,112.334	18,974.936	10,178.46	645.578
LC	Home	85,320.289	19,026.764	10,055.527	647.732
	Away	85,096.246	18,894.818	9803.596	637.998

Table 3. F and p values of the type III tests of fixed effects for the four models that were generated for the corresponding four dependent variables.

	LI		MI		HI		NHI	
	F	**Sig.**	**F**	**Sig.**	**F**	**Sig.**	**F**	**Sig.**
Intercept	63,670.426	0.000	6240.045	0.000	4245.507	0.000	5562.454	0.000
CD	0.005	0.943	3.717	0.055	3.108	0.079	4.350	0.038
CF	0.120	0.729	0.146	0.703	0.241	0.624	0.328	0.567
TQ	0.925	0.348	4.878	0.040	1.333	0.262	1.037	0.321
OQ	0.042	0.839	5.129	0.024	4.195	0.041	2.872	0.091
HP	0.338	0.561	10.213	0.002	8.521	0.004	15.153	0.000
BP	6.855	0.009	0.008	0.927	1.160	0.282	0.318	0.573
CA	0.435	0.510	0.039	0.844	21.412	0.000	0.793	0.374
LC	0.652	0.420	0.940	0.333	6.085	0.014	2.830	0.093

From Tables 2 and 3 it appears that:

- LI is greater for the high BP group compared to the low BP group ($p = 0.009$, d = 0.287).
- MI is greater for the many HP group compared to the few HP group ($p = 0.002$, d = 0.311).
- MI is greater for teams when facing strong opponents compared to when facing weak opponents ($p = 0.024$, d = 0.214).
- MI is greater for strong group compared to weak ($p = 0.04$, d = 0.632).
- HI is greater for home matches compared to away matches ($p = 0.014$, d = 0.228).
- HI is greater for teams in matches with many CA compared to matches with few CA ($p < 0.001$, d = 0.450).
- HI is greater for the many HP group compared to the few HP group ($p = 0.004$, d = 0.303).
- HI is greater for teams when facing strong opponents compared to when facing weak opponents ($p = 0.041$, d = 0.207).
- NHI is greater for the many HP group compared to the few HP group ($p < 0.001$, d = 0.404).
- NHI is greater for teams playing with three central defenders compared to teams playing with two central defenders ($p = 0.038$, d = 0.319).

4. Discussion

The purpose of this study was to investigate the factors influencing the distances covered by soccer players at three different intensity levels, as well as the number of high-intensity runs. Our findings indicate that high-press and opponent team quality affect MI, HI, and NHI; team quality affects MI; location and counterattacks influence HI; the number of central defenders affects NHI; and ball possession impacts LI. Conversely, the number of central forwards does not appear to influence any of the RP metrics. These findings can inform tactical decision making by coaches, taking into account the physical condition of their team and the context of the match.

4.1. Contextual Variables

In this study, we found that location has a statistically significant effect on high-intensity running, with home matches displaying higher HI values. This finding aligns with Gonçalves et al. [20], who observed higher values of high-intensity running in home matches compared to away matches. It appears that the psychological boost from the home crowd motivates players to exert more effort, engaging in more high-intensity actions [15,44]. Other studies have found that in the UEFA Champions League, away matches were associated with increased low-intensity running [18], and in the Croatian first division, higher medium-intensity values were found for away matches [19], differences that do not seem to apply to the Turkish league.

Additionally, our research found that strong teams exhibit higher MI values, which contradicts the findings of Modric et al. [18], who found that team quality was not associated with running performance in the UEFA Champions League. However, a year earlier, another study by Aquino et al. [21] found that the top-ranked teams covered greater total distance and higher acceleration than the bottom-ranked teams in a national league setting (Brazilian 2nd Division League).

Finally, our study found that facing a strong opponent increases the values of MI, HI, and NHI, compared to facing a weak opponent. This finding is consistent with the research by Gonçalves et al. [20] and Gonçalves et al. [22] for the first division of the Brazilian championship and the U20 Brazilian National League, respectively. The former study showed that matches against strong opponents resulted in greater total distance covered, while the latter found that starters playing against strong opponents exhibited higher values of distance in high-speed running. It seems that facing a strong opponent is a factor that increases intrinsic motivation [45].

4.2. Technical–Tactical Variables

In our study, we found that teams with high ball possession percentages exhibit higher LI compared to teams with low ball possession percentages, without statistically significant differences in other RP variables. This finding aligns with da Mota et al. [24], who found that teams with high ball possession covered greater total distances and distances at low intensities compared to teams with low ball possession. Additionally, we discovered that teams involved in matches with many counterattacks (regardless of whether they are performed by themselves or their opponents) have higher values in HI. The results of Külah and Alemdar [46], where the authors found that teams focused on ball possession had a lower average sprint value than teams playing a counterattacking style, agree with our findings. Counterattacks are, indeed, high-intensity actions [47], and high-speed training can be performed within the specific context of counterattacks [48].

Finally, we found that teams engaging in many high-pressing actions exhibit higher values in MI, HI, and NHI compared to teams with fewer high-pressing actions. These findings align with the assertion of Morgans et al. [49] that a defensive tactical strategy that does not promote a "high-press" but maintains a compact defensive shape reduces high metabolic load distance (HMLD), which provides overall information about the soccer players' high-intensity activities (>25.5 W/kg) [50–52]. Additionally, Low et al. [53] showed that using a high-press defending strategy leads to larger dispersion, due to a longer team length and larger interline distances between defenders, midfielders, and forwards. Consequently, covering these larger distances requires greater physical effort. This is further supported by Abreu et al. [54], who found that high-press games in soccer training elicited higher physiological and physical responses than free play.

4.3. Formations

In our study, we found that NHI increases when teams play with three central defenders compared to when they play with two. This finding is consistent with those of Tierney et al. [30] and Modric et al. [29], who also reported greater distances covered at high speeds for teams using three central defenders. These results align with the conclusions drawn from the systematic review of Forcher et al. [55], who found that physical match performance was higher in formations with three defenders (e.g., 3-5-2) compared to formations with four defenders (e.g., 4-4-2).

Additionally, our research did not find any effect of the number of central forwards on RP metrics. This specific aspect has not been directly investigated in previous studies. Indirect conclusions from research that studied overall formations are contradictory; some studies suggest that formations with two central forwards cover greater distances at high intensities [31–33], while others indicate that mean speed and high-intensity activities are greater in the 4-3-3 formation compared to the 4-4-2 formation [34,35].

4.4. Limitations

This study has some limitations that should be acknowledged. Firstly, the sample is exclusively drawn from the Turkish first division during the 2021–2022 season. This geographical and competitive context limits the generalizability of our findings to other leagues or levels of play, where different styles of play [56–58] may influence running performance differently. Secondly, the data collection method used in this study was static, meaning that data were obtained after the completion of matches [59]. This contrasts with a dynamic method, which would involve real-time data acquisition and could account for changes in match status (e.g., goals scored, red cards, substitutions) as they occur [60]. Moreover, while this study included several important factors influencing RP, there are other potential variables (such as weather conditions, playing surface, seasonal variations, mid-season coach change, and fatigue) that were not considered and could also impact running metrics [61–66]. However, to the best of our knowledge, no other study has investigated the effect of so many factors, including formations, technical–tactical, and contextual variables, by simultaneously studying them in multivariate models and using a large sample of 185 high-level matches. In addition, the static method, despite its drawbacks, has been widely used in performance analysis and has provided useful information [37,59].

5. Conclusions

In summary, our study aimed to investigate the factors influencing RP in Turkish soccer teams, focusing on different intensity levels and the number of high-intensity runs. By analyzing a large sample of matches from the Turkish first division during the 2021–2022 season, we identified several key factors that significantly impact RP, including location, team quality, opponent team quality, ball possession, high-press, counterattacks, and the number of central defenders. These findings offer a comprehensive understanding of how various elements interact to affect physical performance in Turkish soccer, providing valuable insights for optimizing team performance.

The primary strengths of our research include the extensive dataset of 185 high-level matches and the multivariate approach that simultaneously examined multiple factors. This holistic methodology allows for a more nuanced analysis of the interactions between different variables influencing RP. However, the study is limited by its focus on a single league, which may restrict the generalizability of the findings. Additionally, the static method of data collection used, while common in performance analysis, does not account for dynamic changes during the match, such as shifts in match status.

The importance of our research lies in its potential impact on both the specialized scientific community and the broader public. For sports scientists and PAs, our findings contribute to the ongoing discourse on the determinants of RP in soccer. For coaches and team managers, understanding these dynamics can inform strategic decisions and training programs, ultimately enhancing team performance and competitive success.

Practically, our results can be applied to improve tactical decision making in soccer. For instance, recognizing that high-pressing actions lead to higher RP metrics can help coaches design training sessions that mimic match conditions and prepare players for the physical demands of competitive play. This can involve specific exercises where players are required to press the opposition in defined zones of the field, followed by rapid counterattacks. Additionally, insights into the effects of opponent quality and match location can guide prematch preparations and in-game adjustments to optimize performance. For example, if a team is playing at home against a strong opponent, the coach might prioritize high-intensity training sessions to boost players' physical readiness and employ strategies to exploit the psychological advantage of the home crowd. Conversely, for away matches against weaker opponents, the focus might shift towards maintaining possession and managing the game's tempo to conserve energy and minimize the physical load on players.

Future research should aim to expand on our findings by incorporating data from multiple leagues and varying levels of play to enhance the generalizability of the results. Furthermore, adopting dynamic data collection methods could provide a more accurate depiction of RP by accounting for real-time changes during matches. Investigating additional variables, such as weather conditions, playing surface, and seasonal variations, could also offer a more comprehensive understanding of the factors affecting RP in soccer. Particular emphasis should be placed by the authors on the players' running under conditions of high temperatures and humidity, as these can have negative consequences, even on the health of the football players [67–69].

In conclusion, our study provides a detailed analysis of the factors influencing RP in Turkish soccer, highlighting the complex interplay between physical, technical–tactical, and contextual variables. By addressing the gaps in the existing literature and offering practical applications, we hope to contribute to the advancement of performance analysis in soccer and support the ongoing efforts to optimize team performance and success.

Author Contributions: S.P. designed the study and provided critical feedback on the manuscript; S.P. and Y.M. collected, processed, and analyzed data and revised the first draft; S.P. conducted the statistical analysis. All authors have read and agreed to the published version of the manuscript.

Funding: This research received no external funding.

Institutional Review Board Statement: The Ethics Committee of the University of Thessaly approves the study (No. 1973. 12 October 2022).

Informed Consent Statement: Not applicable.

Data Availability Statement: Data are available upon request from the corresponding author due to privacy and ethical restrictions.

Conflicts of Interest: The authors declare no conflicts of interest.

References

1. Passos, P.; Araújo, D.; Volossovitch, A. *Performance Analysis in Team Sports*; Routledge, Taylor & Francis Group: London, UK, 2017. [CrossRef]
2. Kirkendall, D.T. Evolution of soccer as a research topic. *Prog. Cardiovasc. Dis.* **2020**, *63*, 723–729. [CrossRef]
3. Martin, D.; O Donoghue, P.G.; Bradley, J.; McGrath, D. Developing a framework for professional practice in applied performance analysis. *Int. J. Perform. Anal. Sport* **2021**, *21*, 845–888. [CrossRef]
4. Martin, D.; O'Donoghue, P.G.; Bradley, J.; Robertson, S.; McGrath, D. Identifying the characteristics, constraints, and enablers to creating value in applied performance analysis. *Int. J. Sports Sci. Coach.* **2024**, *19*, 832–846. [CrossRef]
5. Hughes, M.D.; Bartlett, R.M. The use of performance indicators in performance analysis. *J. Sports Sci.* **2002**, *20*, 739–754. [CrossRef]
6. Herold, M.; Kempe, M.; Bauer, P.; Meyer, T. Attacking key performance indicators in soccer: Current practice and perceptions from the elite to youth academy level. *J. Sports Sci. Med.* **2021**, *20*, 158. [CrossRef]
7. Wright, C.; Carling, C.; Collins, D. The wider context of performance analysis and it application in the football coaching process. *Int. J. Perform. Anal. Sport* **2014**, *14*, 709–733. [CrossRef]
8. Otero-Saborido, F.M.; Aguado-Méndez, R.D.; Torreblanca-Martínez, V.M.; González-Jurado, J.A. Technical-tactical performance from data providers: A systematic review in regular football leagues. *Sustainability* **2021**, *13*, 10167. [CrossRef]
9. Goes, F.; Meerhoff, L.; Bueno, M.; Rodrigues, D.; Moura, F.; Brink, M.; Elferink-Gemser, M.; Knobbe, A.; Cunha, S.; Torres, R. Unlocking the potential of big data to support tactical performance analysis in professional soccer: A systematic review. *Eur. J. Sport Sci.* **2021**, *21*, 481–496. [CrossRef] [PubMed]
10. Mackenzie, R.; Cushion, C. Performance analysis in football: A critical review and implications for future research. *J. Sports Sci.* **2013**, *31*, 639–676. [CrossRef]
11. Kusuma, I.D.M.A.W.; Kusnanik, N.W.; Lumintuarso, R.; Phanpheng, Y. The Holistic and Partial Approach in Soccer Training: Integrating Physical, Technical, Tactical, and Mental Components: A Systematic Review. *Retos* **2024**, *54*, 328–337. [CrossRef]
12. Andrzejewski, M.; Oliva-Lozano, J.M.; Chmura, P.; Chmura, J.; Czarniecki, S.; Kowalczuk, E.; Rokita, A.; Muyor, J.M.; Konefał, M. Analysis of team success based on match technical and running performance in a professional soccer league. *BMC Sports Sci. Med. Rehabil.* **2022**, *14*, 82. [CrossRef] [PubMed]
13. Modric, T.; Versic, S.; Drid, P.; Stojanovic, M.; Radzimiński, Ł.; Bossard, C.; Aftański, T.; Sekulic, D. Analysis of running performance in the offensive and defensive phases of the game: Is it associated with the team achievement in the UEFA Champions League? *Appl. Sci.* **2021**, *11*, 8765. [CrossRef]

14. Paul, D.J.; Bradley, P.S.; Nassis, G.P. Factors affecting match running performance of elite soccer players: Shedding some light on the complexity. *Int. J. Sports Physiol. Perform.* **2015**, *10*, 516–519. [CrossRef] [PubMed]
15. Armatas, V.; Pollard, R. Home advantage in Greek football. *Eur. J. Sport Sci.* **2014**, *14*, 116–122. [CrossRef] [PubMed]
16. Levi, H.R.; Jackson, R.C. Contextual factors influencing decision making: Perceptions of professional soccer players. *Psychol. Sport Exerc.* **2018**, *37*, 19–25. [CrossRef]
17. Lago-Peñas, C. The role of situational variables in analysing physical performance in soccer. *J. Hum. Kinet.* **2012**, *35*, 89–95. [CrossRef] [PubMed]
18. Modric, T.; Versic, S.; Stojanovic, M.; Chmura, P.; Andrzejewski, M.; Konefał, M.; Sekulic, D. Factors affecting match running performance in elite soccer: Analysis of UEFA Champions League matches. *Biol. Sport* **2022**, *40*, 409–416. [CrossRef] [PubMed]
19. Jerkovic, Z.; Modric, T.; Versic, S. Analysis of the associations between contextual variables and match running performance in Croatian First Division Soccer. *Sport Mont* **2022**, *20*, 125–130. [CrossRef]
20. Gonçalves, L.G.C.; Clemente, F.; Vieira, L.H.P.; Bedo, B.; Puggina, E.F.; Moura, F.; Mesquita, F.; Santiago, P.R.P.; Almeida, R.; Aquino, R. Effects of match location, quality of opposition, match outcome, and playing position on load parameters and players' prominence during official matches in professional soccer players. *Hum. Mov.* **2021**, *22*, 35–44. [CrossRef]
21. Aquino, R.; Gonçalves, L.G.; Galgaro, M.; Maria, T.S.; Rostaiser, E.; Pastor, A.; Nobari, H.; Garcia, G.R.; Moraes-Neto, M.V.; Nakamura, F.Y. Match running performance in Brazilian professional soccer players: Comparisons between successful and unsuccessful teams. *BMC Sports Sci. Med. Rehabil.* **2021**, *13*, 93. [CrossRef]
22. Gonçalves, L.G.; Nobari, H.; Rites, A.A.; Nakamura, F.Y.; Garcia, G.R.; Aquino, R. Can contextual factors affect match running performance in elite youth soccer players? A case study in Brazil. *preprint* **2022**. [CrossRef]
23. Modric, T.; Malone, J.J.; Versic, S.; Andrzejewski, M.; Chmura, P.; Konefał, M.; Drid, P.; Sekulic, D. The influence of physical performance on technical and tactical outcomes in the UEFA Champions League. *BMC Sports Sci. Med. Rehabil.* **2022**, *14*, 179. [CrossRef] [PubMed]
24. Da Mota, G.R.; Thiengo, C.R.; Gimenes, S.V.; Bradley, P.S. The effects of ball possession status on physical and technical indicators during the 2014 FIFA World Cup Finals. *J. Sports Sci.* **2016**, *34*, 493–500. [CrossRef]
25. Forcher, L.; Forcher, L.; Wäsche, H.; Jekauc, D.; Woll, A.; Gross, T.; Altmann, S. Is ball-possession style more physically demanding than counter-attacking? The influence of playing style on match performance in professional soccer. *Front. Psychol.* **2023**, *14*, 1197039. [CrossRef]
26. Low, B.; Boas, G.V.; Meyer, L.; Lizaso, E.; Hoitz, F.; Leite, N.; Gonçalves, B. Exploring the effects of deep-defending vs high-press on footballers' tactical behaviour, physical and physiological performance: A pilot study. *Mot. Rev. De Educ.* **2018**, *24*, e1018171. [CrossRef]
27. Plakias, S.; Tsatalas, T.; Moustakidis, S.; Kalapotharakos, V.; Kokkotis, C.; Papalexi, M.; Giakas, G.; Tsaopoulos, D. Exploring the influence of playing styles on physical demands in professional football. *Hum. Mov.* **2023**, *24*, 36–43. [CrossRef]
28. Plakias, S. An integrative review of the game model in soccer: Definition, misconceptions, and practical significance. *Trends Sport Sci.* **2023**, *30*, 85–92. [CrossRef]
29. Modric, T.; Versic, S.; Sekulic, D. Position specific running performances in professional football (soccer): Influence of different tactical formations. *Sports* **2020**, *8*, 161. [CrossRef]
30. Tierney, P.J.; Young, A.; Clarke, N.D.; Duncan, M.J. Match play demands of 11 versus 11 professional football using Global Positioning System tracking: Variations across common playing formations. *Hum. Mov. Sci.* **2016**, *49*, 1–8. [CrossRef]
31. Borghi, S.; Colombo, D.; La Torre, A.; Banfi, G.; Bonato, M.; Vitale, J.A. Differences in GPS variables according to playing formations and playing positions in U19 male soccer players. *Res. Sports Med.* **2021**, *29*, 225–239. [CrossRef]
32. Bradley, P.S.; Carling, C.; Archer, D.; Roberts, J.; Dodds, A.; Di Mascio, M.; Paul, D.; Gomez Diaz, A.; Peart, D.; Krustrup, P. The effect of playing formation on high-intensity running and technical profiles in English FA Premier League soccer matches. *J. Sports Sci.* **2011**, *29*, 821–830. [CrossRef] [PubMed]
33. Arjol-Serrano, J.L.; Lampre, M.; Díez, A.; Castillo, D.; Sanz-López, F.; Lozano, D. The influence of playing formation on physical demands and technical-tactical actions according to playing positions in an elite soccer team. *Int. J. Environ. Res. Public Health* **2021**, *18*, 4148. [CrossRef] [PubMed]
34. Aquino, R.; Vieira, L.H.P.; Carling, C.; Martins, G.H.; Alves, I.S.; Puggina, E.F. Effects of competitive standard, team formation and playing position on match running performance of Brazilian professional soccer players. *Int. J. Perform. Anal. Sport* **2017**, *17*, 695–705. [CrossRef]
35. Vieira, L.H.P.; Aquino, R.; Lago-Peñas, C.; Martins, G.H.M.; Puggina, E.F.; Barbieri, F.A. Running performance in Brazilian professional football players during a congested match schedule. *J. Strength Cond. Res.* **2018**, *32*, 313–325. [CrossRef] [PubMed]
36. FIFA. Instat-Fifa-Epts-Report-Oct-2019. Victoria University. 2021. Available online: https://digitalhub.fifa.com/m/2fd538ffbae39eb2/original/instat-fifa-epts-report-oct-2019.pdf (accessed on 14 November 2023).
37. Plakias, S.; Tsatalas, T.; Armatas, V.; Tsaopoulos, D.; Giakas, G. Tactical Situations and Playing Styles as Key Performance Indicators in Soccer. *J. Funct. Morphol. Kinesiol.* **2024**, *9*, 88. [CrossRef] [PubMed]
38. Morgans, R.; Orme, P.; Michele, R.D. Impact of technical and physical performance on match outcome over five elite European soccer seasons. *J. Sports Med. Phys. Fit.* **2023**, *63*, 417–429. [CrossRef]
39. Castellano, J.; Blanco-Villaseñor, A.; Alvarez, D. Contextual variables and time-motion analysis in soccer. *Int. J. Sports Med.* **2011**, *32*, 415–421. [CrossRef] [PubMed]

40. Castellano, J.; Echeazarra, I. Network-based centrality measures and physical demands in football regarding player position: Is there a connection? A preliminary study. *J. Sports Sci.* **2019**, *37*, 2631–2638. [CrossRef] [PubMed]
41. Gómez, M.-Á.; Mitrotasios, M.; Armatas, V.; Lago-Peñas, C. Analysis of playing styles according to team quality and match location in Greek professional soccer. *Int. J. Perform. Anal. Sport* **2018**, *18*, 986–997. [CrossRef]
42. Rampinini, E.; Coutts, A.J.; Castagna, C.; Sassi, R.; Impellizzeri, F. Variation in top level soccer match performance. *Int. J. Sports Med.* **2007**, *28*, 1018–1024. [CrossRef]
43. Cohen, J. *Statistical Power Analysis for the Behavioral Sciences*; Routledge: London, UK, 2013. [CrossRef]
44. Wolfson, S.; Wakelin, D.; Lewis, M. Football supporters' perceptions of their role in the home advantage. *J. Sports Sci.* **2005**, *23*, 365–374. [CrossRef] [PubMed]
45. Abuhamdeh, S.; Csikszentmihalyi, M.; Jalal, B. Enjoying the possibility of defeat: Outcome uncertainty, suspense, and intrinsic motivation. *Motiv. Emot.* **2015**, *39*, 1–10. [CrossRef]
46. Külah, E.; Alemdar, H. Quantifying the value of sprints in elite football using spatial cohesive networks. *Chaos Solitons Fractals* **2020**, *139*, 110306. [CrossRef]
47. Andrzejewski, M.; Chmura, J.; Pluta, B.; Strzelczyk, R.; Kasprzak, A. Analysis of sprinting activities of professional soccer players. *J. Strength Cond. Res.* **2013**, *27*, 2134–2140. [CrossRef] [PubMed]
48. Asian-Clemente, J.A.; Rabano-Muñoz, A.; Requena, B.; Suarez-Arrones, L. High-speed training in a specific context in soccer: Transition games. *Int. J. Sports Med.* **2022**, *43*, 881–888. [CrossRef] [PubMed]
49. Morgans, R.; Radnor, J.; Fonseca, J.; Haslam, C.; King, M.; Rhodes, D.; Żmijewski, P.; Oliveira, R. Match running performance is influenced by possession and team formation in an English Premier League team. *Biol. Sport* **2024**, *41*, 275–286. [CrossRef] [PubMed]
50. García-Calvo, T.; Ponce-Bordón, J.C.; Pons, E.; Del Campo, R.L.; Resta, R.; Raya-González, J. High metabolic load distance in professional soccer according to competitive level and playing positions. *PeerJ* **2022**, *10*, e13318. [CrossRef]
51. Moreno-Pérez, V.; Malone, S.; Sala-Pérez, L.; Lapuente-Sagarra, M.; Campos-Vazquez, M.A.; Del Coso, J. Activity monitoring in professional soccer goalkeepers during training and match play. *Int. J. Perform. Anal. Sport* **2020**, *20*, 19–30. [CrossRef]
52. Reynolds, J.; Connor, M.; Jamil, M.; Beato, M. Quantifying and comparing the match demands of U18, U23, and 1ST team English professional soccer players. *Front. Physiol.* **2021**, *12*, 706451. [CrossRef]
53. Low, B.; Rein, R.; Raabe, D.; Schwab, S.; Memmert, D. The porous high-press? An experimental approach investigating tactical behaviours from two pressing strategies in football. *J. Sports Sci.* **2021**, *39*, 2199–2210. [CrossRef]
54. Abreu, C.d.O.; Morales, J.C.P.; Greco, P.J.; Praça, G.M. Training defensive high-press in soccer: Physical and physiological responses to different small-sided games played by youth athletes. *Int. J. Perform. Anal. Sport* **2022**, *22*, 749–760. [CrossRef]
55. Forcher, L.; Forcher, L.; Waesche, H.; Jekauc, D.; Woll, A.; Altmann, S. The influence of tactical formation on physical and technical match performance in male soccer: A systematic review. *Int. J. Sports Sci. Coach.* **2023**, *18*, 1820–1849. [CrossRef]
56. Mitrotasios, M.; Gonzalez-Rodenas, J.; Armatas, V.; Aranda, R. The creation of goal scoring opportunities in professional soccer. tactical differences between Spanish La Liga, English Premier League, German Bundesliga and Italian Serie A. *Int. J. Perform. Anal. Sport* **2019**, *19*, 452–465. [CrossRef]
57. Plakias, S.; Moustakidis, E.; Mitrotasios, M.; Kokkotis, C.; Tsatalas, T.; Papalexi, M.; Giakas, G.; Tsaopoulos, D. A Multivariate and cluster analysis of diverse playing styles across European Football Leagues. *J. Phys. Educ. Sport* **2023**, *23*, 1631–1641. [CrossRef]
58. Plakias, S.; Moustakidis, S.; Mitrotasios, M.; Kokkotis, C.; Tsatalas, T.; Papalexi, M.; Giakas, G.; Tsaopoulos, D. Analysis of playing styles in European football: Insights from a visual mapping approach. *J. Phys. Educ. Sport* **2023**, *23*, 1385–1393. [CrossRef]
59. Pratas, J.M.; Volossovitch, A.; Carita, A.I. Goal scoring in elite male football: A systematic review. *J. Hum. Sport Exerc.* **2018**, *13*, 218–230. [CrossRef]
60. Prieto, J.; Gómez, M.Á.; Sampaio, J. From a static to a dynamic perspective in handball match analysis: A systematic review. *Open Sports Sci. J.* **2015**, *8*, 25–34. [CrossRef]
61. Chmura, P.; Konefał, M.; Andrzejewski, M.; Kosowski, J.; Rokita, A.; Chmura, J. Physical activity profile of 2014 FIFA World Cup players, with regard to different ranges of air temperature and relative humidity. *Int. J. Biometeorol.* **2017**, *61*, 677–684. [CrossRef] [PubMed]
62. Dambroz, F.; Clemente, F.M.; Teoldo, I. The effect of physical fatigue on the performance of soccer players: A systematic review. *PLoS ONE* **2022**, *17*, e0270099. [CrossRef]
63. Guerrero-Calderón, B.; Owen, A.; Morcillo, J.A.; Castillo-Rodríguez, A. How does the mid-season coach change affect physical performance on top soccer players? *Physiol. Behav.* **2021**, *232*, 113328. [CrossRef]
64. Illmer, S.; Daumann, F. The effects of weather factors and altitude on physical and technical performance in professional soccer: A systematic review. *JSAMS Plus* **2022**, *1*, 100002. [CrossRef]
65. Meckel, Y.; Doron, O.; Eliakim, E.; Eliakim, A. Seasonal variations in physical fitness and performance indices of elite soccer players. *Sports* **2018**, *6*, 14. [CrossRef] [PubMed]
66. Watanabe, N.; Wicker, P.; Yan, G. Weather conditions, travel distance, rest, and running performance: The 2014 FIFA World Cup and implications for the future. *J. Sport Manag.* **2017**, *31*, 27–43. [CrossRef]
67. Branquinho, L.; Forte, P.; Thomatieli-Santos, R.V.; de França, E.; Marinho, D.A.; Teixeira, J.E.; Ferraz, R. Perspectives on player performance during FIFA World Cup Qatar 2022: A brief report. *Sports* **2023**, *11*, 174. [CrossRef] [PubMed]

68. Ghazzawi, H.A.; Hussain, M.A.; Raziq, K.M.; Alsendi, K.K.; Alaamer, R.O.; Jaradat, M.; Alobaidi, S.; Al Aqili, R.; Trabelsi, K.; Jahrami, H. Exploring the relationship between micronutrients and athletic performance: A comprehensive scientific systematic review of the literature in sports medicine. *Sports* **2023**, *11*, 109. [CrossRef]
69. Heatherly, A.J.; Caputo, J.L.; Johnson, S.L.; Fuller, D.K. Heat acclimation knowledge among recreational runners. *Sports* **2023**, *11*, 49. [CrossRef]

sports

MDPI

Review

Visualization of the Research Panorama of Decision-Making in Soccer: Bibliometric Analysis with VOSviewer and Review of the Most Cited Studies of the Last 15 Years (2010–2024)

Juan David Paucar Uribe [1], Boryi A. Becerra-Patiño [1,2], Jorge Olivares-Arancibia [3], Rodrigo Yáñez-Sepúlveda [4], Aldo Vasquez-Bonilla [5], Daniel Rojas-Valverde [6], José Francisco López-Gil [7,8,*] and Guilherme Machado [9,10]

1 Faculty of Physical Education, National Pedagogical University, Valmaria Cl. 183 # 5199, Bogotá 111166, Colombia; jdpaucaru@upn.edu.co (J.D.P.U.); babecerrap@pedagogica.edu.co or boryialexander.becerrap@um.es (B.A.B.-P.)
2 Programa de Doctorado en Ciencias de la Actividad Física y del Deporte, University of Murcia, 30720 Santiago de la Ribera, Spain
3 Grupo AFySE, Investigación en Actividad Física y Salud Escolar, Escuela de Educación Física, Facultad de Educación, Universidad de las Américas, Santiago 7500975, Chile; jorge.olivares.ar@gmail.com
4 Facultad de Educación y Ciencias Sociales, Universidad Andres Bello, Viña del Mar 2520000, Chile; rodrigoyanezs@unab.cl
5 Grupo de Avances en Entrenamiento Deportivo y Acondicionamiento Físico, Facultad de Ciencias del Deporte, Universidad de Extremadura, 10003 Cáceres, Spain; alvasquezb@unex.es
6 Centro de Investigación y Diagnóstico en Salud y Deporte (CIDISAD-NARS), Clínica de Lesiones Deportivas (Rehab&Readapt), Escuela Ciencias del Movimiento Humano y Calidad Vida (CIEMHCAVI), Universidad Nacional de Costa Rica, Heredia 86-3000, Costa Rica; sofia.gonzalez.rojas@est.una.ac.cr or drojasv@hotmail.com
7 School of Medicine, Universidad Espíritu Santo, Samborondón 092301, Ecuador
8 Vicerrectoría de Investigación y Postgrado, Universidad de los Lagos, Osorno 5290000, Chile
9 Scientific Department and Department of Athletes' Integration and Development, Paulista Football Federation (FPF), São Paulo 05614-060, Brazil; machado.guilhermef@gmail.com
10 Department of Physical Education, Centre of Research and Studies in Soccer (NUPEF), Universidade Federal de Viçosa, Viçosa 36570-900, Brazil
* Correspondence: josefranciscolopezgil@gmail.com

Abstract: Background/Objectives: Various studies have investigated the importance of perceptual–cognitive skills in decision-making and the expert performance of athletes. However, bibliometric study has yet to identify research trends on this topic. The objective of this study was to perform a bibliometric review to identify the research trends in the study of soccer decision-making. Method. A total of 172 studies were included in the databases. Results. The year 2021 was the year with the highest number of published studies (n = 23), and 2016 was the year with the highest number of citations (n = 692). The average number of citations per document was 19.79. The concepts that have the greatest occurrence in the investigations are performance (n = 68), decision-making (n = 54), expertise (n = 32), skill (n = 23), and anticipation (n = 22). The journals with the highest number of published documents are the *Journal of Sport Sciences* (10 documents and 437 citations) and *PLoS One* (11 documents and 349 citations). The countries with the highest number of published documents and citations are England (n = 46 documents and 996 citations), Germany (n = 32 documents and 749 citations), and Spain (n = 38 documents and 597 citations). German Sport University Cologne is the organization that has the most publications and citations (n = 19 and 531). Conclusions. Existing knowledge production on decision-making in soccer has a preference for the study of two major categories: one related to the analysis of the factors associated with perceptual–cognitive skills, mental fatigue, anticipation, creativity, and memory, whereas the second is more related to the study that has decision-making in the manifestations of specific game performance, between experts and novices, in the precision of technical actions, such as the pass, as well as in a methodology for the selection of athletes.

Keywords: assessment; perception; attention; performance; team sport

1. Introduction

Overall, sports are characterized by relationships and interactions between athletes [1], which are manifested in the development of game-changing and unpredictable actions [2]. Soccer is a practice where interpersonal and group cooperation are fundamental in the development of sport [3], so understanding individual and collective decision-making could lead to competition [4]. Research in recent decades has made it possible to identify the importance of the perceptual–cognitive skills associated with the expert performance of athletes [5], including the exploration of the environment to understand the kinematic and positional signals [6–8], the recognition of the game patterns that are specific to football [9], and the perception and intention of deception toward the opponents that is carried out to favor the actions of play [10,11].

Accordingly, players' decision-making is affected by different factors, such as the complexity of the task or action to be solved, the time available, and the contextual background available in the various situations of the game [4]. Among them is understanding and tactical understanding [12], where the player must understand, develop, and identify the most significant amount of information to increase effectiveness [13], quickly restoring his attention [14], and, therefore, cognitive effort is not demanding in the interaction of declarative and procedural tactical knowledge during the game [15]. Likewise, the physical demand of athletes produced by accelerations, decelerations, speeds, and rhythms can increase or decrease according to the group organization and individual understanding [16], so consolidating timely decisions in the total load of fatigue avoids injury levels [17] and increases the capacity of effective passes [18], where it is necessary to implement appropriate pedagogical strategies for the development and acquisition of skills [19]. The consolidation of the sports process in children's and youth stages is vital in developing players' capacities to carry out actions in decision-making [20]. Therefore, the implementation of didactics, such as games in small spaces, has generated interest in the sports science community for the evaluation and detection of talent [21], increasing scientific production to optimize footballers' sports performance [22].

On the other hand, understanding soccer as a sport with open skills [23] is subject to complex challenges in mental fatigue [23,24] as a consequence of the different visual stimuli of the unpredictable trajectory of the ball, the opponents, the equipment, and objects, and limiting logic and understanding, which, as a consequence, constantly predisposes athletes to a state of alertness [14], decreasing sports performance, as various investigations have shown [25,26]. The evolution of the sporty human being and the same sport has increased technological advancement. Technology is not usually useful on some occasions; since it can impair performance, an example of this is that the use of social networks before a competition negatively influences the constant decisions of the players [27], where demanding mental loads must be reduced to establish a better relationship in the understanding of the game [28]. In contrast, the behavior in the individual decisions of footballers has allowed for the creation of instruments through video diagnostics that allow for the recognition of specific actions of football [29], such as the TacticUP video test that comprises offensive and defensive actions in football 11 vs. 11 [13] and tests of the speed of reaction in motor development that are used by neuroscience [30]. This allows for the evaluation of different components, such as measurements of dribbling capacity, support for the dribbling player, and the constant relationship between the ball and the player [31].

Other methods, such as artificial intelligence [32] and three-dimensional multiple object tracking (3D-MOT), were created to develop fundamental and attentional dynamic visualizations during sports to perceive relevant information adequately [33]. Their functions have been associated with dynamic environments and decision-making; despite this, these technologies are still under discussion, generating new challenges in the implementation of technologies in football [34]. For their part, they must consider the specificity of the sport and the level of performance of the athletes [35]. Likewise, characterization and individualization by game positions allow us to understand physical differences [36] and technical–tactical actions [37], which are evident in the investigative interest in decision-making in the goalkeeper, in actions of shots to goal [38], and trajectories from the penalty spot [39,40]; however, in the literature, there is no clarity about the differences in decision-making in the other game positions.

The analysis of the performance factors that influence decision-making is associated with the specific restrictions of time, space, and existing relationships with the receiver or adversary to promote the development of perceptual–cognitive skills, such as anticipation and choice of action [41,42], which help improve the execution carried out by the athlete from complex dynamic motor tasks [43]. In another study, developed by McLoughlin et al. [44] through a qualitative approach through the methodology discussion group, which sought to explore decision-making processes in expert players and almost all expert players, it was concluded that decision-making has four critical points: (1) context prior to the game (coach tactics and instructions, opponent level, and importance of the match or competition); (2) current context of the game (scoreboard and playing time); (3) visual information; and (4) individual differences in the athletes (self-efficacy, perceived pressure, morphofunctional characteristics, fatigue). In this sense, fatigue is a key element to consider in the player's decision-making produced by contextual or environmental variables [4].

With all the above, the scientific evidence continues to focus on different approaches and the consideration of different perceptual–cognitive skills to better understand decision-making. Thus, various studies have concluded that it is necessary to continue developing research that integrates concepts and methodologies from the multiple perspectives with which decision-making has been studied in team sports, such as soccer [4,45]. The same scientific evidence suggests new methodologies to understand the interactions among the different processes that contribute to the development of new research perspectives [46]. These research advances should be put into practice to improve training methods and decision evaluation processes in response to the specificity of the sport and the individuality of the player. To our knowledge, a bibliometric study evaluating decision-making in soccer has not been previously reported in scientific literature. Therefore, the objective of this study was to perform a bibliometric review to identify the trend of the research carried out on decision-making from the use of bibliometrics as a research technique in the Web of Science and PubMed databases, including the documents published between 1 January 2010 and 15 July 2024.

2. Materials and Methods

2.1. Design

This study was developed using bibliometrics as a research technique. Taking as a reference, the theoretical nature of the study and the classification established by Ato et al. [47], a bibliometric analysis is considered a theoretical and retrospective study because it responds to the purpose of systematizing, analyzing, and condensing a large amount of data related to the temporality of the studies and the evolution of the themes addressed over the years [48]. These types of studies analyze trends that are developed in a thematic area to generalize the production of knowledge through specific criteria such as (i) authors; (ii) countries; (iii) institutions; (iv) keywords; (v) document citations; (vi) citations between cited references; and (vii) editorial groups [49].

2.2. Data Extraction

The search for documents was carried out on the Web of Science (WoS) database, especially in the WoS Core Collection. This database was selected because many bibliometric football-related reviews have been conducted there [50–54]. This data platform allows access to a large amount of information from the selected manuscripts and analyzes the influence in the scientific field [48]. Similarly, a search was carried out in PubMed, Scopus database, and SPORTDiscus. When screening the information, 88% of the documents were duplicates. Therefore, it was decided to consider only WoS studies and proceed to add documents that were not present in the other databases consulted, following the guidelines of other bibliometric studies [55,56]. A review based on the WoS database was carried out using the following terms and following the participants, interventions, and outcomes (PIO) strategy: (soccer OR football OR "team sports") AND (knowledge OR intelligence OR "decision making" or "game performance") AND (tactic* OR cognitive OR declarative). Finally, the search equation used was decision-making AND soccer AND players. The search was carried out on July 15 by two leading researchers (J.D.P.-U. and B.A.B.-P.). A systematic process was developed for selecting the included documents based on bibliometric criteria, such as duplication and a direct relationship with the study's objective [57]. Initially, the 1.868 documents submitted to the metadata regulation process were analyzed to eliminate duplicates, lack full access, and no relationships to the study's subject. After searching for documents, 172 documents that met the eligibility criteria established for this study remained (Figure 1).

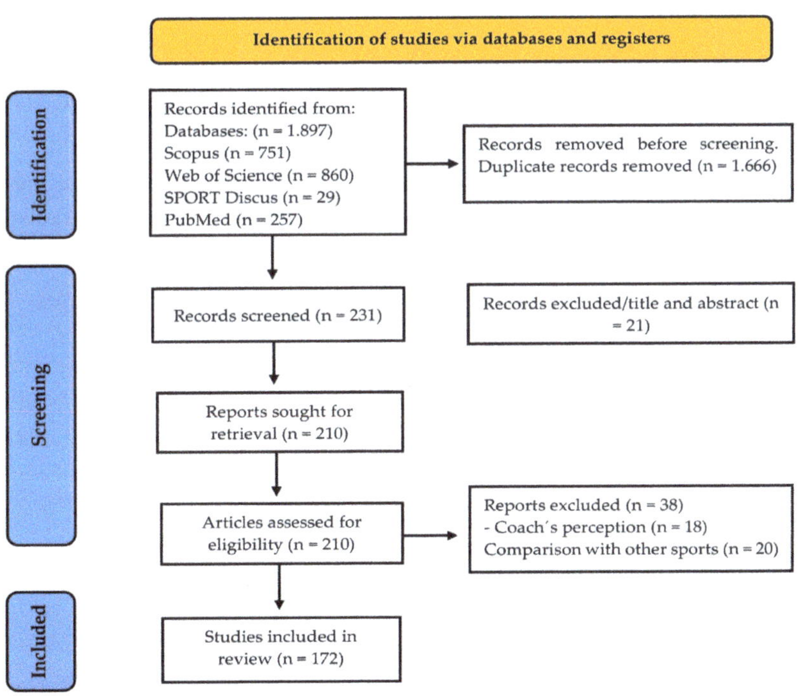

Figure 1. Flow diagram for the selection of studies according to PRISMA guidelines.

2.3. Eligibility Criteria

The inclusion criteria of the studies were as follows: (i) focused on the study of decision-making in child soccer players, adolescents, or adults; (ii) focused on sports samples that aimed to improve training or competition; (iii) were original full-text studies reviewed by academic peers; (iv) focused on studies in soccer players or that included both genders in the study; (v) had access to the complete document to complement the first review; (vi) published between 1 January 2010 and 15 July 2024; and (vii) indexed the journal in the Journal Citation Report (JCR) in the following quartiles: Q1, Q2, Q3, and Q4. The exclusion criteria were as follows: (1) studies that considered the evaluation of team sports where soccer was included; (2) studies that considered the evaluation of robot soccer; (3) studies in sports; and (4) decision-making for the return after injury.

To select the documents, an analysis matrix was developed in Microsoft Excel based on the following categories: (1) year of publication; (2) type of document; (3) most cited articles; (4) name of authors; (5) number of authors by study; (6) keywords; (7) journals and references cited; (8) publishing groups; (9) areas of knowledge; (10) language; (11) countries; and (12) organizations.

2.4. Data Analysis

The identified data were extracted in two different formats: plain text and Excel. The Excel document allows descriptive and percentage analysis of the results via a Microsoft Excel spreadsheet (v. 2006, Microsoft Corporation, Redmond, WA, USA). The plain text format allows the development of analysis by coauthorship for authors, coauthorship by organizations, occurrence by keywords, citation by documents, citation by journals, citation by countries, and citation by authors with the VOSviewer program (v.6.19., Center for Science and Technology Studies, Netherlands). A fragmentation analysis was performed with a value of 2 for attraction and 1 for repulsion. The VOSviewer program allows for the creation of two-dimensional graphs [58] from nodes to establish the central relationships developed from the scientific production stored in the different databases [59].

The following laws were considered to support the bibliometric analysis: (1) Price's law from the coefficient of determination (R^2) coefficient to determine the strength of the linear relationship between two variables [60]; in this case, the number of published documents and citations over the years, as well as the number of citations. (2) Lotka's law allows for the identification of the authors who have published the most studies [61,62], and (3) Zipf's law is oriented to establish the occurrence of the most used keywords [63].

Similarly, the *H*-index was used, which determines academic productivity according to the number of times a document has been cited at least a minimum number of times [64].

3. Results and Discussion

3.1. Evolution of the Number of Documents

The increase in scientific production related to the number of documents published per year between 2010 and 2024 reveals a systematic increase in the number of published studies, with 2023 being the year with the highest production. Similarly, Figure 2 shows that in the middle of 2024, the trend reflects an increase in the number of documents. In terms of the R^2 coefficient of the sample obtained, a substantial increase of 633.33% was identified between the first reference year (2010) and the last reference year (2024).

The number of citations per year slightly increased, and until 2016, there was a significant change of 981.25% compared with the first year (2010). The trend reveals low citation rates for 2017, 2019, and 2022, with decreases of −27.31%, −35.66%, and −55.00%, respectively, compared with 2016, 2018, and 2021 (Figure 3).

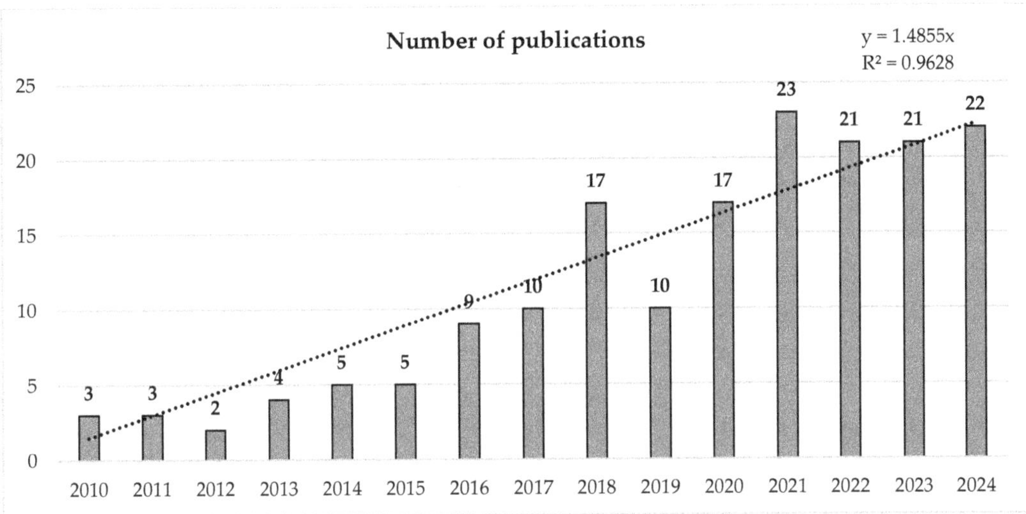

Figure 2. Evolution of the number of annual publications.

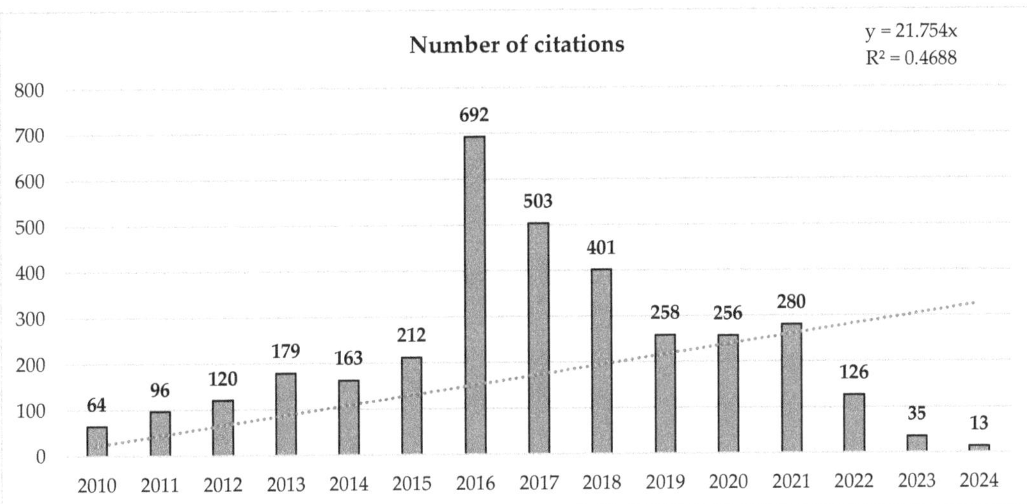

Figure 3. Evolution of the number of annual citations.

3.2. Types of Documents

Different types of documents have been published to socialize studies related to decision-making in football. However, the trend reveals that the most significant number is articles, which account for more than one-third of the total scientific production. In turn, few review studies exist. Research related to the type of documents that are preferably used for the socialization of the research results is empirical research. The low number of review studies for bibliometric analysis is also associated with the scientific development of specific topics (Table 1).

Table 1. Types of documents published.

Type of Document	Number of Documents	Percentage, %
Article	154	89.53
Review	11	6.39
Meeting Abstract	5	2.90
Book Chapter	2	1.16
Total	172	100

3.3. Analysis of the Most Cited Documents

Figure 4 details the behavior of the total number of appointments over nine years. Given the number of documents published per year, for 2016 and 2017, it is also determined as the period that receives the most significant number of citations. The low level of citations in 2018 and 2019 for this type of document is striking, with significant decreases of −89.77 and −79.20 compared with 2016 and 2017, respectively.

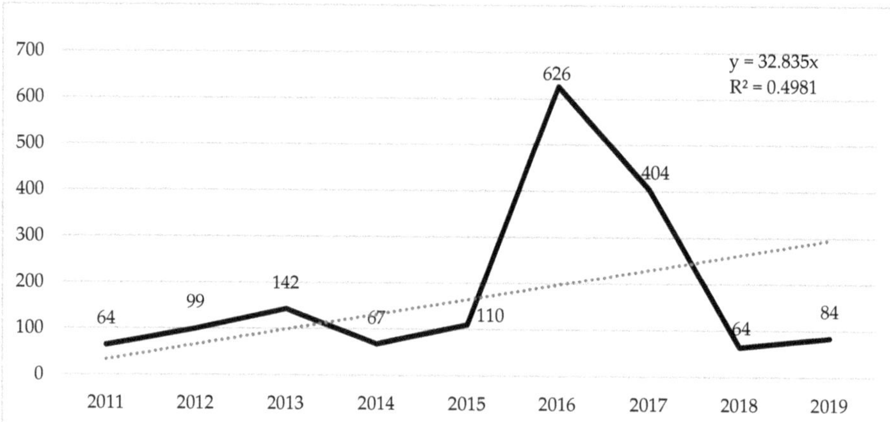

Figure 4. Evolution of the number of citations received per year for the most cited studies.

The analysis of the documents that have received at least 50 citations reveals ten studies (Table 2), of which two are reviewed and the other eight are research articles. Among the ten studies included, only two considered the analysis of physiological, physical, tactical, and technical variables in the decision-making approach of soccer players. All the documents date back to far less than 2017, and in turn, six of these studies were published in journals indexed in the Journal Citation Report (JCR) in the first quartile (Q1). Within the effects that are evaluated, two significant fields can be deduced: one related to the analysis of the factors associated with perceptual–cognitive skills, mental fatigue, anticipation, creativity, and memory, whereas the second is more related to the study that the decision-making in the manifestations of specific performance of the game, between experts and novices, in the precision of technical actions, such as the pass, as well as in a methodology for the selection of athletes. Notably, of the most cited documents, two are reviews [65,66], one is a randomized controlled trial [67], one is a cross-sectional study [68], and, finally, six are experimental studies [7,69–73].

Table 2. Most cited articles.

Author and Publication Year	Type	Journal	Cat Q, Cat Rank JCR, JIC Cat 2023	Effects	Physio Outc	Phys Outc	Tact Outc	Techn Outc	Main Conclusions	Tot Cit	Av Cit per Year *
Rein and Memmert (2016) [65]	Narrative review	*Springerplus*	-	Big data and soccer tactics	Yes	Yes	Yes		The introduction of big data technologies will also require discussions within the research community about how to share data and techniques across research teams. Future soccer research will have to embrace a more robust multidisciplinary approach.	255	31.87
Smith et al. (2016) [67]	Article—randomized controlled Trial	*Journal of Sports Sciences*	Q1 31/127 Sport Sciences	Mental fatigue	Yes		Yes		Mental fatigue had unclear effects on most visual search behavior variables. The results suggest that mental fatigue impairs the accuracy and speed of soccer-specific decision-making. These impairments are unlikely to be related to changes in visual search behavior.	149	18.62
Romeas et al. (2016) [69]	Article—experimental design	*Psychology of Sport and Exercise*	Q1 21/127 Sport Sciences	Precision in passing decision-making			Yes	Yes	Training to process complex and dynamic visual scenes has not only revealed superior learning ability in soccer players but has also improved their passing decision-making accuracy in the field.	149	18.62
Roca et al. (2012) [70]	Article—experimental design	*Journal of Sports Sciences*	Q1 31/127 Sport Sciences	Acquisition of superior anticipation			Yes	Yes	The average hours accumulated per year during childhood in soccer-specific play activity were the strongest predictor of perceptual–cognitive expertise.	142	11.83
Roca et al. (2013) [7]	Article—experimental design	*Journal of Sport and Exercise Psychology*	Q2 59/114 Psychology, Applied	Perceptual–cognitive skills			Yes	Yes	Skilled players reported more accurate anticipation and decision-making than less skilled players, and their superior performance was underpinned by differences in task-specific search behaviors and thought processes.	99	9.00
Gonçalves et al. (2017) [71]	Article—experimental design	*Journal of Strength and Conditioning Research*	Q1 9/127 Sport Sciences	Restrictions on tactical behavior, physical, and physiological performances	Yes	Yes	Yes	Yes	The effects of limiting players' spatial exploration greatly impaired the coadaptation between teammates' positioning while decreasing their physical and physiological performances. These results allow for a better understanding of players' decision-making processes according to specific task rules.	97	13.85

Table 2. *Cont.*

Author and Publication Year	Type	Journal	Cat Q, Cat Rank JCR, JIC Cat 2023	Effects	Physio Outc	Phys Outc	Tact Outc	Techn Outc	Main Conclusions	Tot Cit	Av Cit per Year *
Qader et al. (2017) [66]	Review	*Measurement*	Q1 17/180 Engineering, Multidisciplinary	Methodology for football player selection	Yes	Yes	Yes	Yes	Three main groups of tests were utilized to assess the players: fitness, skills, and anthropometrics. This study improved the understanding of the measures as criteria for player selection. TOPSIS is an effective tool used to solve player selection problems.	67	9.57
Diaz del Campo et al. (2011) [68]	Article—cross-sectional study	*Perceptual and Motor Skills*	Q4 86/99 Psychology, Experimental	Differences between experts and novices			Yes	Yes	Expert players remained superior in decision-making ability when variation in skill execution was controlled. Decision-making differences between levels of expertise decreased with age regarding the first level (skill selection) and increased with age regarding the second level (tactical–context adaptation).	64	4.92
Furley and Memmert (2015) [72]	Article—experimental design	*Frontiers in Psychology*	Q2 62/218 Psychology, Multidisciplinary	Creativity and working memory			Yes	Yes	The pattern of results provided evidence that domain–general working memory capacity is not associated with creativity in a soccer-specific creativity task. Future research on the role of working memory in everyday creative performance needs to distinguish between different types of creative performance while also taking the role of domain-specific experience into account.	60	6.66
Lex et al. (2015) [73]	Article—experimental design	*PLoS One*	Q1 33/135 Multidisciplinary Sciences	Cognitive representations and cognitive processes			Yes	Yes	In contrast to less experienced soccer players, more experienced soccer players possess a functionally organized cognitive representation of team-specific tactics. Moreover, the more experienced soccer players reacted faster to tactical decisions because they needed fewer fixations of similar duration.	50	5.55

Note: The average number of citations per year was calculated from the date of publication to 8 July 2024 *. Cat Q: Category Quartile; Cat Rank JCR: Category Rank in Journal Citation Reports; JIC Cat 2023: Journal Indicator Citation 2023; Physio Outc: Physiological Outcomes; Phys Outc: Physical Outcomes; Tact Outc: Tactical Outcomes; Techn Outc: Technical Outcomes; Tot Cit: Total Citations; Av Cit per year: Average Citation per year; TOPSIS: technique for order performance by similarity to ideal solution.

One hundred seventy-two documents included in this study were identified; thus, to analyze the citations by documents, it was established that each document was cited at least 20 times. Only 48 documents exceeded the requested threshold; only 32 seemed connected. There are seven nodes where the most cited documents are those developed by Roca et al. [70], Romeas et al. [69], and Smith et al. [67] (Figure 5).

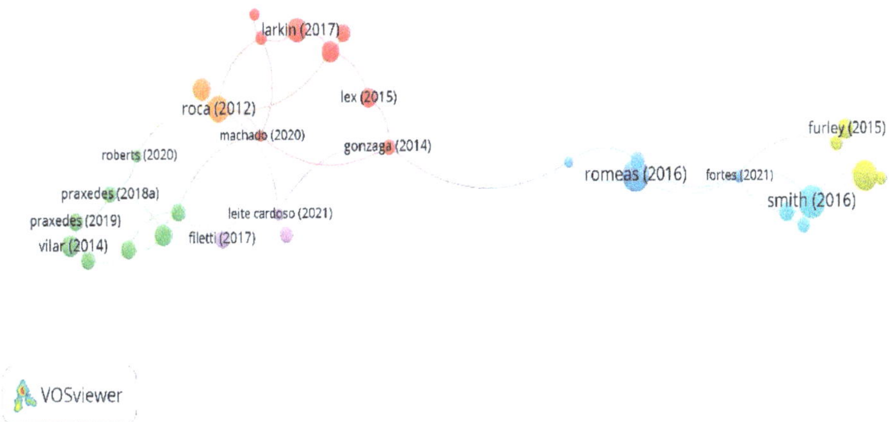

Figure 5. Citation of documents.

3.4. *H-Index*

The average number of citations per document was 19.79 (Figure 6).

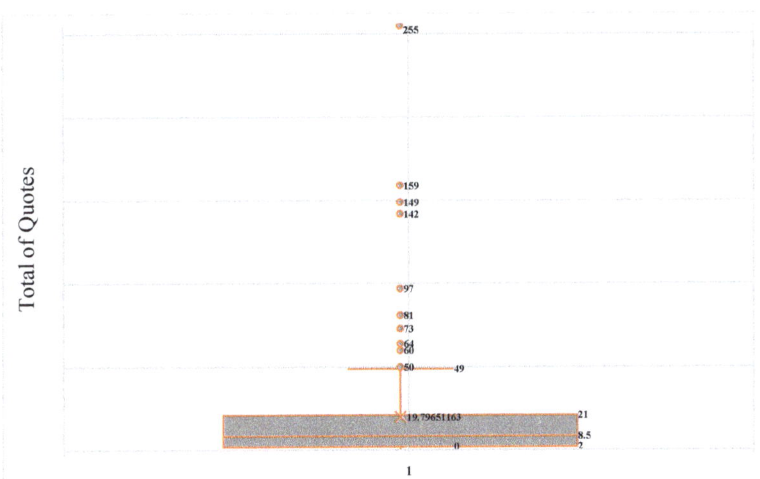

Figure 6. Number of citations as a function of the *H*-index.

3.5. *Author Analysis*

The academic cooperation evaluated in response to the number of authors shows that the most significant number of documents, close to half of the total scientific production, is between three and four authors. Moreover, the scientific production developed by six authors is greater than that carried out by one or two authors, which demonstrates the interest in favoring academic cooperation in search of the production of knowledge in the study of decision-making in football (Table 3).

Table 3. Total number of documents per author.

Number of Authors	Number of Studies	Percentage, %
1–2	28	16.27
3–4	77	44.76
5–6	44	25.58
7–8	17	9.88
≥9	6	3.48

Figure 7 shows the interactions produced between the citations by authors. Five hundred eighty-one authors were established, and only thirty authors have developed three studies with a minimum of 10 citations. The size of the nodes represents the number of documents published, and the color corresponds to the connections established in response to time. There was an intense concentration between the years 2018 and 2019 led by Gonzalez-Víllora, S., while between the years 2020 and 2021, a more significant number of networks were observed, with Teoldo, I., the one that received the highest number of citations in recent years.

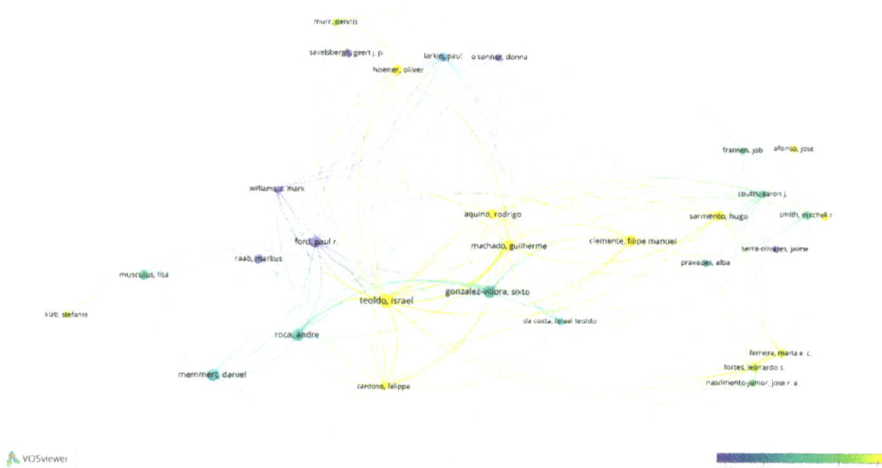

Figure 7. Citation by authors.

3.6. Keyword Analysis

For keyword occurrence, the word was included at least five times in each study. Thus, of the 807 words identified, only 62 met the threshold. The analysis of the most recurrent keywords refers to perceptual processes, anticipation, expertise, and performance. The most referenced concepts were "Anticipation", "Attention"," "Knowledge", "Decision Making", and "Skill". Between 2019 and 2020, the concepts used were "performance", "sport", and "decision-making" (Figure 8).

Finally, between 2020 and 2021, these most referenced concepts were "Talent Identification", "Mental Fatigue", "Cognition", "Visual Search", and "Demands". Thus, the most recent concepts are associated with competition evaluation processes, the development of programs related to game tactics, and the recognition of coaches' perceptions (Figure 8).

Moreover, according to the density map in Figure 9, the concepts related to the number of times that have been cited the most are "*Performance*" ($n = 68$), "*Sport*" ($n = 55$), "*Decision-Making*" ($n = 54$), "*Football*" ($n = 45$), "*Soccer*" ($n = 41$), "*Expertise*" ($n = 32$), "*Skill*" ($n = 23$), and "*Anticipation*" ($n = 22$).

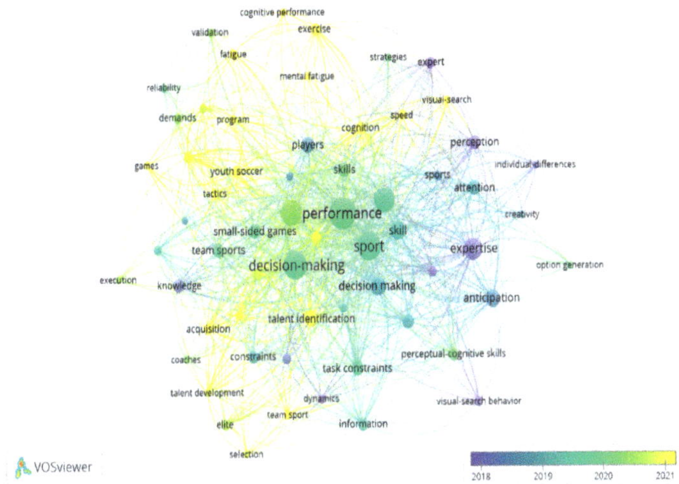

Figure 8. Occurrence by keywords in response to temporality.

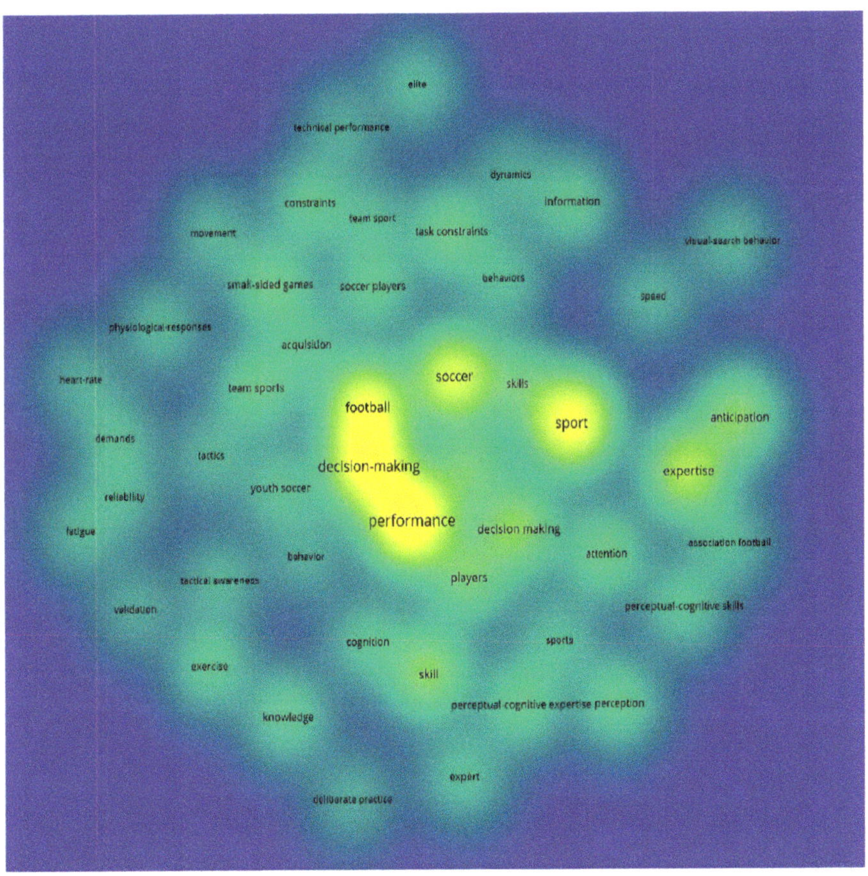

Figure 9. Occurrences by keywords in response to density.

3.7. Analysis of Cited Journals and References

Seventy-seven journals published the 172 documents found for this bibliometric review. To analyze the citations by journals, the journal was considered to have published at least two documents and received at least ten citations. Thus, only 21 magazines met the threshold. Similarly, in the citation map by journal, the journals with the most significant number of published documents are the *Journal of Sport Sciences* (ten documents and 437 citations), *PLoS ONE* (eleven documents and 349 citations), and *Psychology of Sport and Exercise* (seven documents and 259 citations) (Figure 10).

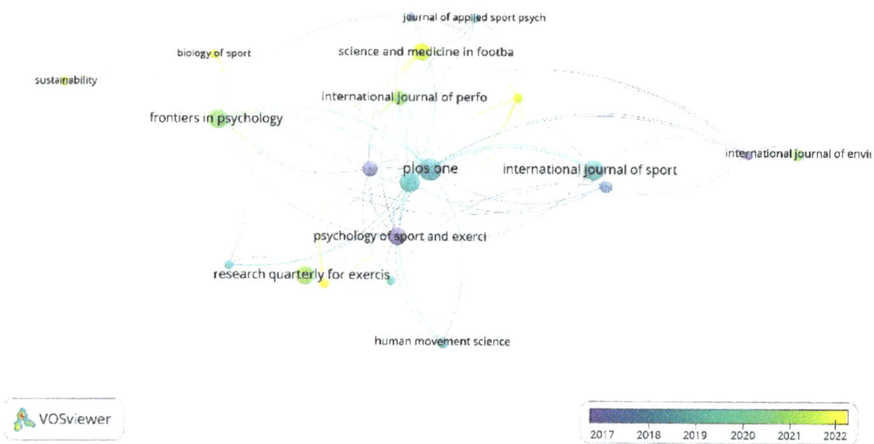

Figure 10. Citations by journal.

Similarly, for the analysis of the cocitations between the journals, 1921 sources were found, where it was established that the minimum number of citations for each journal was 20. Only 49 journals met the requested threshold (Figure 11). The journals with the highest number of citations are the *Journal of Sport Sciences* (n = 615), the *Journal of Sport and Exercise Psychology* (n = 220), *Psychology of Sport and Exercise* (n = 206), and *Sports Medicine* (n = 189).

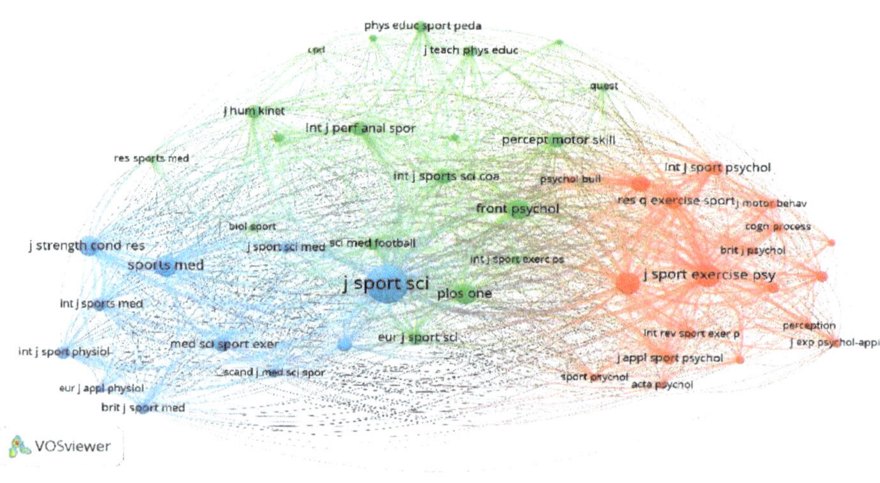

Figure 11. Cocitations by journals.

The analysis of the cited references reveals that there are 5251, 45 of which have been cited at least ten times. These methods were developed by Mann et al. [74], Vaeyens et al. [75], and Roca et al. [76] (Figure 12).

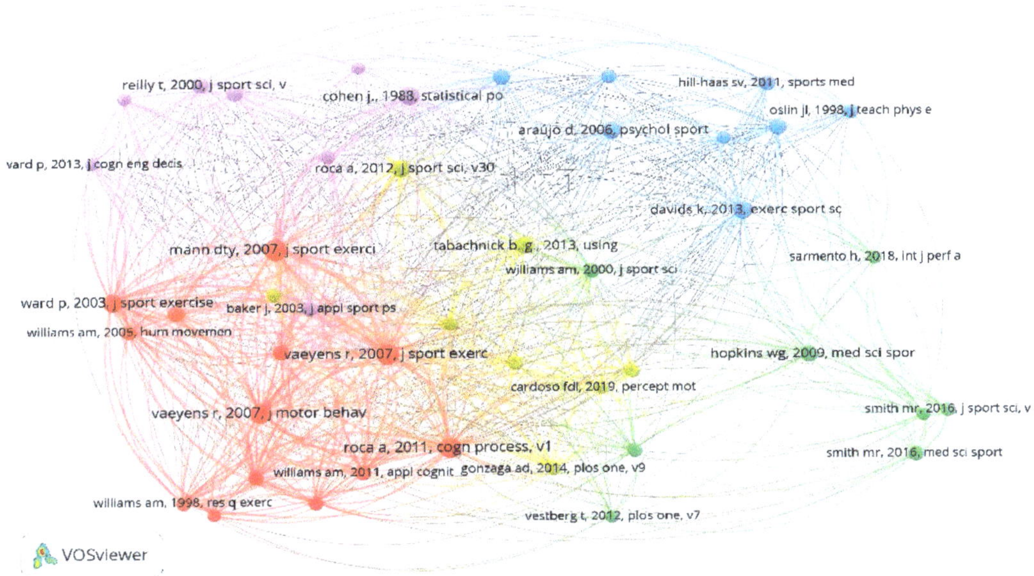

Figure 12. Nodes by cited references.

3.8. Analysis of Publishing Groups

The scientific production by the publishers that publish scientific knowledge on the study of decision-making in football reveals how Taylor & Francis is the publishing group that publishes the most significant number of documents and, in turn, receives the most significant number of citations. It also details how five publishers have received more than 300 citations (Taylor & Francis, Elsevier, Springer, Public Library Science, Human Kinetics). The first four publishers represent half of the total scientific production (51.74%), and in turn, four publishers have received more than 1000 citations (Table 4).

Table 4. Total number of documents published by the editorial groups.

Name	Number of Documents	Number of Citations
Taylor & Francis	42	926
Elsevier	19	454
Frontiers Media SA	15	140
Multidisciplinary Digital Publishing Institute (MDPI)	13	65
Springer	11	407
Public Library Science	11	349
Sage Publications Ltd.a.	11	164
Human Kinetics Publ INC	8	325
Federación Española Asociación Docentes Educación Física	6	7
Termedia Publishing House Ltd.a.	3	24
Total: 10 editorials	139/172	2861

3.9. *Areas of Knowledge*

The analysis of the areas of knowledge where the documents on the study of decision-making in football are published reveals that the most prolific and cited areas are hospitality, leisure, sport, and tourism, with an average of 15.40; sport sciences, with 21.89; and multidisciplinary sciences, with 50.33 citations per published document. Similarly, the first two areas cover more than half of the published documents (55.81%), which reflects the scientific community's interest in developing this type of study associated with specific areas (Table 5).

Table 5. Areas of knowledge according to Web of Science categories.

Areas *	Number of Publications	Number of Citations
Hospitality, Leisure, Sport, and Tourism	49	755
Sport Sciences	47	1029
Psychology	23	403
Multidisciplinary Sciences	12	604
Neurosciences	10	96
5 Areas	141/172	2887

Note: * The same item may be considered in more than one area.

3.10. *Language and Country Analysis*

The analysis by language shows that the most significant production is generated in English (n = 166), with 96.51% of the total scientific production, followed by Spanish (n = 5), with 2.90%, and Portuguese. In addition, among the 172 documents reviewed and included in this bibliometric study, only one study that was different from English and Spanish (Portuguese) was found. Figure 13 establishes the citations of documents by country. Only 40 countries have contributed to the knowledge of decision-making. To establish the threshold, each country was determined to have published at least two studies and received ten citations.

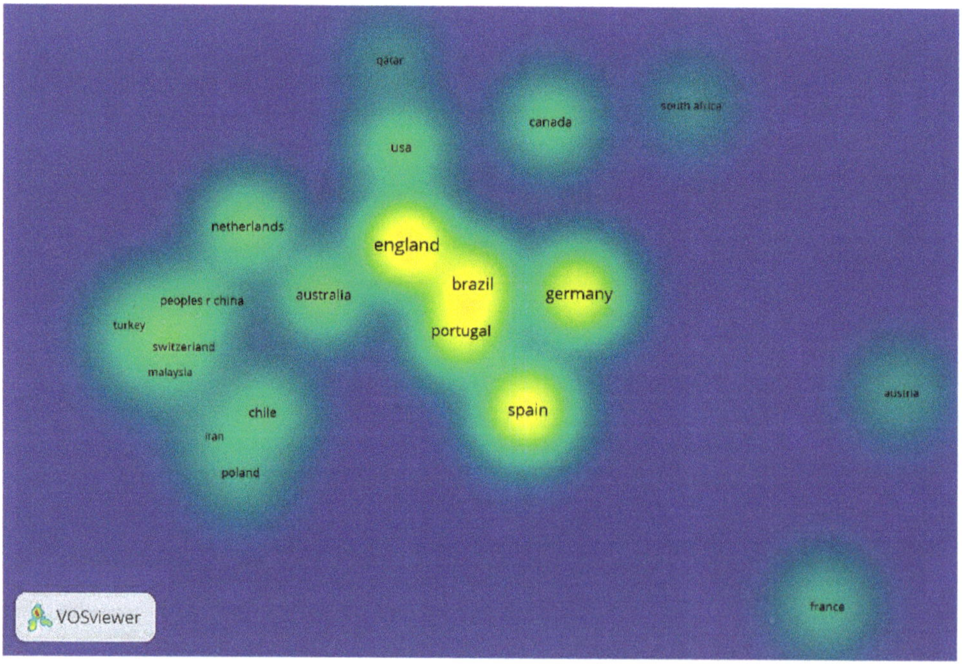

Figure 13. Citation by country.

Thus, only 22 countries met the threshold. The countries that receive the greatest number of documents and citations are England (n = 46 documents and 996 citations), Germany (n = 32 documents and 749 citations), Spain (n = 38 documents and 597 citations), Portugal (n = 27 documents and 481 citations), and Brazil (n = 34 documents and 395 appointments). Specifically, several European countries (Poland, Switzerland, Turkey, Netherlands), Asian countries (China, Malaysia, Iran, Qatar), Africa (South Africa), South America (Chile), North America (Canada, United States), and Oceania (Australia) are increasing their scientific production in the study of decision-making in football. Finally, there are countries on each of the continents, which highlights the importance of this theme among the scientific–academic community.

3.11. Organizations

It is recognized that 313 organizations have been studying decision-making in football. Only 60 organizations have published at least two studies and have received at least ten citations. Specifically, German Sport University Cologne is the organization that has the most publications and citations (n = 19 and 531). Owing to the weather (2016–2018), there is a strong trend among European universities, among which German Sport University Cologne and Liverpool John Moores University stand out. Between 2020 and 2022, there was a strong trend of Brazilian and Portuguese universities, of which the following stand out: the Federal University of Viçosa, the University of São Paulo, the University of Coimbra, and Juiz de Fora Federal University (Figure 14).

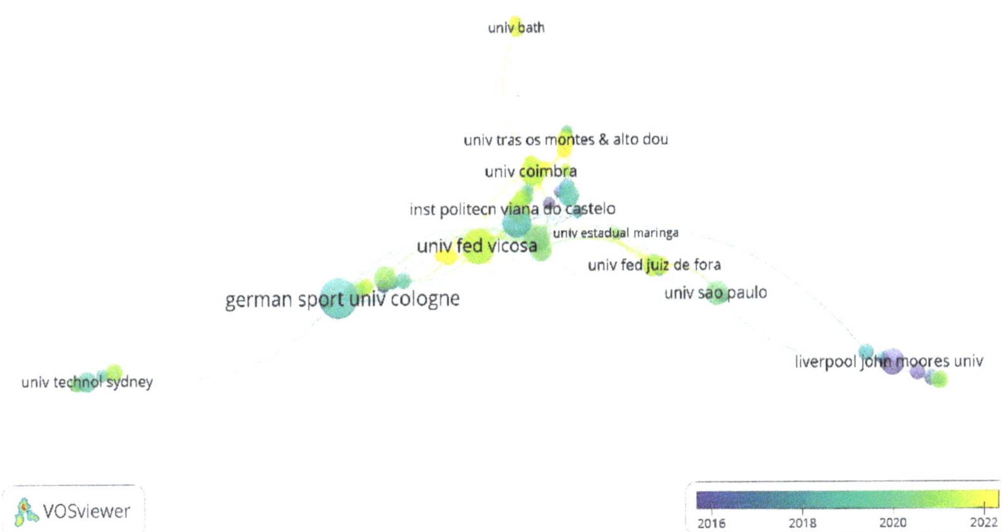

Figure 14. Coauthorship by organizations.

4. Discussion

4.1. Main Findings by Bibliometric Criteria

To our knowledge, this is the first study that performs a bibliometric analysis on scientific publications related to decision-making in soccer. Therefore, by analyzing the evolution and trend of the number of studies related to decision-making in soccer in the last 15 years, the following findings were determined. (1) A total of 172 documents related to the study of decision-making were published between 2010 and July 2024. (2) The number of studies increased by 633.33% between 2010 and 2024, and, in turn, the years with the highest production were between 2021 and 2024. (3) There is a preference for developing research articles (89.53%), with a small percentage of review studies. The years 2016 and 2017 received the most appointments. Documents that have received at least 50 citations are preferably research articles and have been published in Q1 journals. From 2010 to 2024, only two review studies were reported, and no meta-analytical study, scoping review, or bibliometric analysis was reported. At least ten studies have received 50 appointments. (4) The average number of citations per document was 19.79. (5) Half of the total scientific production was carried out by between three and four authors (44.76%). Five hundred eighty-one authors were established; only thirty authors have developed three studies and have a minimum of 10 citations. Between 2018 and 2019, scientific production was led by Gonzalez-Villora, S., whereas between the years 2020 and 2021, there was a greater number of networks. Teoldo, I. is the one who has received the highest number of citations in recent times. (6) The most recent concepts are associated with competition evaluation processes, the development of programs related to game tactics, and the recognition of coaches' perceptions. These are performance, sport, decision-making, football, soccer, expertise, skill, and anticipation. (7) A total of 77 journals published the 172 documents identified in this bibliometric review. The journals that have published the greatest number of documents are the *Journal of Sport Sciences*, *PLoS One*, and *Psychology of Sport and Exercise*. For the analysis of the cocitations between the journals, 1921 sources were found, so the journals with the highest number of citations are the *Journal of Sport Sciences*, the *Journal of Sport and Exercise Psychology*, *Psychology of Sport and Exercise*, and *Sports Medicine*. (8) Taylor & Francis is the publishing group that has published the most documents and received the most citations. (9) The most developed areas, according to the WoS Core, are first, hospitality, leisure, sport, and tourism, and second, sport sciences. (10) Studies on decision-making in soccer have been published in three different languages, with English being the predominant language. (11) A total of 313 organizations have been studying decision-making in football. Only 60 organizations have published at least two studies and have received at least ten citations. The leading institutions are the German Sport University Cologne, Liverpool John Moores University, the Federal University of Viçosa, the University of São Paulo, the University of Coimbra, and the Juiz de Fora Federal University. (12) The evaluated sample mainly consists of studies of professional players, with a low percentage of studies of children (6–12 years) and women's soccer.

4.2. Some Considerations from Major Studies

The increase in studies in specific time windows that study football via bibliometric analyses reveals a preference for the study of research articles over review studies. This is what is detailed in the study developed by García-Angulo and Ortega [77] when studying the scientific production of the soccer goalkeeper. These results are associated with other bibliometric studies that demonstrate similar findings in the studies of small-sided games (SSGs) in soccer [54], youth soccer [52], biomechanics in soccer [78], and research trends and future directions of women's football [79] when the studies between 2010 and 2023 are analyzed. This demonstrates the interest of different professionals in producing knowledge about the study of soccer.

Another of the main findings shows that the number of publications has gradually increased, especially in empirical research studies. In contrast, the number of review studies does not exceed 10% of the total production, like those found in other bibliometric studies on plyometrics in sport [80] and relative age [81]. In this way, the results reported by this bibliometric analysis can be used by different researchers to develop research in less explored themes and fields of study, even more so when the existence of any study related to the development of meta-analytical reviews or scoping reviews on decision-making in football is reported. In contrast, there are different scoping reviews on existing tests to evaluate knowledge and tactical performance in soccer players [82], revealing that there are approximately 29 tests/instruments that allow for the evaluation of the tactical domain beyond the investigative approach and the method of information collection.

A bibliometric study analyzing the 100 most cited articles on sports medicine and exercise revealed that the two most studied anatomical areas were the knee and the brain. At the same time, a narrative review was the most common study [55]. This demonstrates the importance of specificity when studying different areas of knowledge since, for the analysis of decision-making in soccer, the two most studied themes are performance, expertise, and skill. The contribution of bibliometric analyses implies the importance of the findings presented in this type of study because they offer a global overview of the state of the scientific evidence [83].

The studies of the most cited articles also reveal the use of technology [13] for monitoring, and the results are associated with determining the influence of physical, physiological, technical, and tactical variables [71,84]. Among these relationships, game performance is associated with technical–tactical skills (e.g., passing, ball driving, marking, tackling, and intercepting) and decision-making adapted to the context of the game situation [68]. Likewise, the two investigative tendencies found in the study of decision-making in football establish, on the one hand, the study of perceptual–cognitive skills [85], such as mental fatigue, creativity, work memory, and anticipation; on the other hand, the study of decision-making in the technical–tactical performance of athletes is evident, through precision, the factors that condition the pass [86], tactical awareness [87], and tactical decision-making [88].

In the same way as the two investigative trends identified, the study developed by Teoldo et al. [89] relates to fatigue and visual peripheral perception, demonstrating that physical fatigue is conditioning when making faster decisions in association with the tactical actions that players must execute and that, in essence, physical fatigue influences only the response time to make decisions. In this sense, the influence of peripheral perception, physical performance, and tactical behavior in soccer players has been defined so that acute physical fatigue does not influence peripheral perception; however, both physical performance and tactical behaviors are diminished, causing errors in defensive movements and a decrease in offensive tactical actions close to the ball [90]. Moreover, a study by de Souza Fortes et al. [91] revealed that the mental fatigue produced by playing video games before competition affects decision-making in professional players.

By this, studies on the effects of fatigue on performance [92] demonstrate a tendency toward the use of objective indicators for its evaluation, demonstrating that stressful environments produced by heat or stress tend to increase the likelihood that athletes make mistakes in decision-making in situations where they commonly do not perform them [93]. Another systematic and meta-analytical review on the effects of mental fatigue on career performance and tactical behavior concluded that mental fatigue has no effect on the total running distance and tactical behavior expressed by players in the SSG [94]. This is perhaps one of the main contributions of this bibliometric review study because it helps to favor the current panorama of research trends from keywords, the analysis of the most cited studies, the countries that develop the most studies, and the organizations/institutions and authors that have been leading scientific production. With this, it is concluded that there are physical capacities (asymmetries, changes in direction, jumps, accelerations, decelerations), sex (female), population groups (children's soccer, youth soccer), countries of the continents (South American, Asian, African), and concepts that need more excellent research development. All of this is because sports performance is a process through which athletes develop specific psychological behaviors and activities [95,96].

These results highlight the importance of understanding decision-making from different perspectives, so more research is needed to determine the effect and influence of the moment of the competition, the result, the local or visitor play, the title or emergence, age, and sex, among other factors. However, this type of specific knowledge provided by different studies must be adapted to the specific needs of those who guide the preparation process and the transfer of this scientific knowledge to a practical and daily task of the coach and the athlete [97]. Thus, the main gaps in the literature such as greater international cooperation and further development of studies on women's soccer, youth soccer, and children's soccer will allow the establishment of lines of research that focus on the study of decision-making in different contexts of training and competition from observational studies, case studies, and longitudinal studies. It is also necessary to further develop qualitative studies that help us to understand the perceptions of decision-making from the perspective of the coach–athlete.

4.3. Emerging Concepts and Instruments Used for the Evaluation of Decision-Making

Finally, it has been confirmed that a study that deepens a theme can expand the research horizons, revealing that there are emerging concepts associated with decision-making and the identification and selection of sports talent. Among them are "*Constraints*", "*Acquisition*", "*Visual-Search*", "*Program*", "*Cognitive performance*", and "*Tactics*". To carry out different studies related to the evaluation of decision-making in soccer players of different ages, there are scientifically validated technological tools that allow for the evaluation of performance. Among them is the soccer tactical evaluation system (FUT-SAT) that allows for the analysis of the fundamental principles of the game [98]. Other instruments that can be used are the Game Performance Assessment Instrument (GPAI) that allows for the evaluation of four specific domains (game performance, support, decision-making, skill execution) [99], the Performance Assessment in Team Sports (TSAP) [100], the Game Performance Evaluation Tool (GPET) [101], and the TacticUP Video Test for Soccer [13].

4.4. Future Perspectives

The consideration of decision-making as a study theme has increased the research that has been developed to understand soccer's technical–tactical behavior. However, very few studies with multivariate designs allow us to understand the relationships established between decision-making and other skills, characteristics, and processes. Thus, future studies could explore this panorama and provide more significant contributions to the influence that decision-making has on players' sports performance, health, and well being.

Given the future perspectives of studies focused on evaluating, identifying, and recognizing the contributions of the study of decision-making, specifically on perceptual–cognitive skills and technical–tactical components in different population samples, the need arises to carry out a more significant number of review studies, including meta-analyses, scoping reviews, and more specific bibliometric analyses. Similarly, in evaluating athletes, it is necessary to develop a greater number of randomized controlled trials, longitudinal designs, and case studies that provide a greater understanding of the effects of decision-making on other physical, technical, tactical, physiological, psychological capacities, etc.

4.5. Limitations

This study presents different limitations associated with the heterogeneity of population samples and evaluated characteristics, the denomination with which decision-making is studied, and the variables that are related. Another bias of the present study was that only the review of documents in primary databases such as WoS, PubMed, Scopus, and SPORTDiscus were considered; therefore, it is recommended that future bibliometric studies on this topic review the information in other databases to obtain a deeper understanding of the topic under study. In addition, other limitations arise, and to reduce bias, future research should consider the analysis of the language of publication, open-access documents, searching in other databases, and using other search concepts to study decision-making.

5. Conclusions

Literature specializing in the study of decision-making in football prefers the study of technical and tactical variables and, to a lesser extent, physical and physiological variables. By studying the most cited studies, it is confirmed that empirical studies and very few review studies prevail. There is a strong tendency of South American authors and organizations/institutions, mainly Brazilians, to study decision-making. Two critical approaches have been carried out in the study of decision-making: one is related to the perceptual–cognitive skills evaluated in the laboratory and the field through working memory, creativity, and mental fatigue, whereas the second approach is more associated with the manifestation of the technical–tactical behaviors of the players, which are evaluated from the use of video or tests on tactical knowledge. By studying the terms used for the study of decision-making, the investigative trends related to sports performance are oriented as follows: *"Talent identification"*, *"Youth Soccer"*, *"Games"*, *"Coaches"*, *"Cognition"*, *"Speed"*, *"Validation"*, *"Reliability"*, and *"Program"*. Research trends suggest that the study of decision-making should be addressed through interdisciplinary approaches or applied in sport training contexts. On the other hand, the central countries that have been leading in scientific production are also the countries with the most important leagues, among which the following stand out: "England", "Spain", "Germany", "Portugal", and "Brazil". This highlights the importance of interdisciplinary and transdisciplinary research in the study of decision-making in soccer.

The scientific evidence must allow us to glimpse the effects of different training protocols on the induced adaptations for samples identified in the present study as female soccer athletes. In the context of soccer, this type of study could help determine how decision-making helps us to understand the relationship with other variables associated with the physical and mental health of athletes at different ages and levels. The control of training load from the study of decision-making is an essential component in any training process to promote the health and well-being of all athletes. With this, the analysis of decision-making would help coaches and technical staff to consider individualized follow-ups to reduce the stress produced in competition and to think about interdisciplinary support to promote healthy habits and active lifestyles outside the training–competition spaces.

Author Contributions: Conceptualization: J.D.P.U., B.A.B.-P. and G.M.; methodology: J.D.P.U. and B.A.B.-P.; formal analysis: J.D.P.U., B.A.B.-P. and A.V-B.; investigation: J.D.P.U., B.A.B.-P. and J.O.-A.; data curation: J.D.P.U., B.A.B.-P., J.O.-A. and D.R-V; writing—original draft preparation: J.D.P.U., B.A.B.-P., A.V.-B., J.O.-A., R.Y.-S., J.F.L.-G. and G.M.; writing—review and editing: J.D.P.U., B.A.B.-P., J.O.-A., R.Y.-S., A.V.-B., D.R.-V., J.F.L.-G. and G.M.; visualization: J.D.P.U., B.A.B.-P., J.O.-A., R.Y.-S., A.V.-B., D.R.-V., J.F.L.-G. and G.M. All authors have read and agreed to the published version of the manuscript.

Funding: This research received no external funding.

Data Availability Statement: Data supporting the findings of this study are available from the corresponding author upon reasonable request.

Conflicts of Interest: The authors have no conflicts of interest.

References

1. Oh, Y.; Yoo, J.I. Team Cohesion in Individual/Team Sports Athletes: Transformational Leadership and the Role of Social norms. *Healthcare* **2023**, *11*, 792. [CrossRef] [PubMed]

2. Gréhaighne, J.F.; Godbout, P. Tactical Knowledge in Team Sports from a Constructivist and Cognitivist Perspective. *Quest* **1995**, *47*, 490–505. [CrossRef]
3. Wang, X.; Wang, Y.; Zhang, Z. Cultivation Model of Football Training Group Cohesion from the Perspective of Group Psychology. *Entertain. Comput.* **2024**, *49*, 100626. [CrossRef]
4. Ashford, M.; Abraham, A.; Poolton, J. Understanding a Player's Decision-Making Process in Team Sports: A Systematic Review of Empirical Evidence. *Sports* **2021**, *9*, 65. [CrossRef]
5. Williams, A.M.; Jackson, R.C. *Anticipation and Decision-Making in Sport*, 1st ed.; Routledge Ltd.: Milton, FL, USA, 2019. [CrossRef]
6. Abernethy, B.; Gill, D.P.; Parks, S.L.; Packer, S.T. Expertise and the Perception of Kinematic and Situational Probability Information. *Perception* **2001**, *30*, 233–252. [CrossRef]
7. Roca, A.; Ford, P.R.; McRobert, A.P.; Williams, A.M. Perceptual-Cognitive Skills and Their Interaction as a Function of Task Constraints in Soccer. *J. Sport Exerc. Psychol.* **2013**, *35*, 144–155. [CrossRef]
8. Oliva-Lozano, J.M.; Maraver, E.F.; Fortes, V.; Muyor, J.M. Kinematic Analysis of the Postural Demands in Professional Soccer Match Play Using Inertial Measurement Units. *Sensors* **2020**, *20*, 5971. [CrossRef]
9. Beernaerts, J.; De Baets, B.; Lenoir, M.; Van de Weghe, N. Spatial Movement Pattern Recognition in Soccer Based on Relative Player Movements. *PLoS ONE* **2020**, *15*, e0227746. [CrossRef]
10. Güldenpenning, I.; Kunde, W.; Weigelt, M. How to Trick Your Opponent: A Review Article on Deceptive Actions in Interactive Sports. *Front. Psychol.* **2017**, *8*, 917. [CrossRef]
11. Jackson, R.C.; Barton, H.; Bishop, D.T. Knowledge is Power? Outcome Probability Information Impairs Detection of Deceptive Intent. *Psychol. Sport Exer.* **2020**, *50*, 101744. [CrossRef]
12. Gonçalves, E.; Noce, F.; Barbosa, M.A.M.; Figueiredo, A.J.; Hackfort, D.; Teoldo, I. Correlation of the Peripheral Perception With the Maturation and the Effect of the Peripheral Perception on the Tactical Behaviour of Soccer Players. *Int. J. Sport Exerc. Psychol.* **2020**, *18*, 687–699. [CrossRef]
13. Machado, G.; da Costa, I.T. TacticUP Video Test for Soccer: Development and Validation. *Front. Psychol.* **2020**, *11*, 1690. [CrossRef] [PubMed]
14. Sun, H.; Soh, K.G.; Xu, X. Nature Scenes Counter Mental Fatigue-Induced Performance Decrements in Soccer Decision-Making. *Front. Psychol.* **2022**, *13*, 877844. [CrossRef]
15. Cardoso, F.D.S.L.; González-Villora, S.; Guilherme, J.; Teoldo, I. Young Soccer Players With Higher Tactical Knowledge Display Lower Cognitive Effort. *Percept. Mot. Ski.* **2019**, *126*, 499–514. [CrossRef]
16. Dambroz, F.; Teoldo, I. Better Decision-Making Skills Support Tactical Behaviour and Reduce Physical Wear Under Physical Fatigue in Soccer. *Front. Physiol.* **2023**, *14*, 1116924. [CrossRef]
17. Raya-González, J.; Pulido, J.J.; Beato, M.; Ponce-Bordón, J.C.; López Del Campo, R.; Resta, R.; García-Calvo, T. Analysis of the Effect of Injuries on Match Performance Variables in Professional Soccer Players: A Retrospective, Experimental Longitudinal Design. *Sports Med. Open* **2022**, *8*, 31. [CrossRef]
18. Barte, J.C.M.; Nieuwenhuys, A.; Geurts, S.A.E.; Kompier, M.A.J. Motivation Counteracts Fatigue-Induced Performance Decrements in Soccer Passing Performance. *J. Sports Sci.* **2019**, *37*, 1189–1196. [CrossRef]
19. Roca, A.; Ford, P.R. Decision-Making Practice During Coaching Sessions in Elite Youth Football Across European Countries. *Sci. Med. Footb.* **2020**, *4*, 263–268. [CrossRef]
20. Machado, G.; González-Villora, S.; Teoldo, I. The Relationship Between Deliberate Practice, Play, and Futsal in Childhood and Adolescence and the Development of Different Decision-Making Skills in Professional Female Soccer Players. *Psychol. Sport Exerc.* **2023**, *68*, 102470. [CrossRef]
21. Fenner, J.; Doncaster, G.; McRobert, A.; Ford, P.; Iga, J.; Unnithan, V. A Preliminary Investigation into the Evaluation of Possession-Based Small-Sided Games and the Influence of Decision-Making Ability in Identifying Talented Pre-Pubertal Soccer Players. *Apunt. Sports Med.* **2022**, *57*, 100378. [CrossRef]
22. DE Dios-Álvarez, V.; Lorenzo-Martínez, M.; Padrón-Cabo, A.; Rey, E. Small-Sided Games in Female Soccer Players: A Systematic Review. *J. Sports Med. Phys. Fit.* **2022**, *62*, 1474–1480. [CrossRef] [PubMed]
23. Holfelder, B.; Klotzbier, T.J.; Eisele, M.; Schott, N. Hot and Cool Executive Function in Elite- and Amateur- Adolescent Athletes from Open and Closed Skills Sports. *Front. Psychol.* **2020**, *11*, 694. [CrossRef] [PubMed]
24. Heppe, H.; Kohler, A.; Fleddermann, M.T.; Zentgraf, K. The Relationship Between Expertise in Sports, Visuospatial, and Basic Cognitive Skills. *Front. Psychol.* **2016**, *7*, 904. [CrossRef] [PubMed]
25. Gantois, P.; Caputo Ferreira, M.E.; Lima-Junior, D.; Nakamura, F.Y.; Batista, G.R.; Fonseca, F.S.; Fortes, L.S. Effects of Mental Fatigue on Passing Decision-Making Performance in Professional Soccer Athletes. *Eur. J. Sport Sci.* **2020**, *20*, 534–543. [CrossRef]
26. Soylu, Y.; Ramazanoglu, F.; Arslan, E.; Clemente, F. Effects of Mental Fatigue on the Psychophysiological Responses, Kinematic Profiles, and Technical Performance in Different Small-Sided Soccer Games. *Biol. Sport* **2022**, *39*, 965–972. [CrossRef]

27. Fortes, L.S.; De Lima-Junior, D.; Fiorese, L.; Nascimento-Júnior, J.R.A.; Mortatti, A.L.; Ferreira, M.E.C. The Effect of Smartphones and Playing Video Games on Decision-Making in Soccer Players: A Crossover and Randomised Study. *J. Sport Sci.* **2020**, *38*, 552–558. [CrossRef]
28. Trecroci, A.; Boccolini, G.; Duca, M.; Formenti, D.; Alberti, G. Mental Fatigue Impairs Physical Activity, Technical and Decision-Making Performance During Small-Sided Games. *PLoS ONE* **2020**, *15*, e0238461. [CrossRef]
29. Bennett, K.J.M.; Novak, A.R.; Pluss, M.A.; Coutts, A.J.; Fransen, J. Assessing the Validity of a Video-Based Decision-Making Assessment for Talent Identification in Youth Soccer. *J. Sci. Med. Sport* **2019**, *22*, 729–734. [CrossRef]
30. Calle-Jaramillo, G.A.; Gonzalez-Palacio, E.V.; Perez-Mendez, L.A.; Rojas-Jaramillo, A.; Gonzalez-Jurado, J.A. Design and Validation of a Test to Evaluate the Execution Time and Decision-Making in Technical-Tactical Football Actions (Passing and Driving). *Behav. Sci.* **2023**, *13*, 101. [CrossRef]
31. Iuliano, E.; Bonavolontà, V.; Ferrari, D.; Bragazzi, N.; Capasso, B.; Kuvačić, G.; De Giorgio, A. The Decision-Making in Dribbling: A Video Analysis Study of U10 Soccer Players' Skills and Coaches' Quality Evaluation. *Front. Psychol.* **2023**, *14*, 1200208. [CrossRef]
32. Pu, Z.; Pan, Y.; Wang, S.; Liu, B.; Chen, M.; Ma, H.; Cui, Y. Orientation and Decision-Making for Soccer Based on Sports Analytics and AI: A Systematic Review. *J. Autom. Sin.* **2024**, *11*, 37–57. [CrossRef]
33. Romeas, T.; Chaumillon, R.; Labbé, D.; Faubert, J. Combining 3D-MOT With Sport Decision-Making for Perceptual-Cognitive Training in Virtual Reality. *Percep. Mot. Ski.* **2019**, *126*, 922–948. [CrossRef]
34. Harenberg, S.; McCarver, Z.; Worley, J.; Murr, D.; Vosloo, J.; Kakar, R.S.; McCaffrey, R.; Dorsch, K.; Höner, O. The Effectiveness of 3D Multiple Object Tracking Training on Decision-Making in Soccer. *Sci. Med. Footb.* **2022**, *6*, 355–362. [CrossRef] [PubMed]
35. Gou, Q.; Li, S. Study on the Correlation Between Basketball Players' Multiple-Object Tracking Ability and Sports Decision-Making. *PLoS ONE* **2023**, *18*, e0283965. [CrossRef] [PubMed]
36. Slimani, M.; Nikolaidis, P.T. Anthropometric and Physiological Characteristics of Male Soccer Players According to their Competitive Level, Playing Position and Age Group: A Systematic Review. *J. Sports Med. Phys. Fit.* **2019**, *59*, 141–163. [CrossRef]
37. Arjol-Serrano, J.L.; Lampre, M.; Díez, A.; Castillo, D.; Sanz-López, F.; Lozano, D. The Influence of Playing Formation on Physical Demands and Technical-Tactical Actions According to Playing Positions in an Elite Soccer Team. *Int. J. Environ. Res. Public Health* **2021**, *18*, 4148. [CrossRef]
38. Piechota, K.; Majorczyk, E. Decision-Making Time and Neuromuscular Coordination in Youth and Senior Soccer Goalkeepers. *Sensors* **2023**, *23*, 4483. [CrossRef]
39. Furley, P.; Noël, B.; Memmert, D. Attention Towards the Goalkeeper and Distraction During Penalty Shootouts in Association Football: A Retrospective Analysis of Penalty Shootouts from 1984 to 2012. *J. Sports Sci.* **2017**, *35*, 873–879. [CrossRef]
40. Van der Kamp, J.; Dicks, M.; Navia, J.A.; Noël, B. Goalkeeping in the Soccer Penalty Kick. *Ger. J. Exerc. Sport Res.* **2018**, *48*, 169–175. [CrossRef]
41. Gréhaighne, J.F.; Godbout, P.; Bouthier, D. The Teaching and Learning of Decision Making in Team Sports. *Quest* **2001**, *53*, 59–76. [CrossRef]
42. Baker, J.; Cote, J.; Abernethy, B. Learning from the Experts: Practice Activities of Expert Decision Makers in Sport. *Res. Q. Exerc. Sport.* **2003**, *74*, 342–347. [CrossRef] [PubMed]
43. van Maarseveen, M.J.J.; Oudejans, R.R.D.; Mann, D.L.; Savelsbergh, G.J.P. Perceptual-Cognitive Skill and the in Situ Performance of Soccer Players. *Q. J. Exp. Psychol.* **2018**, *71*, 455–470. [CrossRef] [PubMed]
44. McLoughlin, E.J.M.; Broadbent, D.P.; Kinrade, N.P.; Coughlan, E.K.; Bishop, D.T. Factors Affecting Decision-Making in Gaelic Football: A Focus Group Approach. *Front. Psychol.* **2023**, *14*, 1142508. [CrossRef] [PubMed]
45. Silva, A.F.; Conte, D.; Clemente, F.M. Decision-Making in Youth Team-Sports Players: A Systematic Review. *Int. J. Environ. Res. Public Health* **2020**, *17*, 3803. [CrossRef]
46. Gleeson, E.; Kelly, S. Phenomenal Decision-Making in Elite Soccer: Making the Unseen seen. *Sci. Med. Footb.* **2020**, *4*, 1–9. [CrossRef]
47. Ato, M.; López-García, J.J.; Benavente, A. A Classification System for Research Designs in Psychology. *Ann. Psychol.* **2013**, *57429*, 1038–1059. [CrossRef]
48. Hernández-Torrano, D.; Ho, Y.S. A Bibliometric Analysis of Publications in the Web of Science Category of Educational Psychology in the Last Two Decades. *Psicol. Educ.* **2021**, *27*, 101–113. [CrossRef]
49. Becerra Patiño, B.A.; Paucar Uribe, J.D.; Martínez-Benítez, C.F.; Gamonales, J.M. Determination of the Scientific Productivity of the Spanish Journal Retos According to Bibliometric Indicators: (2016–2024). *Retos* **2024**, *58*, 670–682. [CrossRef]
50. Adán, L.; García-Angulo, A.; Gómez-Ruano, M.A.; Sainz de Baranda, P.; Ortega-Toro, E. Bibliometric Analysis of Scientific Production in Female Football. *J. Sport Health Res.* **2020**, *12*, 302–317.
51. Clemente, F.M. Bibliometric Analysis of Scientific Production in Small-Sided Games. *Hum. Mov.* **2023**, *24*, 1–17. [CrossRef]
52. Liu, B.; Zhou, C.J.; Ma, H.W.; Gong, B. Mapping the Youth Soccer: A Bibliometrix Analysis Using R-tool. *Digit. Health.* **2023**, *9*, 20552076231183550. [CrossRef] [PubMed]

53. Martínez-Benítez, C.F.; Becerra-Patiño, B. A comprehensive bibliometric analysis of small-sided games in soccer: 20 years (2003–2023) of scientific exploration. *J. Phys. Educ. Sport* **2023**, *23*, 2620–2631. [CrossRef]
54. Martínez Benítez, C.F.; Becerra-Patiño, B.; Rada-Perdigon, D.A. Mapping the Research Trend in the Web of Science on Small-Sided Games in Soccer: A Bibliometric Study Between 2010–2023. *Retos* **2024**, *55*, 363–378. [CrossRef]
55. Khatra, O.; Shadgan, A.; Taunton, J.; Pakravan, A.; Shadgan, B. A Bibliometric Analysis of the Top Cited Articles in Sports and Exercise Medicine. *Orthop. J. Sports Med.* **2021**, *9*, 2325967120969902. [CrossRef]
56. Becerra-Patiño, B.A.; Paucar-Uribe, J.D.; Olivares-Arancibia, J.; Ojeda-Aravena, A.; Yáñez-Sepúlveda, R.; Gamonales, J.M.; López-Gil, J.F.; Hernández-Beltrán, V. Mapping the Knowledge of Research Trends in Sports Performance Asymmetries from 2015 to 2024: A Bibliometric Study and Analysis of the Most-Cited Papers. *Sports* **2025**, *13*, 93. [CrossRef]
57. Salinas-Ríos, K.; García-López, A. Bibliometrics, a Useful Tool Within the Field of Research. *J. Basic Appl. Psychol. Res.* **2022**, *3*, 10–17. [CrossRef]
58. Van Eck, N.J.; Waltman, L. Visualizing Bibliometric Networks. In *Measuring Scholarly Impact*; Ding, Y., Rousseau, R., Wolfram, D., Eds.; Springer International Publishing: Berlin/Heidelberg, Germany, 2014; pp. 285–320. [CrossRef]
59. McAllister, J.T.; Lennertz, L.; Atencio Mojica, Z. Mapping a Discipline: A Guide to Using VOSviewer for Bibliometric and Visual Analysis. *Sci. Technol. Libr.* **2022**, *41*, 319–348. [CrossRef]
60. Price, D.D.S. A General Theory of Bibliometric and Other Cumulative Advantage Processes. *J. Am. Soc. Inf. Sci.* **1976**, *27*, 292–306. [CrossRef]
61. Coile, R.C. Lotka's Frequency Distribution of Scientific Productivity. *J. Am. Soc. Inf. Sci.* **1977**, *28*, 366–370. [CrossRef]
62. Bufrem, L.; Prates, Y. Recorded Scientific Knowledge and Information Measuring Practices. *Ciência Informação* **2005**, *34*, 9–25. [CrossRef]
63. Vega-Muñoz, A.; Salazar-Sepúlveda, G.; Contreras-Barraza, N.; Araya-Silva, L. Scientific Mapping of Coastal Governance: Global Benchmarks and Trends. *J. Mar. Sci. Eng.* **2022**, *10*, 751. [CrossRef]
64. Hirsch, J.E. An Index to Quantify an Individual's Scientific Research Output. *Proc. Natl. Acad. Sci. USA* **2005**, *102*, 16569–16572. [CrossRef] [PubMed]
65. Rein, R.; Memmert, D. Big Data and Tactical Analysis in Elite Soccer: Future Challenges and Opportunities for Sports Science. *Springerplus* **2016**, *5*, 1410. [CrossRef] [PubMed]
66. Qader, M.A.; Zaidan, B.B.; Zaidan, A.A.; Ali, S.K.; Kamaluddin, M.A.; Radzi, W.B. A Methodology for Football Players Selection Problem Based on Multi-Measurements Criteria Analysis. *Measurement* **2017**, *111*, 38–50. [CrossRef]
67. Smith, M.R.; Zeuwts, L.; Lenoir, M.; Hens, N.; De Jong, L.M.; Coutts, A.J. Mental Fatigue Impairs Soccer-Specific Decision-Making Skill. *J. Sports Sci.* **2016**, *34*, 1297–1304. [CrossRef]
68. Diaz del Campo, D.G.; Gonzalez Villora, S.; Garcia Lopez, L.M.; Mitchell, S. Differences in Decision-Making Development between Expert and Novice Invasion Game Players. *Percept. Mot. Ski.* **2011**, *12*, 871–888. [CrossRef]
69. Romeas, T.; Guldner, A.; Faubert, J. 3D-Multiple Object Tracking Training Task Improves Passing Decision-Making Accuracy in Soccer Players. *Psychol. Sport Exerc.* **2016**, *22*, 1–9. [CrossRef]
70. Roca, A.; Williams, A.M.; Ford, P.R. Developmental Activities and the Acquisition of Superior Anticipation and Decision Making in Soccer Players. *J. Sports Sci.* **2012**, *30*, 1643–1652. [CrossRef]
71. Gonçalves, B.; Esteves, P.; Folgado, H.; Ric, A.; Torrents, C.; Sampaio, J. Effects of Pitch Area-Restrictions on Tactical Behavior, Physical, and Physiological Performances in Soccer Large-Sided Games. *J. Strength. Cond. Res.* **2017**, *31*, 2398–2408. [CrossRef]
72. Furley, P.; Memmert, D. Creativity and Working Memory Capacity in Sports: Working Memory Capacity is not a Limiting Factor in Creative Decision Making Amongst Skilled Performers. *Front. Psychol.* **2015**, *6*, 115. [CrossRef]
73. Lex, H.; Essig, K.; Knoblauch, A.; Schack, T. Cognitive Representations and Cognitive Processing of Team-Specific Tactics in Soccer. *PLoS ONE* **2015**, *10*, e0118219. [CrossRef] [PubMed]
74. Mann, D.T.; Williams, A.M.; Ward, P.; Janelle, C.M. Perceptual-Cognitive Expertise in Sport: A Meta-Analysis. *J. Sport Exerc. Psychol.* **2007**, *29*, 457–478. [CrossRef] [PubMed]
75. Vaeyens, R.; Lenoir, M.; Williams, A.M.; Philippaerts, R.M. Mechanisms Underpinning Successful Decision Making in Skilled Youth Soccer Players: An Analysis of Visual Search Behaviors. *J. Mot. Behav.* **2007**, *39*, 395–408. [CrossRef] [PubMed]
76. Roca, A.; Ford, P.R.; McRobert, A.P.; Williams, A.M. Identifying the Processes Underpinning Anticipation and Decision-Making in a Dynamic Time-Constrained Task. *Cogn. Process.* **2011**, *12*, 301–310. [CrossRef]
77. García-Angulo, A.; Ortega, E. Análisis Bibliométrico de la Producción Científica Sobre el Portero en Fútbol. *Rev. Iberoam. Psicol. Ejerc. Deporte* **2014**, *10*, 205–214.
78. Plakias, S.; Tsatalas, T.; Mina, M.A.; Kokkotis, C.; Kellis, E.; Giakas, G. A Bibliometric Analysis of Soccer Biomechanics. *Appl. Sci.* **2024**, *14*, 6430. [CrossRef]
79. Cherappurath, N.; Shamshadali, P.; Elayaraja, M.; Azeezul Kabber, D. Mapping the Field: A Bibliometric Analysis of Women's Football Research Trends and Future Directions. *Apunt. Sports Med.* **2024**, *59*, 100448. [CrossRef]

80. Becerra Patiño, B.A.; Varón-Murcia, J.J.; Cárdenas-Contreras, S.; Castro-Malaver, M.A.; Ávila-Martínez, J.D. Scientific Production on the Relative Age Effect in Sport: Bibliometric Analysis of the Last 9 Years (2015–2023). *Retos* **2024**, *52*, 623–638. [CrossRef]
81. Becerra Patiño, B.A.; Paucar-Uribe, J.D.; Montilla-Valderrama, V. Bibliometric Analysis of Plyometrics in Sport: 40 Years of Scientific Production. *Retos* **2024**, *53*, 183–195. [CrossRef]
82. Rechenchosky, L.; Menegassi, V.M.; Jaime, M.O.; Borges, P.H.; Sarmento, H.; Mancha-Triguero, D.; Serra-Olivares, J.; Rinaldi, W. Scoping Review of Tests to Assess Tactical Knowledge and Tactical Performance of Young Soccer Players. *J. Sports Sci.* **2021**, *39*, 2051–2067. [CrossRef]
83. Sheng, Y.; Huiting, Z.; Qiang, Z.; Chenhui, L. A Corpus-Based Bibliometric Study of Highly Cited Papers in Sport Sciences. *Sage Open* **2024**, *14*, 21582440231225856. [CrossRef]
84. Machado, G.; González-Villora, S.; Roca, A.; Teoldo, I. Developing cognitive and Motor Decision-Making Skills Through Tactical Principles and Small-Sided Games in Youth Soccer. *Int. J. Perform. Anal. Sport* **2024**, *24*, 444–463. [CrossRef]
85. Larkin, P.; O'Connor, D.; Williams, A.M. Does Grit Influence Sport-Specific Engagement and Perceptual-Cognitive Expertise in Elite Youth Soccer? *J. Appl. Sport Psychol.* **2015**, *28*, 129–138. [CrossRef]
86. Fortes, L.S.; Nascimento-Júnior, J.R.A.; Mortatti, A.L.; Lima-Júnior, D.R.A.A.; Ferreira, M.E.C. Effect of Dehydration on Passing Decision Making in Soccer Athletes. *Res. Q. Exerc. Sport* **2018**, *89*, 332–339. [CrossRef]
87. González-Villora, S.; García-López, L.-M.; del Campo, D.; Contreras-Jordán, O.-R. Tactical Awareness and Decision Making in Youth Football Players (12 years): A Descriptive Study. *J. Study Educ. Dev.* **2010**, *33*, 489–501. [CrossRef]
88. Machado, G.; González-Villora, S.; Sarmento, H.; Teoldo, I. Development of Tactical Decision-making Skills in Youth Soccer Players: Macro- and Microstructure of Soccer Developmental Activities as a Discriminant of Different Skill Levels. *Int. J. Perform. Anal. Sport* **2020**, *20*, 1072–1091. [CrossRef]
89. Teoldo, I.; Dambroz, F.; González-Villora, S. Exploring the Effects of Physical Fatigue on Cognitive Performance of Youth Soccer Players. *Int. J. Sport Exerc. Psychol.* **2022**, *22*, 290–305. [CrossRef]
90. Teoldo, I.; Dambroz, F.; Brito, J. Performance of soccer players under acute physical fatigue: An approach based on cognitive, tactical and physical aspects. *Heliyon* **2024**, *10*, e30516. [CrossRef]
91. de Sousa Fortes, L.; Barbosa, B.T.; Mortatti, A.L.; Moreira, A.; Ferreira, M. Effect of Mental Fatigue on Decision-Making Skill During Simulated Congested Match Schedule in Professional Soccer Athletes. *Curr. Psychol.* **2024**, *43*, 1785–1793. [CrossRef]
92. Chen, X.X.; Ji, Z.G.; Wang, Y.; Xu, J.; Wang, L.Y.; Wang, H.B. Bibliometric Analysis of the Effects of Mental Fatigue on Athletic Performance from 2001 to 2021. *Front. Psychol.* **2023**, *13*, 1019417. [CrossRef]
93. Donnan, K.J.; Williams, E.L.; Stanger, N. The Effect of Exercise-Induced Fatigue and Heat Exposure on Soccer-Specific Decision-Making During High-Intensity Intermittent Exercise. *PLoS ONE* **2022**, *17*, e0279109. [CrossRef] [PubMed]
94. Clemente, F.M.; Ramirez-Campillo, R.; Castillo, D.; Raya-González, J.; Silva, A.F.; Afonso, J.; Sarmento, H.; Rosemann, T.; Knechtle, B. Effects of Mental Fatigue in Total Running Distance and Tactical Behavior During Small-Sided Games: A Systematic Review With a Meta-Analysis in Youth and Young Adult's Soccer Players. *Front. Psychol.* **2021**, *12*, 656445. [CrossRef] [PubMed]
95. Ávila-Martínez, J.D.; Castro-Malaver, M.A.; Becerra-Patiño, B.A.; Varón-Murcia, J.; Cárdenas-Contreras, S.; Pino-Ortega, J. Gender Differences for the Relative Age Effect on Physical Skills and Emotional Intelligence in Child Volleyball and Soccer Athletes. *J. Funct. Morphol. Kinesiol.* **2024**, *9*, 244. [CrossRef]
96. Montenegro Bonilla, A.D.; Rodríguez Pachón, S.D.; Hernández-Beltrán, V.; Gamonales, J.M.; Rico-González, M.; Pino-Ortega, J.; Olivares-Arancibia, J.; Yánez-Sepúlveda, R.; López-Gil, J.F.; Becerra Patiño, B.A. Comparative Analysis of the Physical, Tactical, Emotional, and Mood Characteristics of Under-13 Soccer Players by Performance Level. *J. Funct. Morphol. Kinesiol.* **2024**, *9*, 237. [CrossRef] [PubMed]
97. Becerra Patiño, B.A.; Escorcia-Clavijo, J.B. The Transfer and Dissemination of Knowledge in Sports Training: A Scoping Review. *Retos* **2023**, *50*, 79–90. [CrossRef]
98. Borges, P.H.; Guilherme, J.; Rechenchosky, L.; da Costa, L.C.A.; Rinadi, W. Fundamental Tactical Principles of Soccer: A Comparison of Different Age Groups. *J. Hum. Kinet.* **2017**, *58*, 207–214. [CrossRef]
99. Oslin, J.L.; Mitchell, S.A.; Griffin, L.L. The game performance assessment instrument (GPAI): Development and preliminary validation. *J. Teach. Phys. Educ.* **1998**, *17*, 231–243. [CrossRef]
100. Grehaigne, J.F.; Godbout, P.; Bouthier, D. Performance assessment in team sports. *J. Teach. Phys. Educ.* **1997**, *16*, 500–516. [CrossRef]
101. García-López, L.M.; González-Villora, S.; Gutiérrez, D.; Serra, J. Development and validation of the game performance evaluation tool (GPET) in soccer. *Rev. Euroam. De Cienc. Del Deporte* **2013**, *2*, 89–99.

sports

MDPI

Review

A Narrative Review of the Velocity and Acceleration Profile in Football: The Influence of Playing Position

Charles Cotteret [1], Ángel González-de-la-Flor [1], Jaime Prieto Bermejo [2], Jaime Almazán Polo [1] and Sergio L. Jiménez Saiz [3,*]

[1] Department of Physiotherapy, Faculty of Medicine, Health and Sports, European University of Madrid, 28670 Villaviciosa de Odón, Spain; charles.cotteret@universidadeuropea.es (C.C.); angel.gonzalez@universidadeuropea.es (Á.G.-d.-l.-F.); jaime.almazan@universidadeuropea.es (J.A.P.)

[2] Faculty of Economic and Business Sciences, Universidad Rey Juan Carlos, 28032 Madrid, Spain; jaime.prieto@urjc.es

[3] Sport Sciences Research Centre, Universidad Rey Juan Carlos, 28943 Fuenlabrada, Spain

* Correspondence: sergio.jimenez.saiz@urjc.es

Abstract: To enhance athletic performance and reduce the risk of injury, load quantification has allowed for a better understanding of the individual characteristics of the physical demands on soccer players during training or competition. In this regard, it appears crucial to summarize scientific evidence to provide useful information and future directions related to the speed and acceleration profiles of male soccer players. This review aims to evaluate the findings reflected in the available literature on both profiles in football, synthesizing and discussing data from scientific articles, while providing insights into quantification methods, employed thresholds, tracking systems, terminology, playing position, and microcycle day. Therefore, it is hoped that this narrative review can support objective decision-making in practice for coaches, sports scientists, and medical teams regarding individualized load management and the appropriate selection of metrics, to explore current trends in soccer player profiles.

Keywords: GPS technology; initial speed; playing positions; acceleration profile; speed running

1. Introduction

1.1. Characteristics and Evolution of Physical Demands in Soccer, Technology

Soccer is a complex team sport influenced by a multitude of contextual variables that interact at both the player and team levels [1]. Due to this complexity, the assessment of players' and teams' physical, technical, and tactical abilities cannot be understood in isolation [2,3]. From a physical demand's perspective, soccer is primarily an intermittent aerobic sport, where players alternate between high-intensity, multidirectional efforts and numerous low-intensity rest periods [4,5]. During competition, while most efforts occur at low speeds, several critical aspects of successful performance outcomes require high-speed actions [5].

The literature over the last decade provides consensus on the significant increase in high-intensity actions in soccer without an accompanying rise in the total distance covered [6–9]. Longitudinal studies over several seasons in the English and Spanish leagues show notable increases in high-intensity and sprint distances. This change in the game's intensity is partly attributed to evolving tactical strategies that prioritize quick transitions, high pressing, and rapid counterattacks. These strategies demand more frequent high-intensity accelerations, which allow players to cover shorter distances at higher speeds.

Alongside this, there are longer rest periods between actions, enabling greater recovery and sustaining a more intense style of play. This shift highlights the importance of players' ability to perform high-intensity actions intermittently and repeatedly, a critical factor for physical performance in soccer [10–13].

1.2. Load Monitoring and Technology

Monitoring athletes in team sports is increasingly important to understand individual responses to load, with the goal of optimizing physical performance and minimizing injury risk (Figure 1) [14,15]. Individual adaptations to physical exercise can vary significantly among players and are related to individual fitness levels, as well as the intensity and duration of training loads. Therefore, it is essential to tailor training programs in an individualized manner [14,16–19]. There are various methods for load individualization, and studies show a strong interest in investigating these methods [14,20,21].

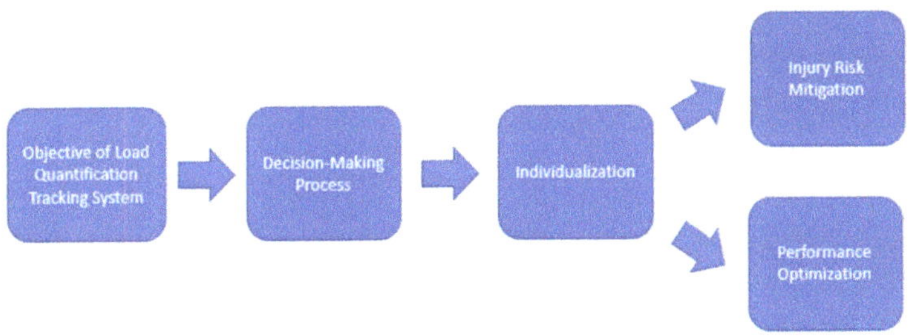

Figure 1. Objective of Load Quantification in Football.

In contemporary soccer, load indicators need to be interpretable in real time so that coaches can make decisions without sacrificing training time for assessments or load monitoring [22,23].

The three most commonly used analysis devices in soccer are multi-camera optical sensor video systems, local positioning systems (LPS) based on radar, and global positioning systems (GPS) (Table 1) [18,24–27]. One of the major drawbacks, apart from the fixed and costly installation like LPS, is the inability to use these systems for real-time training monitoring. This limitation arises because LPS typically require a controlled environment with a fixed setup, making them impractical for dynamic training conditions where mobility is essential [28,29]. In the past decade, there has been an increase in the use of GPS technology, making it the most widely used system in current soccer (Table 1) [12,30–32]. GPS offers the possibility of objectively measuring a wide range of variables, allowing coaches to understand players' conditioning needs according to playing position during training sessions or competitions [4,10,20,33].

Table 1. An Overview of Tracking Systems in Soccer: Technologies, Models, and Applications in Performance Monitoring.

	TRACKING SYSTEMS		
Instrument	**Model**	**Frequency**	**N° of Papers**
GPS	WIMU PRO™	18 Hz	1
	WIMU PRO™	10 Hz	2
	Catapult OptimEye S5	10 Hz	2
	Catapult Vector S7	10 Hz	4
	Catapult Player Tek	10 Hz	1
	GPSports SPI PRO X	15 Hz	3
	GPSports SPI PRO X II	15 Hz	2
	GPSports SPI HPU	15 Hz	1
	GPSports SPI Elite	1 Hz	1
	STATSports Apex	18 Hz	2
	STATSports Apex ProSeries	10 Hz	2
	STATSports Viper	10 Hz	4
	GPEXE Pro	18 Hz	1

Table 1. *Cont.*

TRACKING SYSTEMS			
Instrument	**Model**	**Frequency**	**N° of Papers**
LPM	Inmotiotec GmbH	45 Hz	1
OTS	Second Spectrum®	25 Hz	2
	Mediacoach	ND	1
	TRACAB	ND	1
	InStat Fitness	25 Hz	1
RFID	RadioEye™	40 Hz	1
Video Analysis	ProZone Version 3.0	-	2

GPS global positioning system, LPM local position measurement, OTS optical tracking system, RFID radio frequency identification.

1.3. External Load Monitoring

External load monitoring is valuable in selecting the appropriate load indicators. However, given the complexity of soccer, it is not possible to assess the impact of a single performance indicator when analyzing external load [4,34]. The most commonly used indicators for quantifying external load in soccer include total distance, distances covered in specific speed zones, number of sprints, maximum speed, number of accelerations-decelerations, and exposure time during training and matches, as we can observe in Figure 2 [4,15,20,35,36]. Several authors link these variables to session duration in minutes, which becomes significant when different exposure times exist, such as in a match or a post-match session. Consequently, it is necessary to prorate this load to the exposure time to account for session density [4,37].

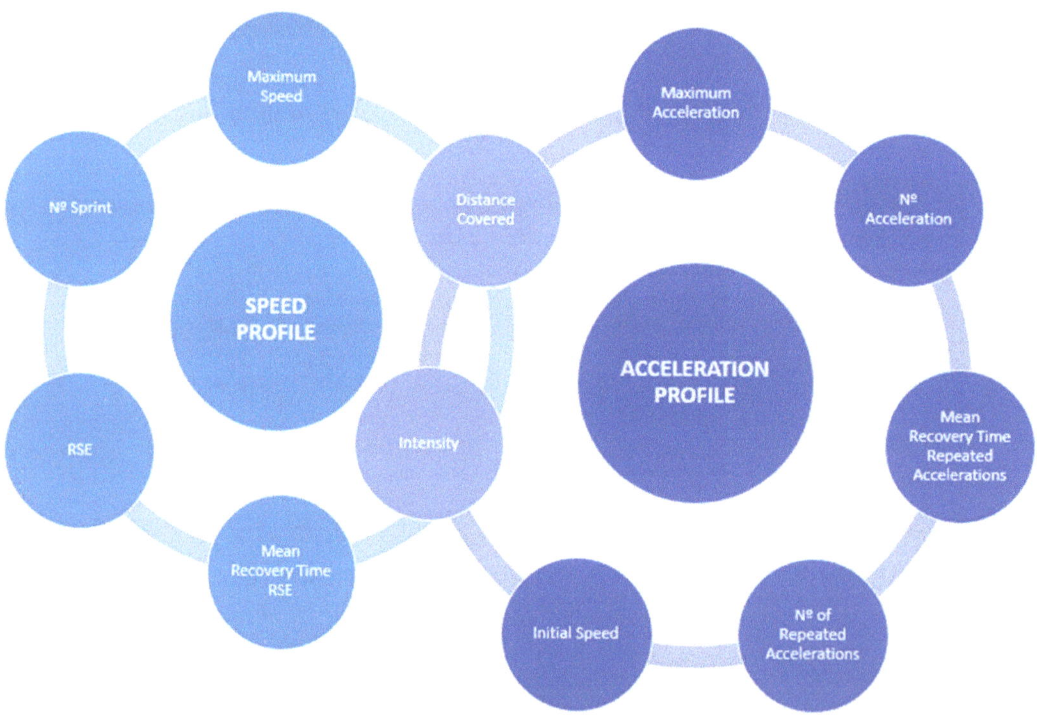

Figure 2. Variables of the Speed and Acceleration Profile in Football.

1.4. Load Distribution and Injuries

In the updated model of injury etiology, training and match loads contribute, along with intrinsic and extrinsic factors, to the multifactorial model of injury etiology [38]. Research on injury prevention in soccer has focused on the relationships between external and internal load indicators to better understand how to prevent them [39]. It has been demonstrated that training load is a modifiable risk factor for overuse injuries [40]. This information becomes even more relevant considering that overuse injuries, which are prevalent in soccer, are often due to errors in load perception and programming [39].

From a preventive perspective, the current literature has established that the injury rate in soccer is higher during competition, with a greater impact on the lower limb due to overuse injuries (66%), particularly muscle injuries, with hamstrings being the most frequently affected [41,42]. Analyzing injury load and economic cost in professional players from European clubs, hamstring injuries had an injury load of 15.4 days/1000 h with an economic cost of €90,367/1000 h, figures that are significant in terms of club performance [43].

In a recent study, Perez et al. demonstrated the impact of weekly external training load and matches as risk factors for muscle overuse injuries. Current data suggest that the combination of a high external training load during the week and a short high-intensity running period during the match could increase the risk of muscle injuries in professional soccer players [44].

Similar to training load, playing position could substantially influence football players' injury rates [45]. According to Swart et al., midfielders experienced the highest absolute number of injuries (50%), followed by defenders (33%) and forwards (17%) [46]. Likewise, Leventer et al. found that midfielders suffer the highest number of injuries (38%), followed by defenders (30%) and forwards (21%) [45].

2. Speed Profile

2.1. Maximum Velocity

Among load indicators, the maximum running speed or peak velocity that a soccer player can reach during a match has become one of the most popular variables for assessing a player's physical talent [30]. Additionally, optimizing maximum speed enables players to respond more effectively to the demands of the game [4]. It is essential to consider each player's position, as faster players tend to reach a lower percentage of their Vmax during matches compared to slower players [47,48]. Generally, forwards are faster than defenders, and both are faster than midfielders. Many contextual variables can influence the analysis of individual speed reached in matches, and caution is needed when making inter- or intra-player comparisons [20,30,49].

The average maximum speeds reached throughout the season tend to remain stable around 30.7 km/h. Therefore, all teams have players capable of reaching top speeds > 30 km/h, which limits the discriminatory usefulness of maximum speeds to distinguish between higher- and lower-ranked teams. Most players (56%) reached a maximum speed between 32.0 and 33.9 km/h, and only 0.6% of players (three individuals) reached speeds above 35 km/h [30,50]. Besides categorizing players as fast, moderate, or slow with maximum speeds > 32.70 km/h, between 31.70–32.69 km/h, and <31.69 km/h, respectively, another major advantage of maximum speed is its use in defining intensity zones (Figure 3) [20,51].

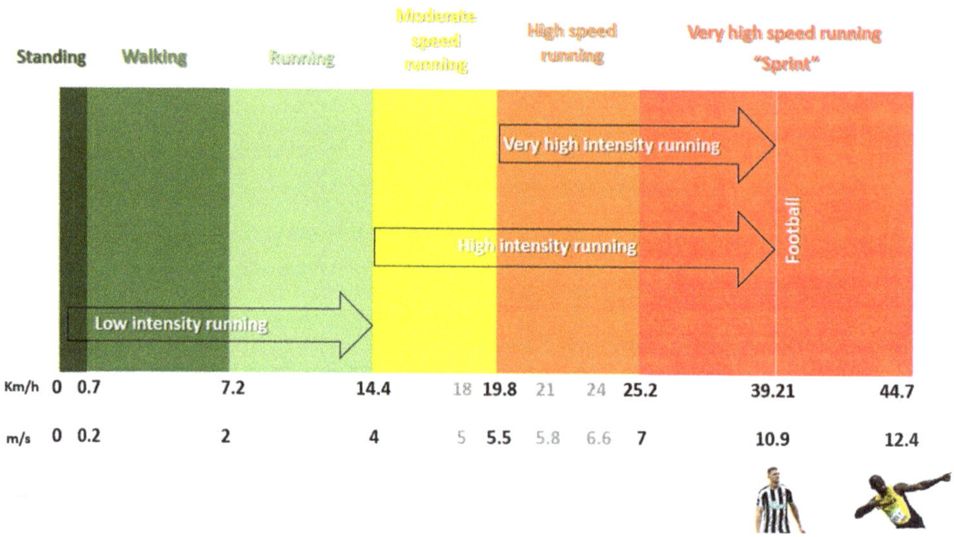

Figure 3. Speed and Intensity Zones: Colored Segments Represent Commonly Used Speed Zones; Arrows Indicate Intensity Zones.

2.2. Absolute Threshold

As shown in Figure 3, player activity is classified into different speed or intensity zones ranging from 0 to 36 km/h, but there are no standardized speed zones. The lack of a universal definition leads to confusion about speed-level thresholds, which can result in erroneous conclusions based on a fixed speed threshold [24,52]. Using a fixed threshold determines absolute speed ranges, that is, arbitrary speed zones independent of players' fitness levels. Absolute ranges appear to be commonly adopted in soccer; however, interpreting arbitrary speed zones has the disadvantage of masking individual capabilities [20,35,53]. Intensity zones based on absolute ranges are typically divided into six zones, measuring the distance covered according to the speed attained.

- Standing 0–0.6 km/h [34]
- Walking > 0.7–7.2 km/h [34]
- Running > 7.2–14.3 km/h [34]
- Medium-speed running (MSR) 14.4–19.8 km/h [34,49]
- High-speed running (HSR) 19.8–25.1 km/h [10,33,34,49,54–58]
- Sprint or very-high-speed running (VHSR) > 25.2 km/h [10,33,34,49,55–57,59]

The lack of consensus in defining absolute thresholds leads to the use of five other predetermined thresholds [52]:

- Walking 0–7 km/h [5,52]
- Running 7–13 km/h [5,52]
- MSR > 13–18 km/h [5,52,60]
- HSR > 18–21 km/h [5,52,60]
- Sprint > 21 km/h [5,52,60]

In a more isolated manner, some authors describe only four zones, using the following thresholds: <6 km/h (low), 6–18 km/h (moderate), 18–24 km/h (high), and >24 km/h (very high). In addition to the described ranges, it is important to analyze the terminology used; some authors employ the term HSR to denote speeds > 14.4 km/h (MSR) and VHSR for speeds > 20 km/h (HSR) [51,61,62].

In soccer, research often focuses on the distance covered at high intensity, and several authors assert that high-intensity actions are considered the best indicator of performance [24,52,54]. Although some studies consider an absolute threshold around 18 km/h to determine the distance covered at high speed, others use a threshold of 19.8 km/h, indicating a clear lack of consensus in the current literature regarding the categorization of these actions [4,10,63–66]. Some researchers use the term "high intensity" to encompass both high-intensity and sprint segments, combining the distances covered in both ranges, which further complicates potential comparisons among authors [55]. Within high intensity, the distance covered during sprints is even less defined, with differences of more than 4 km/h in the two most commonly used fixed thresholds of 21 and 25.2 km/h; some authors even use a threshold of 24 km/h [8,9,12,64,66–69]. The lack of clarity in sprint thresholds arises from how they are recorded; they can be counted numerically or by the distance covered. Generally, a sprint is recorded as an effort that involves a minimum movement of 1 m, maintained for at least 1 s, and reaching a defined speed [66]. Therefore, when sprints are recorded numerically, an action can fall into the high-intensity zone (speed > 21 km/h) or very-high-intensity zone (>24 or 25 km/h, depending on the authors) [55]. Confusion arises when a high-intensity threshold is defined as distance covered during a sprint, as it would actually refer to the distance covered at very high intensity [12]. When comparing results across various studies, it is essential to differentiate between the number of sprints at high or very high intensity and the distance covered during sprints, which would be equivalent to the distance covered at very high intensity [70].

2.3. RSE and RSA

In the context of speed profiles, performing high-intensity actions intermittently and repeatedly is a key factor for physical performance [71]. The ability to repeat efforts, referred to as "repeated sprint ability" (RSA), is a fitness requirement that quantifies maximal or near-maximal efforts such as sprinting or accelerating, interspersed with brief recovery intervals consisting of either complete rest or low- to moderate-intensity activity [72,73]. Repeated sprint exercise (RSE) and intermittent sprinting differ in recovery times, with almost complete recovery of 60 to 300 s for intermittent sprints and recovery periods of less than 60 s for RSE [74,75]. Buchheit et al. classified high-intensity actions based on recovery duration between repeated efforts, with times of 30 s, 31 to 60 s, and >61 s [76]. Recovery time is a critical factor in the onset of fatigue and has been linked to the ability to reproduce sprints [71,72]. Moreover, the energy cost of intermittent activities is 3.1 to 6.3 times greater than that of running at a constant speed, resulting in increased internal load during intermittent running exercises, such as shuttle runs or near-maximal accelerations [77]. The physiological demands during repeated sprint exercise are primarily affected by the intensity of accelerations [78,79].

Significant differences were found between field positions, with forwards exhibiting significantly better RSA compared to defenders and midfielders. However, no differences were observed in high-intensity activity across positions [80]. Conversely, Carling et al. reported that midfielders performed more high-intensity actions separated by short recovery times (20 s), and running intensity was higher during recovery periods. Regarding full-backs (FB), the number of high-intensity RSEs was statistically greater than in other playing positions [71].

2.4. Relative Threshold of Velocity

When the importance and relevance of high-intensity actions in match outcomes have been described, the use of relative speed ranges could address this issue [51,81]. The arbitrary method is commonly employed in professional football to quantify external load data, while the use of individualized methods is on the rise [20]. Utilizing absolute thresholds may underestimate or overestimate the intensity of actions during matches [54,82]. Although activity profiles have been extensively studied, a common methodological limitation is the exclusive use of absolute values. Recent findings suggest that the specific demands of each player should be considered individually [51]. An individualized threshold based on a player's maximum speed allows for the evaluation of each player's specific demands, reducing error in quantifying physical performance at different intensities [52].

Given the significant variability in running capacity among different players, it is logical to individualize sprint thresholds, high-speed runs, and moderate speeds [51]. This approach of using a relative threshold compared to an absolute threshold could reduce the risk of underestimating or overestimating the players' effort, as it has been shown that the distance covered can be misinterpreted based on the maximum speed each player is capable of achieving [51,52]. To establish relative thresholds, it is essential to consider each player's maximum speed, enabling the calculation of thresholds as percentages based on their attained Vmax (Table 2) [68,83,84]. In 2015, Reardon et al. set a value of 60% of maximum speed to define a high-intensity threshold [48]. This was further supported and expanded in 2016 by Castellano et al., who described three relative thresholds: >40% of maximum speed for low intensity, 40-60% for moderate intensity, and >60% for high intensity [85]. Subsequently, even more refined relative thresholds were defined based on intensity: low (0% to 19.99%), moderate (20% to 54.99%), high (55% to 74.99%), and sprint (>75%). These relative zones correspond to the previously defined absolute intensity zones: low (<6 km/h), moderate (6–18 km/h), high intensity (18–24 km/h), and sprint (>24 km/h), thereby adapting to each player's individual capabilities [51]. Similar thresholds were used for youth football players to define speed and intensity zones: low < 34%, moderate 34–61%, and high > 61% [86].

Table 2. Speed and Intensity Zones in Football: Absolute and Relative Threshold with Corresponding Literature Frequency.

SPEED PROFILE			
	Absolute	**Relative**	**N° of Papers**
Very-Low-Speed Walking	0–5.9 km/h		1
Standing	0–0.7 km/h 0–0.6 km/h		1 3
Walking	<7.1 km/h 0.7–7.2 km/h 0.1–8 km/h		2 4 1
Low-Speed Walking	6–11.9 km/h		1
Jogging	7.2–14.3 km/h 8.1–13 km/h		6 1
Low-Speed Jogging	12–13.9 km/h		1
Low-Speed Running	0–10.8 km/h 13.1–16 km/h <14 km/h		1 1 1
Medium-Speed Running	14–17.9 km/h		2
Moderate-Speed Running	>14.4 km/h		1
Intermediate-Speed Running	>10.8–19.8 km/h 16.1–19 km/h		1 1

Table 2. *Cont.*

SPEED PROFILE			
	Absolute	**Relative**	**N° of Papers**
Running	14.4–19.8 km/h		10
High-Speed Running	4–5.5 m/s >5.5 m/s 5.5–7 m/s 18–23.9 km/h 18–21 km/h 19.8–25.2 km/h 19.1–22 km/h >19.8 km/h	70% Peak Match Speed 75% Peak Match Speed >Maximal Aerobic Speed >30% Anaerobic Reserve	1 + 1 2 + 1 1 + 2 1 + 2 1 11 1 4
Very-High-Speed Running	5.5–7 m/s 21–24 km/h >25.2 km/h		1 1 1
Maximum-Speed Running	>22.1 km/h		1
Sprint	>24 km/h >25.2 km/h >7 m/s	80% Peak Match Speed 85% Peak Match Speed 90% Peak Match Speed >85% Peak Speed	5 + 1 14 + 1 4 + 1 1
Very-Low-Intensity Running	0–7 km/h	<10–20% Peak of velocity	1 + 1
Low-Intensity Running	<14.3 km/h	<40% Maximum Speed	2 + 1
	7–13 km/h	20–40% Peak of velocity	1 + 1
Moderate-Intensity Running	<19.8 km/h 13–18 km/h	40–60% Maximum Speed	1 + 2 1
High-Intensity Running	>5.5 m/s 5.5–7 m/s >14.4 km/h 17–23.99 km/h 18–21 km/h >19.8 km/h	>60–75% Maximum Speed 60–80% Peak of velocity	2 + 1 1 + 1 3 1 1 2
Very-High-Intensity Running	>19.8 km/h >21 km/h	>75% Maximum Speed >80% Peak of velocity	2 + 1 1 + 1

2.5. Comparison Relative and Absolute Threshold

The high-intensity running distance is significantly overestimated in faster players when compared with their relative thresholds. Similarly, in slower players, the high-intensity distance is underestimated relative to their own thresholds [51,87]. Faster players can operate at a relatively lower percentage of their maximum capacity compared to slower players, who may be performing at a relatively higher percentage of their maximum. Likewise, sprint distance is overestimated for faster players, while it is underestimated for slower players [51]. This is because, for a very fast player capable of reaching a maximum speed of 36 km/h, attaining a speed of 24 km/h is less demanding than for a player with a maximum speed of 31 km/h. Thus, it is easier for the faster player to accumulate distance above that speed than for a slower player, a discrepancy not present with a relative threshold, as it adapts to each player's individual capability. According to Gabbett et al., comparing positions using an absolute HSR threshold (>21 km/h) versus a relative threshold (>60% Vmax), forwards can cover a distance of 269 m or 354 m, respectively. In contrast, defenders cover 697 m or 570 m, respectively [87]. Therefore, high-intensity distance can vary between 3% and 5% of the total distance covered, depending on the chosen threshold, which is an important consideration when high intensity represents 2% to 15% of total distance [48,51,87].

If there is a discrepancy between the absolute and relative quantification of workload, such a discrepancy will have significant implications for planning individualized training programs. It is essential to accurately quantify each individual's workload, relative stress, and recovery status to achieve an effective training program [51]. So far, studies have not provided a rationale for the use of an absolute threshold over a relative threshold [52]. In conclusion, for any intensity range, an individualized threshold based on the maximum speed a player can reach could be more specific and precise for assessing physical demands than an absolute threshold [47,52,54]. In addition to the chosen threshold, a soccer player's workload indicators may vary according to age [76], position [13,67,76,88] and the accumulated fatigue during the match [63,89].

2.6. According to Playing Position

It is important to remember that soccer players have individual roles within the team, as each has specific tactical tasks and distinct physical needs during matches [10,47]. There are countless positional possibilities depending on the tactical model adopted by the coach. However, positions are generally grouped for programming purposes into goalkeepers (GK), central defenders (CD), full-backs (FB), central midfielders (MF), wide midfielders (WMF), and forwards (FW) (Table 3) [8,31,67,90,91].

Table 3. Distribution of Playing Positions, Abbreviations, and Frequency in the Literature.

	PLAYING POSITION		
	Position	**Abbreviation**	**N° of Papers**
Defender	Center Back	CB	6
	Central Defender	CD	24
	Full-Back	FB	24
	Extreme Defender	ED	1
	Wide Defender	WD	7
	Wing Back	WB	1
Midfielder	Central Midfielder	CM	18
	Midfielder	MF/MD	12/4
	Wide Midfielder	WMF/WMD/WM	7/2/15
	Offensive Midfielder	OM/OMF	1/3
Forward	Forward	FW/F/FO	17/4/1
	Stricker	S/ST	3/1
	Attacker	A/ATT/AT	1/1/3
	Wide Attacker	WA/W	1/2
	Offensive Attacker	OA	1
	Center Forward	CF	3

Currently, there are divergences regarding the influence of the tactical system and the individual demands of each playing position. Recent studies have shown that FW and MF experienced greater physical demands when playing in a 1-4-2-3-1 tactical formation compared to a 1-4-4-2 formation [92]. In a comparison of eight different formations, the results revealed that the extent to which tactical formation affects match performance depends on the position. In terms of physical performance, CDs and FBs showed greater sprint distances when playing in a formation with only three defenders at the back (1-3-4-3, 1-3-5-2) compared to all other formations [93].

Conversely, Bradley et al. found no significant differences in high-intensity distance covered between the 1-4-4-2, 1-4-3-3, and 1-4-5-1 formations. However, an interesting finding was that FW performed 30% more high-intensity running in a 1-4-3-3 tactical formation compared to the 1-4-4-2 and 1-4-5-1 formations [94]. Higher high-speed distance was observed when the match was tied for midfielders, when losing for defenders, and when winning for attackers [85]. Bradley and Noakes similarly reported 17% less high-intensity running for defenders and 15% more for FW in won matches compared to lost ones [95]. Additionally, a Bundesliga study found that the likelihood of winning a match increased by 31.7% when midfielders increased their sprint distance by 100 m (>24 km/h). For FB, increasing the number of sprints improved the probability of winning a match by 8.6% [96]. While this is a reductionist approach that does not reflect the complexity of all game characteristics, it highlights the influence of playing position on multiple physical and technical variables for players [97–99].

Regarding high-speed performance across different playing positions, research indicates that CDs engage in considerably less high-speed activity compared to other positional roles (excluding goalkeepers) [70]. Numerous authors support these findings, reporting that CDs perform fewer sprints than any other position [70,100–103]. In addition to performing fewer high-intensity actions, CDs generally accumulate the lowest total distance [10,25,70,104,105]. Using relative thresholds, Javier et al. found similar results, with distances between 30–60% and 70–80% of Vmax lower than other positions [52]. In terms of low-intensity time, it accounts for 74.9% to 79.6% of total time based on playing position, with CDs and FWs spending the most time walking or jogging [67,100].

Similarities exist between CD and FW profiles, with FWs running less frequently than CDs [70,100–103] yet often covering 10% more distance between 60–80% of Vmax than other positions [52]. Redwood-Brown et al. reported that FWs typically cover more high-intensity or sprint distances than defenders and, in some cases, midfielders. However, no significant differences were found between playing positions for high-intensity or sprint distance [106]. Thus, there is evidence that FWs cover less distance in low- or medium-intensity actions, although some authors found no significant differences in high-intensity match demands [105,106]. Considering total weekly load, FWs cover a total distance of 20,330 m and FB 17,862 m, with no significant differences between positions in terms of weekly total distance covered [107].

During training sessions, wide players (FB and WMF) and FW cover the most high-intensity distance, which is consistent with match patterns [107]. It is well-documented that wide players, whether defenders or midfielders, accumulate greater high-intensity and sprint distances than central players [47,48,56,67,70,100–104,108]. Recent studies reveal that WMFs spend more time in high-intensity zones, covering greater distances between 18–21 km/h and >21 km/h than all other positions [52,109]. Many other authors define FB as the position that covers the most sprint and high-speed distance (>19.6 km/h), whereas MF is the position that accumulates the least distance at these intensities [47,64,67,100,104].

Overall, MFs cover the highest absolute and relative total distances, achieving greater low-intensity activities and a higher number of efforts, yet accumulating less high-speed and sprint distances compared to other positions [25,34,47,48,52,109]. In terms of total distance covered, the literature is consistent in identifying MFs as those who cover the greatest distance [70,100–103,105]. They cover double the distance of CDs [10,25,104] and cover more meters per minute than FWs or defenders, both at home and away matches [106]. Their performance is characterized by high total distance, particularly at moderate speeds such as jogging and running [67,100,110].

Regarding maximum speed, offensive players were the fastest, with maximum speeds of 30.6 km/h for FW and WMF [70]. Recent studies have found similar results, with higher speed peaks for WMFs, but the attained speed was higher, between 8.82 and 8.88 $m{\cdot}s^{-1}$ (31.75 km/h and 31.96 km/h). The slowest players were MFs, with a maximum speed of

7.96 m·s^{-1} (28.65 km/h) [90,111]. Regarding average speed during matches, MFs or WMFs showed significantly higher values [56].

Physical requirements are specific to each playing position, and players develop their profiles according to these positional demands, which may explain the variability in speed profiles by position [90,112]. This implies that improving team success requires a higher level of physical activity in certain positions and greater technical activity in others. Furthermore, the interpretation of speed profile variables during matches must consider the influence of contextual, environmental, or situational factors, such as match location, opponent quality, and match result [98,113–117].

3. Acceleration Profile

Interest in accelerometry variables has been growing over the years, and in professional football, they are now considered some of the most commonly used metrics for monitoring players [35,118,119]. This shift in focus may be explained by the fact that players rarely have the time and space to reach maximum speeds and therefore rely heavily on their ability to accelerate maximally [120]. For a more valid measurement of workload, it is essential to include accelerometry-related parameters, such as distance, time, or the number of actions across various zones, as these provide complementary information to the more commonly used speed profile variables [121,122].

The incorporation of accelerometry-related factors into workload monitoring has highlighted a 6% to 10% difference in workload estimation compared to monitoring techniques that rely solely on speed-based metrics [123–126].

In football, having a greater acceleration capacity can be decisive in critical moments, and it is estimated that during a match, a player performs between 1000 and 1400 short actions, including changes in direction and intensity, approximately every 60 s. This represents about 7% to 10% of the player's total workload [101,118,127,128]. During matches, English players perform around 656 accelerations, Croatian players around 600, while Spanish players accumulate 581 [31,67,121]. Other studies have found a total of 76 accelerations [126] and 115 accelerations [118]. The variation in methods, tracking systems, and the classification of accelerations makes it challenging to conclude the potential reasons behind these differences [126].

3.1. Absolute Threshold and Initial Velocity

To account for the total number of accelerations performed by a player, changes in speed greater than 0.5 m·s^{-2} are generally quantified without differentiating the intensity of each effort [31,100,121]. One of the methods for classifying accelerometry is the absolute method, which categorizes the intensity of the effort based on a predetermined fixed threshold (Table 4).

Varley et al. defined a single threshold > 2.78 m·s^{-2} to classify accelerations as maximum [118]. Other authors used a similar threshold (>3 m·s^{-2}) to classify both high-intensity accelerations and decelerations, expanding the terminology with a low threshold for accelerations between 1 and 2 m·s^{-2} and a moderate threshold for accelerations between 2 and 3 m·s^{-2} [34,70,101,121,123,128–130]. Isolated studies have reported other thresholds for high-intensity accelerations above 3.5 m·s^{-2} [65]. Lastly, Bradley et al. used two thresholds, considering moderate accelerations between 2.5 and 4 m·s^{-2} and high-acceleration efforts with a threshold > 4 m·s^{-2} [60,64,131]. Ultimately, there is no consensus on defining the absolute threshold for high-intensity accelerations, with data ranging from 2.78, 3, 3.5, and even 4 m·s^{-2} [31,55,56,60,64,65,123,128].

Table 4. Acceleration Zones in Football: Absolute and Relative Thresholds with Corresponding Literature Frequency.

ACCELERATION PROFILE			
	Absolute	**Relative**	**N° of Papers**
Total Accelerations	>0.5 m·s^{-2}		3 + 0
Very-Low-Intensity Accelerations	<1.0 m·s^{-2}	<25% ACCmax	1 + 1
Low-Intensity Accelerations	0–1 m·s^{-2} 1.1–1.5 m·s^{-2} 1–2 m·s^{-2} >1.5 m·s^{-2} <3 m·s^{-2}	<50% ACCmax	1 + 1 1 2 1 1
Moderate-Intensity Accelerations	1.6–2 m·s^{-2} >2 m·s^{-2} 2.1–2.5 m·s^{-2} >2–3 m·s^{-2} 2–4 m·s^{-2} >2.5 m·s^{-2}	<75% ACCmax	1 + 1 2 1 2 4 1
Intermediate-Intensity Accelerations	1–2 m·s^{-2}		1
High-Intensity Accelerations	>2.78 m·s^{-2} 2–3 m·s^{-2} >3 m·s^{-2} 3–4 m·s^{-2} >4 m·s^{-2}	>75% ACCmax	1 + 2 1 9 1 4
Maximal Accelerationns	>3 m·s^{-2}		1
Total Decelerations	>(−) 0.5 m·s^{-2}		3
Low-Intensity Decelerations	(−) 0–1 m·s^{-2} <(−) 3 m·s^{-2} (−) 1–1.9 m·s^{-2}		1 2 1
Moderate-Intensity Decelerations	>(−) 2 m·s^{-2} (−) 2–2.9 m·s^{-2} (−) 2–4 m·s^{-2}		1 1 4
Intermediate-Intensity Decelerations	(−) 1–2 m·s^{-2}		1
High-Intensity Decelerations	>(−) 3 m·s^{-2} (−) 2–3 m·s^{-2} (−) 3–4 m·s^{-2} >(−) 4 m·s^{-2}		7 1 1 3
Maximal Decelerations	>(−) 3 m·s^{-2}		1
Initial Running	ND 0–7 km/h 7.1–14 km/h >14.1 km/h	ND	1 2 2 2

3.2. *Initial Velocity*

However, this approach does not consider that the ability to accelerate largely depends on the player's initial velocity (Vini), with a correlation coefficient of 0.98 between the two variables [34]. As illustrated in Figure 4, the maximum possible acceleration for each player progressively decreases as the initial running speed increases [111,132] and most efforts involving high accelerations reach low or moderate peak speeds [34]. Similarly, Aughey and Varley demonstrated that 85% of accelerations do not exceed speeds of 15.84 km/h, and 98% of maximum accelerations (ACCmax) occur from a standstill or at speeds below

14.4 km/h [118]. De Hoyo et al. found that over two-thirds of high-intensity accelerations reach peak speeds below 19.8 km/h, while previous research reported that 40% reach speeds between 7 and 15 km/h, and high-intensity accelerations that end at sprint speeds account for 19% [133].

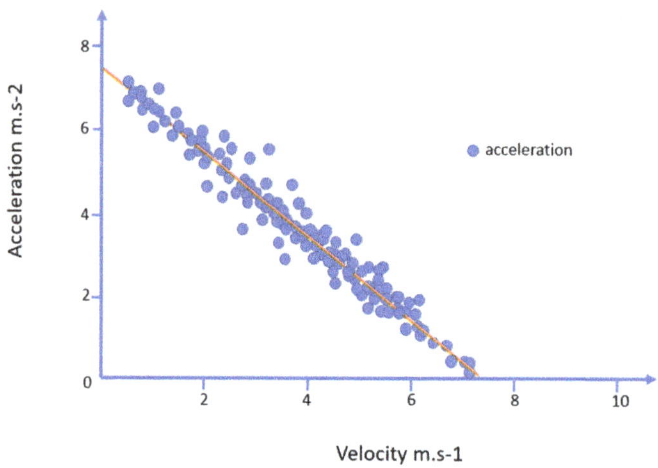

Figure 4. Acceleration Intensity Based on Initial Velocity.

It is common to mistakenly categorize acceleration as low or high intensity based solely on an absolute numerical value, without considering the initial velocity, which does not always accurately reflect the actual intensity of the effort. When using absolute acceleration thresholds, accelerations starting at higher running speeds can be misclassified [132]. Energy and muscle loads are underestimated when efforts begin at a relatively high initial running speed, classifying an acceleration as low intensity when it is actually high intensity [134]. For example, efforts starting from 16.7 km/h have maximum accelerations of 2.29 $m{\cdot}s^{-2}$ and would therefore be classified with an absolute threshold of 3 $m{\cdot}s^{-2}$ as a submaximal effort, despite being very demanding. Indeed, when starting a running effort, few players can reach accelerations of 3 $m{\cdot}s^{-2}$ [111,132]. Conversely, actions with a low starting speed are overestimated, as an acceleration of 3 $m{\cdot}s^{-2}$ represents only 50% of the maximum acceleration when starting from a standstill [124]. Ultimately, it is correct to consider the initial speed when categorizing an acceleration as high or low intensity, but it is necessary to go further by using different absolute thresholds based on the initial speed [34,132]. Subsequently, absolute thresholds for high-intensity accelerations based on initial running speed were defined: above 4.51 $m{\cdot}s^{-2}$ from a standstill, >3.25 $m{\cdot}s^{-2}$ from walking, >2.4 $m{\cdot}s^{-2}$ from jogging, >1.72 $m{\cdot}s^{-2}$ from running [132]. As soccer players are often in motion before initiating an acceleration effort, to anticipate a game situation or follow an opponent, it seems logical to find a significant number of efforts starting from a speed that exceeds being stationary or walking [34]. All of this indicates that the ability to accelerate decreases as running speed increases, and maximum acceleration occurs at the beginning of the action. For these reasons, it is important to use relative thresholds that take into account the initial speed and each player's individual acceleration capabilities [132,133].

3.3. Relative Threshold of Acceleration

To date, the classification of acceleration data based on movement intensity has primarily relied on previously cited absolute thresholds. While the use of these thresholds allows for comparison of physical performance across different cross-sectional and longitudinal studies, their main disadvantage is that they do not take into account the player's relative individual capacity [120,124,135].

The percentage acceleration method classifies the intensity of an effort based on the ratio of the measured acceleration of that specific effort to the maximum acceleration the individual can achieve (Table 4) [132]. Sonderegger et al. propose four different intensity zones: a high-intensity zone with accelerations > 75% of ACCmax, a moderate-intensity zone with accelerations between 50–75% of ACCmax, a low-intensity zone with accelerations between 25–50% of ACCmax, and a very-low-intensity zone with accelerations below 25% of ACCmax [34]. Using an absolute threshold of >3 m·s^{-2}, another of >4 m·s^{-2}, and finally a relative threshold of > 75% ACCmax, they found a number of high-intensity accelerations of 120, 59, and 84, respectively [34]. Additionally, these relative thresholds can be applied based on initial speed across three ranges: from walking (0–7 km/h), from jogging (7.1–14.3 km/h), and from running (>14.4 km/h). According to initial speed, the ACCmax values reached were 6.01 m·s^{-2} from a standstill, 4.33 m·s^{-2} while walking, 3.20 m·s^{-2} while jogging, and 2.29 m·s^{-2} while running [34,132,133].

Ultimately, the relative method could avoid the biases introduced by absolute methods, and calculating intensity thresholds based on individual results would be more convenient for counting and categorizing accelerations [132]. Additionally, the acceleration percentage allows for the determination of individual intensity thresholds specific to a single player or a playing position [34,133].

3.4. Position and Intensity

Analyzing the initial speed and acceleration intensity by playing position, Oliva-Lozano et al. (2020) found that initial speed was significantly higher for low-intensity accelerations compared to high-intensity accelerations only for WMF and FW positions. No significant differences were found in initial speed and acceleration intensity for CD, FB, and MF. Therefore, it is essential to evaluate the acceleration profile by playing position, as it influences acceleration intensity and initial speed [111].

Previous studies have shown significant differences between playing positions and maximum acceleration capacity [90,111,133,136]. In general, footballers with higher maximum acceleration rates can jump higher, run faster (over short distances), and achieve changes of direction at higher speeds [137].

When total accelerations are counted, the most commonly used threshold in current literature refers to an intensity > 0.5 m·s^{-2} [31,100]. During matches, the highest number of accelerations was found for CDs with 743 total accelerations, while FWs recorded the lowest with 610 accelerations. However, analysis of the total weekly number of accelerations in training showed no differences between the different playing positions [100]. Using the same threshold, Sekulic et al. found 517 accelerations for midfielders and 451 for FWs, again the position with the fewest accelerations. The total number of accelerations does not consider the intensity or initial speed of each acceleration, preventing an accurate interpretation of the actual load represented by these accelerations [31].

CDs have more accelerations in low (1–2 m·s^{-2}) and moderate (2–3 m·s^{-2}) thresholds; however, MFs covered the most distance accelerating within the low-intensity threshold compared to CDs and FWs. FBs and WMFs had an acceleration density 10 to 20% higher than central positions (MFs and CDs) [138].

Using an absolute high-intensity threshold of >2.78 m·s^{-2}, Mallo et al. found that CDs recorded the highest number of accelerations, while FWs had the fewest [67]. The most commonly used threshold for high-intensity accelerations is an absolute value of >3 m·s^{-2}. FBs and FWs were the positions that recorded the highest number of accelerations at this intensity, averaging seven and six accelerations per match, respectively. The position with the fewest high-intensity accelerations was midfielders, with an average of 1.9 accelerations [56,100]. Using the same threshold, Sekulic et al. found similar results, with FWs performing the most accelerations, totaling 39. Other positions recorded around 20 maximum accelerations per match [31]. Alonso-Callejo et al. were the only authors to find higher values for acceleration-related variables in CDs, while the lowest ACCmax values on match day were observed for WMFs [90].

Oliva-Lozano et al. defined WMF as the most demanding position for acceleration profiles, with 34.9 high-intensity accelerations (>3 m·s^{-2}), 36 m covered while accelerating, and a maximum acceleration of 4.7 m·s^{-2}, WMF covered the most distance accelerating, reached the highest maximum acceleration, and performed the greatest number of accelerations compared to other positions. On the other hand, MF covered the least distance (260 m), had the lowest maximum acceleration (4.4 m·s^{-2}), and performed the fewest high-intensity accelerations. Regarding accelerations of intensity < 3 m·s^{-2} MF had the highest number of actions [111].

By analyzing three acceleration-intensity thresholds (low, moderate, high) simultaneously, Barrera et al. suggest that the number of accelerations performed at different speeds varies according to the positional demands. For game roles, the highest number of low-intensity accelerations (1–1.9 m·s^{-2} was performed by MFs, who had substantially higher values compared to all other positions. For moderate-intensity accelerations (2–2.9 m·s^{-2}), attacking players (OAs) performed the most actions, showing differences with all positions except FBs, who also differed from CDs, FWs and MFs. For high-intensity accelerations (3–4.0 m·s^{-2}), OAs and FWs had the highest performance, significantly different from other positions (MFs, CDs, and FBs) [70].

Using a relative threshold of 70% of maximum acceleration, CDs had fewer accelerations, while lateral positions (FBs and WMFs) accelerated more often than any other position [126]. De Hoyo et al. took it a step further with a relative acceleration profile based on initial speed. De Hoyo et al. went further by analyzing relative acceleration profiles based on initial speed. With an intensity of 75% of maximum acceleration (high intensity), CDs showed more accelerations from walking (0–7 km/h) compared to jogging (7.1–14.3 km/h). FWs and WMFs accelerated more from running (>14.4 km/h) than from walking or jogging. FBs completed more accelerations from walking and running than from jogging. Finally, MFs performed a greater number of high-intensity accelerations from walking, and their accelerations from running were greater than from jogging. Comparing the total number of high-intensity accelerations regardless of initial speed, FW, WMF, and FB performed more accelerations than CD and MF. Additionally, MF performed more high-intensity accelerations than CD [133].

With an intensity threshold of >2 m·s^{-2}, wide players accelerated significantly more than central players, but these results were only found during the first half of the game, with no differences in the second half or during a full match. Therefore, the ability to accelerate depends on the position and the microcycle day [90,108].

The theoretical maximum acceleration ranged from 5.73 m·s^{-2} for FBs on the day before the match to 8.68 m·s^{-2} for CDs on match day, while the recorded maximum acceleration was 3.27 m·s^{-2} for MFs the day before the match and 5.35 m·s^{-2} for CDs on match day. Both theoretical and recorded data agreed that the least intense day was the day before the match, and the most intense was match day. Additionally, the recorded data showed that the most intense training day in terms of acceleration throughout the week was the first loading day (Wednesday), except for MFs, for whom it was Thursday [90]. Stevens et al. found similar data, with the most intense acceleration load occurring on Wednesday, close to matching the game load, with a 90% overlap [122]. This highlights the importance of recording accelerations during both matches and training [4].

3.5. RAA and RHAA

The ability to repeat accelerations, known as "repeated acceleration ability" (RAA), is defined as the capacity to accelerate repeatedly (three or more accelerations) with short recovery times (less than 45 s) [139]. RAA has been proposed as an alternative physical capability that may be more relevant to performance than repeated sprint ability (RSA), since high-intensity accelerations require significant energy expenditure and are up to eight times more frequent than sprints. The results showed that RAA profiles were relatively homogeneous, with no significant differences between playing positions or between different parts of the game [140]. The use of absolute thresholds of 1.5 $m{\cdot}s^{-2}$ to define RAA efforts might not accurately reflect what happens during matches, as this threshold could be too low and might overestimate high-intensity runs. The ability to repeat submaximal efforts may not be as critical for performance, and several authors have defined the ability to repeat high-intensity accelerations (RHAA) [139–141]. RHAA is defined as a minimum of three consecutive high-intensity actions with an average recovery duration of 20 s or less between efforts [71]. High-intensity accelerations were measured using relative thresholds of 70% and 80% of the ACCmax obtained during a 40-m sprint test. An average of eight RHAA efforts were detected with a 70% threshold and 5.1 with an 80% threshold. The average number of efforts within each RHAA was four and 3.6 for the 70% and 80% thresholds, respectively [139].

Regarding RHAA by playing position and game timing, there was a slight decrease in the average number of RHAA efforts in the second half for all positions except midfielders (MF), using a 70% ACCmax threshold. With a higher threshold (80% ACCmax), midfielders showed a moderate decrease in RHAA in the second half, with no significant effects for FWs, FBs, or WMFs. For wide players (FBs and WMFs), a longer RHAA effort duration was recorded compared to other positions [139]. In conclusion, RHAA occurs frequently in football, with small but significant differences between playing positions, as well as between the first and second halves of the game [139,140].

4. Conclusions and Future Directions

There is no evident consensus due to the lack of homogeneity in intensity thresholds. Furthermore, the relationships between the two profiles are unclear; faster players do not necessarily achieve the maximum acceleration values [90,111,133]. Monitoring acceleration and velocity profiles more comprehensively not only appears important from a training load and injury-prevention perspective but also provides the coaching staff with specific information necessary to develop and prescribe training protocols that are replicable to match demands [120]. The abundance of external load measures requires a thorough selection of the most useful variables for the specific demands of each playing position. Standardizing the classification of these various measures is of vital importance for organizing this task, as well as when attempting to compare the results obtained in different studies [56].

The use of GPS devices in football players' daily routines provides a virtually inexhaustible source of individualized data. Their emergence is in response to the growing need to monitor training loads, prevent overload and fatigue, and identify and combat the most common muscular injuries among football players. GPS devices also allow for the assessment of an individual player's response in various positions on the field. These results can assist sports scientists, medical staff, and coaches in understanding the variability of relative speed and acceleration profiles, thereby aiding the design of individualized training programs tailored to the positional demands of each player.

When referring to an "individualized" load quantification, a methodology based on relative thresholds adapted to the player's maximum physical capacities should be applied, rather than merely categorizing variables by playing position. Additionally, relative individualization uses percentages that could enable direct comparison of external load variables across different devices. This data could be even more relevant for accelerometry variables, given the variability that exists between devices or different brands.

The positional differences between the speed profile and acceleration profile are distinct; therefore, it is recommended to collect variables from both profiles. In addition to quantifying across various intensities, it is suggested to quantify at least the number of actions performed and the distance covered for both profiles, as discrepancies exist between these variables depending on the playing position. The initial speed should also be taken into account when assessing the acceleration profile.

Quantifying these variables using relative thresholds in both profiles could also be highly beneficial throughout the entire rehabilitation process of an injured player. During the gradual return of the player to the field, physiotherapists and physical trainers alike often question whether the player is ready to engage in group training sessions and subsequently compete. Measuring external load in an individualized manner, based on the player's current maximum physical capacities, could optimize load quantification at each stage of rehabilitation, aiming to ensure performance and minimize the risk of recurrence or relapse. The initial group sessions are part of the reconditioning process, and the player's maximum acceleration or speed capacities are not yet fully restored. Therefore, each session will be more demanding for the player, and the use of absolute thresholds or the lack of consideration for the initial acceleration speeds could lead to erroneous load quantification, underestimating the actual external load of the session and increasing the risk of recurrence. Additionally, controlling training load and preventing injuries are essential components in promoting public health and well-being. Maintaining an appropriate training load helps to improve physical condition without overburdening the body, which reduces the risk of injuries and contributes to both physical and mental well-being. This practice not only protects athletes but also benefits anyone engaging in physical activity, from recreational participants to those with specific health goals.

In the context of public health, preventing injuries through controlled training reduces the incidence of musculoskeletal issues, which are a leading cause of work absenteeism and medical expenses. This means that proper management of exercise load not only prevents individual health problems but also optimizes healthcare resources, reducing the demand for medical services and promoting a more active, healthy society.

Furthermore, focusing on injury prevention and load management fosters a culture of safe and sustainable physical activity, which enhances overall population well-being by making exercise accessible and safe. Our results could provide male football players with reference information on the maximum physical capacities to achieve before returning to training or competition.

Thus, the most relevant studies related to Variables and Playing Position for Velocity and Acceleration Profiles in Football will be detailed in Table 5 for better understanding and clarity.

Table 5. Summary of Study Characteristics Variables and Playing Position for Velocity and Acceleration Profiles in Football.

Article	Type of Study	Aim of Study	Sample Size	Competition Category	Speed Profile	Acceleration Profile	Term	Threshold	Playing Position	Tracking Systems
Alonso-Callejo 2022 [90]	Observational retrospective study	To analyse the differences in the A–S profile of elite football players induced by playing position and the microcycle day	$n = 25$ elite male football players six consecutive microcycles 2021	Spanish Second division	Maximal theoretical speed (abscissa axis intercept (x) in A–S linear regression) Maximmal speed (m/s) Linear slope. Calculated: -A0/S0	Maximal theoretical acceleration Maximal acceleration (m/s^2)	S0 Smax AS-slope A0 ACC-max	Absolute	CD ($n = 5$) FB ($n = 3$) MF ($n = 6$) WMF ($n = 6$) FW ($n = 5$)	GPS, WIMU PRO™, RealTrack System SL, Almeria, Spain 18 Hz
Modric 2019 [100]	Observational	To identify associations between RP and GPI in professional soccer players and to compare RP and GPI among soccer playing positions	$n = 101$ professional soccer players 14 matches 2018/2019	Croatian Soccer League	Total distance covered (m) Walking (<7.1 km/h) (m) Jogging (7.2–14.3 km/h) (m) Running (14.4–19.7 km/h) (m) High speed running (19.8–25.1 km/h) (m) Sprinting (≥25.2 km/h) (m)	Total accelerations (>0.5 m/s^2) (count) High-intensity accelerations (>3 m/s^2) (count) Total decelerations (<[−]0.5 m/s^2) (count) High-intensity decelerations (<[−]3 m/s^2) (count)	HSR HIA HID	Absolute	CD ($n = 26$) FB ($n = 24$) MF ($n = 33$) WMF ($n = 10$) FW ($n = 8$)	GPS, Catapult S5 and X4 devices, Melbourne, Australia. 10 Hz
Modric 2020 [107]	Observational	To examine the position-specific associations between running performance (RP) during the training and match in professional-level male soccer	$n = 15$ professional soccer players, 15 matches, and 75 training sessions	Croatian Soccer League	Total distance covered (m) Low-intensity running (<14.3 km/h) (m) Running (14.4–19.7 km/h) (m) High-speed running (19.8–25.1 km/h) (m) Sprinting (≥25.2 km/h) (m) High-intensity running (>19.8 km/h) (m)	Total accelerations (>0.5 m/s^2) (count) High-intensity accelerations (>3 m/s^2) (count) Total decelerations (<[−]0.5 m/s^2) (count) High-intensity decelerations (<[−]3 m/s^2) (count)	LIR HSR HIR HIA HID	Absolute	CD ($n = 22$ sessions) FB ($n = 23$ sessions) MF ($n = 29$ sessions) WMF ($n = 6$ sessions) FW ($n = 12$ sessions)	GPS, Optim-Eye S5 & X4, Catapult, Melbourne, Australia 10 Hz
Sekulic 2021 [31]	Observational	To evaluate position-specific match running performance (MRP) to determine the effect of COVID-19 lockdowns on the physical performance of professional football players	$n = 21$ professional football players 17 matches 2019/2020	Croatian Soccer League	Total distance covered (m) Low-intensity running (≤ 14.3 km/h) (m) Running (14.4–19.7 km/h) (m) High-intensity running (≥ 19.8 km/h) (m)	Total accelerations (>0.5 m/s^2) (count) High-intensity accelerations (>3 m/s^2) (count) Total decelerations (less than −0.5 m/s^2) (count) High-intensity decelerations (less than −3 m/s^2) (count)	LIR HIR HIA HID	Absolute	CD ($n = 38$ sessions) FB ($n = 20$ sessions) MF ($n = 46$ sessions)	GPS, Vector S7, Catapult, Catapult Sports Ltd., Melbourne, Victoria, Australia 10 Hz

Table 5. *Cont.*

Article	Type of Study	Aim of Study	Sample Size	Competition Category	Speed Profile	Acceleration Profile	Term	Threshold	Playing Position	Tracking Systems
Sondereg-ger 2018 [34]	Observational	To investigate the strengths and limitations of different indicators to measure physical load	n = 139 junior players (n = 70 elite and n = 69 sub elite) 14 matches (n = 7 elite, n = 7 sub elite) and 181 files (n = 90 elite, n = 91 sub elite)	National under-18 (U18) Switzerland	Total distance (m) Standing (0.0–0.7 km·h^{-1}) (m) Walking (>0.7–7.2 km·h^{-1}) (m) Jogging (>7.2–14.4 km·h^{-1}) (m) Running (>14.4–19.8 km·h^{-1}) (m) High-speed running (>19.8–25.2 km·h^{-1}) (m) Sprinting (>25.2 km·h^{-1}) (m)	Initial running speed (km/h) Low acceleration (>1–2 m·s^{-2}) (n°) Moderate acceleration (>2–3 m·s^{-2}) (n°) High acceleration (>3 m·s^{-2}) (n°) High acceleration (>4 m·s^{-2}) (n°) Very low (<25% amax) (n°) Low (<50% amax) (n°) Moderate (<75% amax) (n°) High (≥75% amax) (n°)	HSR Vinit Amax	Absolute And Relative	CD (n = 15, (files n = 22) FB (n = 18, (files n = 24) MF (n = 17, (files n = 21) WMF (n = 7, (files n = 8) FW (n = 13, (files n = 15)	LPM (local position measurement) Inmotiotec GmbH, Regau, Austria 45 Hz
Martínez-Cabrera 2017 [91]	Observational	To compare metabolic power (MP) and the traditional approach using speed running during soccer matches in absolute values and in zones of intensity in function of the playing positions	n = 38 professional soccer players 18 friendly matches 2013/2014	Romanian First League	Walking (0.1 to 8 km/h) (m) Jogging (8.1 to 13 km/h) (m) Low-speed running (13.1 to 16 km/h) (m) Intermediate-speed running (16.1 to 19 km/h) (m) High-speed running (19.1 to 22 km/h) (m) Maximum-speed running (>22.1 km·h^{-1}) (m)	ND	LSR ISR HSR MSR	Absolute	CD (n = 64 files) WD (n = 55 files) CM (n = 58 files) WA (n = 70 files) A (n = 53 files)	GPS, GPSports SPI PRO X II, Canberra, Australia 15 Hz
Martínez-Cabrera 2021 [134]	Observational	To analyze the characteristics of acceleration efforts using individual relative thresholds according to the initial speed during official matches in elite young soccer players according to player position	n = 26 young soccer players 18 matches (n = 108 match files)	Spanish soccer club (La Liga BBVA)	Walking (S1 = 6 km/h), Jogging (S2 = 10.8 km/h), Running (S3 = 15 km/h)	Initial speed (km/h) 0–7 km/h 7.1–14 km/h >14.1 km km/h Acceleration maximum (m·s^{-2}) Number of high accelerations (>75% Accmax) Number of high accelerations (>3 m·s^{-2})	Sinit Amax	Absolute And Relative	CD (n = 40 files) FB (n = 23 files) MD (n = 18 files) W-MD (n = 20 files) S (n = 7 files)	GPS, SPI Pro X; GPSports Canberra, Australia 15 Hz
De Hoyo 2018 [133]	Cross-sectional design	To analyse the acceleration profile in elite professional soccer players according to their initial speed but also considering players' position	n = 24 professional male soccer players 35 competitive matches 2015/2016	Spanish soccer club (La Liga BBVA)	ND	Initial speed (km/h) 0–7 km/h 7.1–14 km/h >14.1 km km/h Maximum acceleration (m·s^{-2}) Number of accelerations (>75% Accmax)	Vinit Amax	Relative	CB (n = 14 files) FB (n = 20 files) MD (n = 20 files) W-MD (n = 16 files) S (n = 11 files)	GPS, SPI Pro X; GPSports Canberra, Australia 15 Hz

Table 5. *Cont.*

Article	Type of Study	Aim of Study	Sample Size	Competition Category	Speed Profile	Acceleration Profile	Term	Threshold	Playing Position	Tracking Systems
Oliva-Lozano 2020 [111]	Observational	To describe positional differences in the acceleration and sprint profiles of professional football players in match-play, and analyse start speeds required based on the intensity of accelerations and decelerations	$n = 23$ professional male football players 30 competitive microcycles	Spanish Second Division (LaLiga 123)	Total sprint actions (above 24 km/h) (count) Total distance covered by sprinting (above 24 km/h) (m) Average distance covered per sprint (above 24 km/h) (m) Maximum speed reached in the match (km/h) Duration of sprint (s)	Total distance covered accelerations (m) Total distance covered decelerations (m) Total number of low-intensity accelerations (below 3 m/s^2) Total number of high-intensity accelerations (above 3 m/s^2) Total number of low-intensity decelerations (above −3 m/s^2) Total number of high-intensity decelerations (below −3 m/s^2) ACCHIGH—DECHIGH Average magnitude of accelerations (m/s^2) Average magnitude of decelerations (m/s^2) Maximum magnitude of accelerations (m/s^2) Maximum magnitude of decelerations (m/s^2)	SPA SPD SPD-avg Vmax ACC-dis DEC-dis ACC-low ACC-high DEC-low DEC-high DIFF-acdc ACC-avg DEC-avg ACC-max DEC-max	Absolute	CD ($n = 4$) FB ($n = 5$) MF ($n = 5$) WMF ($n = 4$) FW ($n = 5$)	GPS, WIMU Pro, Real Track Systems, Almería, Spain 10 Hz
Barrera 2021 [70]	Quasi-experimental design	To evaluate the activity profile of different positional roles in competitive professional soccer matches	$n = 25$ professional soccer players 11 official matches 2019/2020	Portugueses LigaPro	Maximum speed (km/h) Total distance (m) Very-low-speed walking (0–5.9 $km{\cdot}h^{-1}$) (m) Low-speed walking (6–11.9 $km{\cdot}h^{-1}$) (m) Low-speed jogging (12–13.9 $km{\cdot}h^{-1}$) (m) Medium-speed running (14–17.9 $km{\cdot}h^{-1}$) (m) High-speed running (18–23.9 $km{\cdot}h^{-1}$) (m) Sprinting (24 $km{\cdot}h^{-1}$) (m)	Number of low acceleration (1.0–1.9 $m{\cdot}s^{-2}$) Number of moderate acceleration (2–2.9 $m{\cdot}s^{-2}$) Number of high acceleration (3–4 $m{\cdot}s^{-2}$) Number of low deceleration (1.0–1.9 $m{\cdot}s^{-2}$) Number of moderate deceleration (2–2.9 $m{\cdot}s^{-2}$) Number of high decelerations (3–4 $m{\cdot}s^{-2}$)	ND	Absolute	CD ($n = 42$) WD ($n = 31$) CM ($n = 34$) OA ($n = 28$) CF ($n = 14$)	GNSS, SPI HPU, GPSports, Canberra, Australia 15 Hz
Arjol-Serrano 2021 [92]	Observational	To examine the differences in the physical demands and technical-tactical actions encountered by soccer players between two playing formations (1-4-2-3-1 and 1-4-4-2) for each playing position	$n = 23$ professional male soccer players 31 official matches	Spanish Second Division	Total distance (m) Distance covered (14.4 $km{\cdot}h^{-1}$) (m) Distance covered (19.8. $km{\cdot}h^{-1}$) (m) Distance covered (25.0 $km{\cdot}h^{-1}$) (m)	Number of accelerations (2–4 $m{\cdot}s^{-2}$) Number of accelerations (>4 $m{\cdot}s^{-2}$) Number of decelerations (2–4 $m{\cdot}s^{-2}$) Number of decelerations (>4 $m{\cdot}s^{-2}$)	TD Acc Dec	Absolute	CD ($n = 48$ files) WD ($n = 44$ files) CM ($n = 28$ files) WM ($n = 27$ files) OM ($n = 28$ files) FW ($n = 29$ files)	GPS, APEX pod accelerometer, MAPPS Technology and Bluetooth LE; STATSports, Newry, North Ireland 18 Hz

Table 5. *Cont.*

Article	Type of Study	Aim of Study	Sample Size	Competition Category	Speed Profile	Acceleration Profile	Term	Threshold	Playing Position	Tracking Systems
Mallo 2015 [67]	Observational	To examine the physical demands imposed on professional soccer players	17 pre-season friendly matches (n = 111 files) 2011/2012–2012/2013	Spanish First Division "La Liga"	Total distance (m) Standing still (0–0.6 km·h^{-1}) (m) Walking (0.7–7.1 km·h^{-1}) (m) Jogging (7.2–14.3 km·h^{-1}) (m) Running (14.4–19.7 km·h^{-1}) (m) High-speed running (19.8–25.1 km·h^{-1}) (m) Sprinting (>25.1 km·h^{-1}) (m) High-intensity running (>14.4 km.h^{-1}) (m) Very-high-intensity running (>19.8 km.h^{-1}) (m) Maximal running speed (km/h)	Number of accelerations (<1.0 m·s^{-2}) Number of accelerations (1.1–1.5 m·s^{-2}) Number of maximal accelerations (1.6–2.0 m·s^{-2}) Number of accelerations (2.1–2.5 m·s^{-2}) Number of accelerations (>2.5 m·s^{-2}) Number of accelerations (>2.78 m·s^{-2})	HSD HIR VHIR	Absolute	CD (n = 23 files) FB (n = 20 files) CM (n = 22 files) WM (n = 26 files) FW (n = 20 files)	GPS, SPI Elite, GPSports Systems, Camberra, Australia 1 Hz.
Coutinho 2024 [112]	Observational	To compare the microcycle load distribution between teams from different competitive levels	n = 78 professional outfield football players, 22 training microcycles, three teams 2022/2023	First, Second, and Third Portugal division	Total distance covered (m/min), Running (14.4 km·h^{-1}–19.7 km·h^{-1}) (m/min) High-speed running (>19.8 km·h^{-1}) (m/min) Sprinting distance (>25.2 km·h^{-1}) (m/min)	Number of high accelerations (>3 m/s) (counts/min) Number of high decelerations (>3 m/s) (counts/min)	HSR	Absolute	CB (n = 16) FB (n = 12) MF (n = 22) W (n = 16) S (n = 12)	GPS, Catapult, Vector S7, Catapult Sports, Melbourne, Australia 10 Hz
Martín-García 2018 [10]	Observational	To determine the external load of a football team across playing position and relative to competition for a structured microcycle	n = 24 players and 42 training weeks and 37 competitive 2015–2016	Reserve Squad of a Spanish La Liga club	Total (m), High-speed running (>19.8 km/h) (m) Sprint distances (>25.2 km/h) (m)	Number of Accelerations (>3.m·s^{-2}) Number of Decelerations (>3 m·s^{-2})	TD HSR SPR ACC DEC	Absolute	CD (n = 3) (GPS = 104) FB (n = 6) (GPS = 145) MF (n = 3) (GPS = 45) OMF (n = 5) (GPS = 121) FW (n = 7) (GPS = 90)	GPS, Viper Pod, 50 gr, 88 × 33 mm; STATSports Viper; Northern Ireland 10 Hz
Díez 2021 [62]	Observational	To analyse the physical demands and technical-tactical actions for each playing position according to game location and final outcome in professional soccer players	n = 21 professional male soccer players 30 official matches 2017/2018	Spanish Second Division	Total distance (m) Moderate speed running distance (>14.4 km/h) (m) High-speed running distance (>19.8 km/h) (m) Sprint distance (>25 km/h) (m)	Number of Accelerations (between 2–4 m·s^{-2}) Number of Accelerations (>4 m·s^{-2}) Number of Decelerations (between 2–4 m·s^{-2}) Number of Decelerations (>4 m·s^{-2})	TD MSR HSR SPR	Absolute	CD (n = 5) WD (n = 4) MD (n = 8) F (n = 4)	GPS, APEX pod accelerometer, MAPPS Technology and Bluetooth LE; STATSports; North Ireland 18 Hz

Table 5. *Cont.*

Article	Type of Study	Aim of Study	Sample Size	Competition Category	Speed Profile	Acceleration Profile	Term	Threshold	Playing Position	Tracking Systems
Kavanagh 2024 [84]	Observational	To examine the relationships between high-intensity distances covered above generic and relative speed thresholds in English Premier League (EPL) matches across two consecutive seasons	n = 16 elite male soccer players and 38 matches two consecutive seasons 2019–2020/2021–2021	English Premier League	Total distance (m) High-speed running distance (>5.5 m/s) (m) High-intensity running distance (5.5–7 m/s) (m) Sprint distance (>7 m/s) (m) Total distance covered >Maximal Aerobic Speed Distance covered > 85% peak speed (m) Distance > 30% Anaerobic Speed Reserve (m)	ND	TD HSRD HIRD MAS PS ASR	Absolute And Relative	Defender (n = 7) Midfielders (n = 6) Forwards (n = 3)	Optical Tracking System Second Spectrum®, Los Angeles, CA, USA 25 Hz
Duthie 2018 [37]	Observational Longitudinal	To examine differences between the peak running speed, acceleration, and metabolic power of elite youth soccer across a range of age levels by position	n = 96 Elite junior soccer players 61 games within the 2015, 2016, and 2017 season, for a total of 441 individual match observations	-	Distance covered per unit of time (m·min^{-1})	Absolute instantaneous acceleration (m·s^{-2}) (count)	ND	Absolute	Attacker ATT Defender DEF Midfielder MID Wide WIDE	GPS, VIPER Units; STATSports Newry, UK 10 Hz
Kim 2023 [116]	Observational	To establish differences between positions and other contextual factors (match location, match outcome, playing formation, and score line) for both external and internal MIP variables	n = 24 male outfield players 31 matches 338 individual match observations	English Football League Championship Academy	Average speed (m·min^{-1}) High-speed running (m·min^{-1}; 5.5 to 7 m·s^{-1}) Sprinting (m·min^{-1}; >7 m·s^{-1})	Average acceleration/deceleration (m·s^{-2})	HSR Ave-Acc	Absolute	CD (n = 4) (GPS n = 52) WD (n = 5) (GPS n = 54) CM (n = 8) (GPS n = 89) WM (n = 5) (GPS n = 54) ST (n = 2) (GPS n = 28)	GPS, Vector S7, Catapult Innovations, Melbourne, Australia 10 Hz
Miguel 2022 [131]	Observational Cohort Study	To describe and characterize the daily and weekly external load in an amateur soccer team and based on the weighting factors determined by the match reference, compare the external loads between playing positions	n = 24 amateur soccer players 19 competitive microcycles 132 individual match observations 2018/2019	Portuguese regional competition	Total distance covered (m) High-speed running distance (4.0–5.5 m/s) (m) Very-high-speed running distance (5.5–7.0 m/s) Sprint distance (>7.0 m/s) (m)	Total number of accelerations "moderate intensity" (2.0–4.0 m/s^2) Total number of accelerations "high intensity" (>4.0 m/s^2) Total number of decelerations "moderate intensity" (2.0–4.0 m/s^2) Total number of accelerations "high intensity" (>4.0 m/s^2)	TDC HSRD VHSRD SpD MIAcc HIAcc MIDec HIDec	Absolute	CD (n = 4) (GPS n = 30) FB (n = 4) (GPS n = 30) CM (n = 6) (GPS n = 38) WM (n = 5) (GPS n = 24) F (n = 3) (GPS n = 10)	GPS, PlayerTek, Catapult Innovations, Melbourne, Australia 10 Hz

Table 5. *Cont.*

Article	Type of Study	Aim of Study	Sample Size	Competition Category	Speed Profile	Acceleration Profile	Term	Threshold	Playing Position	Tracking Systems
Kavanagh 2023 [135]	Retrospective study	To analyze the positional distances covered above generic and individualized speed thresholds within the most demanding phases of match play	n = 17 male professional soccer players 76 official league matches 2019–2020/2020–2021	English Premier League	Total distance covered (m) High speed running distance (5.5 m/s) (m) Total distance covered > Maximal Aerobic Speed Sprint distance (7 m/s) (m) Distance > 30% Anaerobic Speed Reserve (m)	ND	HSR MAS ASR	Absolute and Rela-tive	FB (n = 4) CD (n = 4) CM (n = 3) WM (n = 3) F (n = 3)	Optical Tracking System Second Spectrum®, Los Angeles, CA, USA 25 Hz
Casamich-ana 2021 [130]	Observational	To compare weekly accumulative load during the in-season competitive period by professional soccer players according to the amount of time played in official matches (90-min, > 60-min, < 60-min, and 0-min) regarding the players' position	n = 24 professional football players 42 training weeks and 37 official matches 2015–2016	Reserve squad of a Spanish La Liga	Total distance (m) High speed running (>19.8 km·h^{-1}) (m) Sprint meters (>25.2 km·h^{-1}) (m) High metabolic load distance (>25.5 W·kg^{-1}) (m)	Number of accelerations (ACC; >3 m·s^{-2}) Number of decelerations (DEC; <−3 m·s^{-2}).	TD HSR SPR HMLD ACC DEC	Absolute	FB (GPS n = 34) CD (GPS n = 26) MF (GPS n = 12) OMF (GPS n = 30) FW (GPS n = 20)	GPS, Viper Pod, 50 g, 88 × 33 mm, STATSports Viper, Northern Ireland 10 Hz
Djaoui 2022 [119]	Observational	To analyse the influence of congested periods of matches on the acceleration (Acc) and deceleration (Dec) profiles of elite soccer players	n = 23 elite male professional soccer players 31 official matches 2016 Two consecutive season (March–December)	National Premier League Swiss	Total distance covered (m) Low-speed running (0–10.8 km.h^{-1}) (m) Intermediate-speed running (>10.8–19.8 km.h^{-1}) High-speed running (>19.8–25.2 km.h^{-1}) (m) Sprint (>25.2 km.h^{-1}) (m)	Total distance decelerating (m) Maximal Deceleration (<−3 m·s^{-2}) (m) High Deceleration (−3 to <−2 m·s^{-2}) (m) Intermediate Deceleration (−2 to <−1 m·s^{-2}) (m) Low Deceleration (−1 to <0 m·s^{-2}) (m) Total distance acccelerating (m) Low Acceleration (>0 to 1 m·s^{-2}) (m) Intermediate Acceleration (>1 to 2 m·s^{-2}) (m) High Acceleration (>2 to 3 m·s^{-2}) (m) Maximal Acceleration (>3 m·s^{-2}) (m)	TDC LSR ISR HSR Tdec MDec MAcc HDec HAcc IDec IAcc LDec LAcc	Absolute	CB (n = 5) (GPS = 58) FB (n = 5) (GPS = 65) CM (n = 6) (GPS = 72) WF (n = 4) (GPS = 36) CF (n = 4) (GPS = 39)	GPS, Viper, STATSports, Ireland 10 Hz

Table 5. *Cont.*

Article	Type of Study	Aim of Study	Sample Size	Competition Category	Speed Profile	Acceleration Profile	Term	Threshold	Playing Position	Tracking Systems
Guerrero-Calderón 2022 [58]	Observational	To compare the training and match load of professional soccer players according to the playing position, and analyse the relationship between the metabolic and running speed metrics	n = 30 professional male soccer players n = 33 training weeks and n = 38 matches 2015–2016	Spanish First Division	Total distance (m) Low-speed running distance (<14 km/h) (m) Medium-speed running distance (14 to 18 km/h) High-speed running distance (18 to 21 km/h) (m) Very-high-speed running distance (21 to 24 km/h) Sprint running distance (>24 km·h^{-1}) (m)	Number of accelerations (2 m·s^{-2}) Number of decelerations (<2 m·s^{-2})	LSRD MSRD HSRD VHSRD SPD	Absolute	CD (GPS n = 89) ED (GPS n = 61) CM (GPS n = 71) WM (GPS n = 76) FO (GPS n = 36)	GPS, GPEXE Pro 18, GPEXE, Udine, Italy 18 Hz
Caro 2022 [59]	Observational	To analyse sub-maximum intensity periods (SubMIP's) manifested by professional soccer players during official matches according to the player position	n = 14 professional soccer players, n = 247 individual records, during 15 official matches 2019–2020	Azerbaijan Premier League	Total distance (m) High-speed running (>19.8 km/h) (m) Very-high-speed running or sprint (>25.2 km/h) Mean metabolic power metres per minute High metabolic load distance (>25.5 W/kg)	Number of accelerations (>3.m·s^{-2}) Number of decelerations (<−3 m·s^{-2}) Acceleration density (%)	HSR VHSR HMLD Met-Pow Acc-Dens	Absolute	CD (GPS = 76) WD (GPS = 50) MF (GPS = 36) OMF (GPS = 26) FW (GPS n = 59)	GPS, STATSports APEX ProSeries; STATSports, Newry, Northern Ireland 10 Hz
Garcïa-Calvo 2022 [27]	Observational	To examine the Spanish professional soccer players' high metabolic load distance profile, comparing competitive level and playing positions	n = 1321 players n = 18,131 individual match observations 2018/2019–2019/2020	First and Second Spanish Professional Soccer Leagues	High Metabolic Load Distance: Distance covered with a power consumption above 25.5 W·kg^{-1} Running at a constant velocity of 5.5 m·s^{-1} or 19.8 km·h^{-1}	High Metabolic Load Distance: Accelerations or decelerations (2 to 4 m·s^{-2})	HMLD	Absolute	CB FB CM WM FW	Mediacoach
Forcher 2022 [93]	Observational	To examine to what extent the physical match performance of professional soccer players is both position and player-specific	n = 25 players across 15 clubs 25 matchdays n = 163 matches 2019–2020	German Bundesliga	Total distance (m) High-intensity distance (17–23.99 km/h) (m) Sprinting distance (>24 km/h) (m)	Number of accelerations (>1.5 s^{-2})	ND	Absolute	CD n = 658 WD (n = 244 files) WB (n = 122 files) CM (n = 538 files) WM (n = 187 files) FW (n = 215 files)	Tracking system TRACAB, Chyron Hego, Melville, NY, USA
Modric 2023 [110]	Observational	To provide a comparative analysis of RP of professional soccer match-play across two highest-level soccer competitions: UCL and WC	Professional soccer players UCL n = 244 matches n = 20 WC n = 581 matches n = 55	Union of European Football Associations Champions League AND Fédération Internationale De Football Association World Cup	Total distance (m) High-intensity running (>5.5 m/s) (m)	ND	TD HIR	Absolute	FB (GPS n = 189) CD (GPS n = 300) CM (GPS n = 195) WM (GPS n = 87) FW (GPS n = 54)	Optical systems: InStat Fitness InStat Limited, Limerick, Republic of Ireland 25 Hz

Table 5. *Cont.*

Article	Type of Study	Aim of Study	Sample Size	Competition Category	Speed Profile	Acceleration Profile	Term	Threshold	Playing Position	Tracking Systems
Silva 2024 [81]	Retrospective study	To analyse the relations and differences between distances covered during official matches of the Portuguese first division, according to specific thresholds	n = 20 elite level soccer players n = 34 matches (111 observations) 2021–2022	First division of the Portuguese League	Distance covered > 25.2 km/h (m) Distance covered > 70% peak match speed (m) Distance covered > 75% peak match speed (m) Distance covered > 80% peak match speed (m) Distance covered > 85% peak match speed (m) Distance covered > 90% peak match speed (m)	ND	ND	Absolute And Relative	FB (n = 3) CD (n = 6) CM (n = 5) WM (n = 4) FW (n = 2)	GPS, Catapult Vector S7—Catapult Sports, Melbourne, Australia 10 Hz
Morgans 2023 [117]	Observational	To examine the impact of playing position (PP), match location (ML), and opposition standard (OS) on team and individual acceleration (ACC) and deceleration (DEC) efforts	n = 50 elite football players U23 24 matches 2020/21	English Premier Development League	ND	High-intensity acceleration (>+3 m·s^{-2}) (count) Highintensity deceleration (<−3 m·s^{-2}) (count)	ND	Absolute	CB (GPS n = 68) FB (GPS n = 24) CM (GPS n = 54) WM (GPS n = 15) CF (GPS n = 27)	GPS, Apex, STATSports Software; version 4.3.8, Northern Ireland, UK 10 Hz
Oliva-Lozano 2023 [36]	Observational	To investigate the periods in which sprints occurred during official matches and analyze these sprints considering the effect of the playing position and different contextual variables	n = 20 male soccer players n = 252 sprints n = 6 matches	Spanish semi-professional club	Maximum velocity (km/h) Starting Velocity (km/h) Distance covered sprinting (>24 km/h (m)	Maximum acceleration (m·s^{-2}) Maximum deceleration (m·s^{-2})	Vmax V0 SPD ACC-max DEC-max	Absolute	FB CD MF WMF FW	GPS, WIMU Pro systems RealTrack Systems, Almeria, Spain

Table 5. *Cont.*

Article	Type of Study	Aim of Study	Sample Size	Competition Category	Speed Profile	Acceleration Profile	Term	Threshold	Playing Position	Tracking Systems
Ingebrigts-en 2015 [108]	Observational	To characterise the acceleration and sprint profiles of elite football match play	$n = 15$ professional players ($n = 101$ observations) 15 home game	Norwegian elite football team (Rosenborg FC)	Total distance covered (m) Walking (from 0 to 7.1 km·h^{-1}) (m) Jogging (from 7.2 to 14.3 km·h^{-1}) (m) Running (from 14.4 to 19.7 km·h^{-1}) (m) High-speed running (from 19.8 to 25.2 km·h^{-1}) Sprinting (≥25.2 km·h^{-1}) (m) Low- and moderate-intensity activities (locomotion <19.8 km·h^{-1}) (m) High-intensity activities (locomotion (≥19.8 km·h^{-1}) (m)	Number of acceleration (>2 m·s^{-2})	ND	Absolute	CD ($n = 3$) FB ($n = 4$) CM ($n = 2$) WM ($n = 4$) AT ($n = 2$)	Tracking system RadioEye™ technology (ZXY SportTracki-ng AS, Radionor Communica-tions AS, Trondheim, Norway) 40 Hz
Bradley 2009 [69]	Observational	To determine the activity profiles of a large sample of English FA Premier League soccer players and examine high-intensity running during elite-standard soccer matches for players in various playing positions	$n = 370$ players 28 games competitive season 2005/2006	English FA Premier League	Total distance (m) Standing (0–0.6 km/h) (m) Walking (0.7–7.1 km/h) (m) Jogging (7.2–14.3 km/h) (m) Running (14.4–19.7 km/h) (m) High-speed running (19.8–25.1 km/h) (m) Sprinting (>25.1 km/h) (m) High-intensity running (>14.4 km/h) (m) Very-high-intensity running (>19.8 km/h) (m)	ND	HSR HIR VHIR	Absolute	CD ($n = 92$) FB ($n = 84$) CM ($n = 80$) WM ($n = 52$) AT ($n = 62$)	Tracking system ProZone Version 3.0, ProZone Sports Ltd.1, Leeds, UK

Table 5. *Cont.*

Article	Type of Study	Aim of Study	Sample Size	Competition Category	Speed Profile	Acceleration Profile	Term	Threshold	Playing Position	Tracking Systems
Núñez-Sánchez 2017 [52]	Observational	To compare the relative running demands ($m \cdot min^{-1}$), among different soccer players positions, coded by an absolute threshold vs. an individualized threshold based on splits of 10% of peak velocity, during friendly games, with the same tactical system and monitoring with a GPS	n = 20 semiprofessional soccer players four friendly matches	Spanish soccer league	Very-low-intensity running (0–7 $km \cdot h^{-1}$) (m) Low-intensity running (7–13 $km \cdot h^{-1}$) (m) Medium-intensity running (13–18 $km \cdot h^{-1}$) (m) High-intensity running (18–21 $km \cdot h^{-1}$) (m) Very-high-intensity running (>21 $km \cdot h^{-1}$) (m) <10% Peak of velocity (m) 10–20% Peak of velocity (m) 20–30% Peak of velocity (m) 30–40% Peak of velocity (m) 40–50% Peak of velocity (m) 50–60% Peak of velocity (m) 60–70% Peak of velocity (m) 70–80% Peak of velocity (m) 80–90% Peak of velocity (m) >90% Peak of velocity (m)	ND	VLIR LIR MIR HIR VHIR PV	Absolute and Relative	CB n = 4 FB n = 4 CM n = 4 WM n = 4 F n = 4	GPs, SPI-pro W2b, GPSport, Canberra, Australia 15 Hz
Bradley 2013 [95]	Observational	To examine the effects of high (HPBPT) and low-percentage ball possession teams (LPBPT) on physical and technical profiles in elite soccer matches	n = 810 players 54 matches	English FA Premier League	Total distance (m) Standing (0–0.6 km/h) (m) Walking (0.7–7.1 km/h) (m) Jogging (7.2–14.3 km/h) (m) Running (14.4–19.7 km/h) (m) High-speed running (19.8–25.1 km/h) (m) Sprinting (>25.1 km/h) (m) High-intensity running (>19.8 km/h) (m)	ND	HIR	Absolute	CD (n = 199) FB (n = 177) CM (n = 191) WM (n = 110) AT (n = 133)	Tracking system ProZone Version 3.0, ProZone Sports Ltd.1, Leeds, UK

Author Contributions: Conceptualization, C.C., J.A.P., J.P.B. and S.L.J.S.; Methodology, C.C., J.A.P., J.P.B., Á.G.-d.-l.-F. and S.L.J.S.; Validation, C.C., J.A.P., J.P.B. and S.L.J.S.; Investigation, C.C., Á.G.-d.-l.-F. and S.L.J.S.; Writing—original draft preparation, C.C., J.A.P., J.P.B. and S.L.J.S.; Writing—review and editing, C.C., J.A.P., J.P.B., Á.G.-d.-l.-F. and S.L.J.S.; Supervision, C.C., J.A.P., J.P.B., Á.G.-d.-l.-F. and S.L.J.S.; Project administration, S.L.J.S. All authors have read and agreed to the published version of the manuscript.

Funding: This research received no external funding.

Institutional Review Board Statement: Not applicable.

Informed Consent Statement: Not applicable.

Data Availability Statement: Data is contained within the article.

Conflicts of Interest: The authors declare no conflicts of interest.

References

1. Salmon, P.; Mclean, S. Complexity in the beautiful game: Implications for football research and practice. *Sci. Med. Footb.* **2020**, *4*, 162–167. [CrossRef]
2. Carling, C.; Bloomfield, J.; Nelsen, L.; Reilly, T. The role of motion analysis in Elite Soccer. *Sports Med.* **2008**, *38*, 839–862. [CrossRef]
3. Sal de Rellán-Guerra, A.; Rey, E.; Kalén, A.; Lago-Peñas, C. Age-related physical and technical match performance changes in elite soccer players. *Scand. J. Med. Sci. Sports* **2019**, *29*, 1421–1427. [CrossRef]
4. Bendala, F.J.T.; Vázquez, M.A.C.; Suarez-Arrones, L.J.; Sánchez, F.J.N. Comparison of external load in high speed actions between friendly matches and training sessions. *Retos Nuevas Tend. Educ. Física Deporte Y Recreación* **2018**, *33*, 54–57.
5. Coker, N.A.; Wells, A.J.; Ake, K.M.; Griffin, D.L.; Rossi, S.J.; McMillan, J.L. Relationship between running performance and RECOVERY-STRESS state in collegiate soccer players. *J. Strength Cond. Res.* **2017**, *31*, 2131–2140. [CrossRef]
6. Barnes, C.; Archer, D.T.; Hogg, B.; Bush, M.; Bradley, P.S. The evolution of physical and technical performance parameters in the English Premier League. *Int. J. Sports Med.* **2014**, *35*, 1095–1100. [CrossRef] [PubMed]
7. Zhou, C.; Gómez, M.Á.; Lorenzo, A. The evolution of physical and technical performance parameters in the Chinese Soccer Super League. *Biol. Sport* **2020**, *37*, 139–145. [CrossRef] [PubMed]
8. Bush, M.; Barnes, C.; Archer, D.T.; Hogg, B.; Bradley, P.S. Evolution of match performance parameters for various playing positions in the English Premier League. *Hum. Mov. Sci.* **2015**, *39*, 01–11. [CrossRef] [PubMed]
9. Bush, M.; Archer, D.T.; Barnes, C.; Hogg, B.; Bradley, P.S. Longitudinal match performance characteristics of UK and non-UK players in the English Premier League. *Sci. Med. Footb.* **2017**, *1*, 2–9. [CrossRef]
10. Martín-García, A.; Gómez Díaz, A.; Bradley, P.S.; Morera, F.; Casamichana, D. Quantification of a Professional Football Team's External Load Using a Microcycle Structure. *J. Strength Cond. Res.* **2018**, *32*, 3511–3518. [CrossRef]
11. Wallace, J.L.; Norton, K.I. Evolution of World Cup soccer final games 1966–2010: Game structure, speed and play patterns. *J. Sci. Med. Sport* **2014**, *17*, 223–228. [CrossRef]
12. Pons, E.; Ponce-Bordón, J.C.; Díaz-García, J.; Del Campo, R.L.; Resta, R.; Peirau, X.; García-Calvo, T. A longitudinal exploration of match running performance during a football match in the spanish la liga: A four-season study. *Int. J. Environ. Res. Public Health* **2021**, *18*, 1133. [CrossRef] [PubMed]
13. Buchheit, M.; Simpson, B.M.; Mendez-Villanueva, A. Repeated high-speed activities during youth soccer games in relation to changes in maximal sprinting and aerobic speeds. *Int. J. Sports Med.* **2013**, *34*, 40–48. [CrossRef]
14. Arcos, A.L.; Martínez-Santos, R.; Yanci, J.; Mendiguchia, J.; Méndez-Villanueva, A. Negative associations between perceived training load, volume and changes in physical fitness in professional soccer players. *J. Sports Sci. Med.* **2015**, *14*, 394–401.
15. Jaspers, A.; De Beéck, T.O.; Brink, M.S.; Frencken, W.G.P.; Staes, F.; Davis, J.J.; Helsen, W.F. Predicting Future Perceived Wellness in Professional Soccer: The Role of Preceding Load and Wellness. *Int. J. Sports Physiol. Perform.* **2019**, *14*, 1074–1080. [CrossRef]
16. Pearce, L.; Woods, C.; Sinclair, W.; Leicht, A. Officiating Role Influences the Physical Match Activity Profiles of Rugby League Touch Judges and Referees. *J. Hum. Kinet.* **2017**, *58*, 225–231. [CrossRef] [PubMed]
17. Djaoui, L.; Haddad, M.; Chamari, K.; Dellal, A. Monitoring training load and fatigue in soccer players with physiological markers. *Physiol. Behav.* **2017**, *181*, 86–94. [CrossRef] [PubMed]
18. Casamichana, D.; Castellano, J.; Calleja-Gonzalez, J.; RomaN, J.S.; Castagna, C. Relationship between indicators of training load in soccer players. *J. Strength Cond. Res.* **2013**, *27*, 369–374. [CrossRef]
19. Ward, P.; Coutts, A.J.; Pruna, R.; McCall, A. Putting the i back in team. *Int. J. Sports Physiol. Perform.* **2018**, *13*, 1107–1111. [CrossRef] [PubMed]

20. Rago, V.; Brito, J.; Figueiredo, P.; Krustrup, P.; Rebelo, A. Relationship between External Load and Perceptual Responses to Training in Professional Football: Effects of Quantification Method. *Sports* **2019**, *7*, 68. [CrossRef]
21. Fanchini, M.; Ghielmetti, R.; Coutts, A.J.; Schena, F.; Impellizzeri, F.M. Effect of training-session intensity distribution on session rating of perceived exertion in soccer players. *Int. J. Sports Physiol. Perform.* **2015**, *10*, 426–430. [CrossRef] [PubMed]
22. Foster, C.; Rodriguez-Marroyo, J.A.; de Koning, J.J. Monitoring Training Loads: The Past, the Present, and the future. *Int. J. Sports Physiol. Perform.* **2017**, *12*, S2-2. [CrossRef] [PubMed]
23. Thorpe, R.T.; Atkinson, G.; Drust, B.; Gregson, W. Monitoring fatigue status in elite team-sport athletes: Implications for practice. *Int. J. Sports Physiol. Perform.* **2017**, *12*, S2-27. [CrossRef] [PubMed]
24. Cummins, C.; Orr, R.; O'Connor, H.; West, C. Global Positioning Systems (GPS) and Microtechnology Sensors in Team Sports: A Systematic Review. *Sports Med.* **2013**, *43*, 1025–1042. [CrossRef] [PubMed]
25. Strauss, A.; Sparks, M.; Pienaar, C. The use of GPS analysis to quantify the internal and external match demands of semi-elite level female soccer players during a tournament. *J. Sports Sci. Med.* **2019**, *18*, 73–81. [PubMed]
26. Azcárate, U.; Yanci, J.; Los Arcos, A. Influence of match playing time and the length of the between-match microcycle in Spanish professional soccer players' perceived training load. *Sci. Med. Footb.* **2018**, *2*, 23–28. [CrossRef]
27. García-Calvo, T.; Ponce-Bordón, J.C.; Pons, E.; del Campo, R.L.; Resta, R.; Raya-González, J. High metabolic load distance in professional soccer according to competitive level and playing positions. *PeerJ* **2022**, *10*, e13318. [CrossRef] [PubMed]
28. Impellizzeri, F.M.; Marcora, S.M.; Coutts, A.J. Internal and external training load: 15 years on. *Int. J. Sports Physiol. Perform.* **2019**, *14*, 270–273. [CrossRef]
29. Gallo, T.F.; Cormack, S.J.; Gabbett, T.J.; Lorenzen, C.H.; Gallo, T.F.; Cormack, S.J.; Gabbett, T.J.; Lorenzen, C.H. Pre-training perceived wellness impacts training output in Australian football players. *J. Sports Sci.* **2015**, *34*, 1445–1451. [CrossRef] [PubMed]
30. Del Coso, J.; Brito de Souza, D.; Moreno-Perez, V.; Buldú, J.M.; Nevado, F.; Resta, R.; López-Del Campo, R. Influence of players' maximum running speed on the team's ranking position at the end of the Spanish Laliga. *Int. J. Environ. Res. Public Health* **2020**, *17*, 8815. [CrossRef] [PubMed]
31. Sekulic, D.; Versic, S.; Decelis, A.; Castro-Piñero, J.; Javorac, D.; Dimitric, G.; Idrizovic, K.; Jukic, I.; Modric, T. The effect of the COVID-19 lockdown on the position-specific match running performance of professional football players; preliminary observational study. *Int. J. Environ. Res. Public Health* **2021**, *18*, 12221. [CrossRef] [PubMed]
32. Schulze, E.; Julian, R.; Skorski, S. The Accuracy of a Low-Cost GPS System during Football-Specific Movements. *J. Sports Sci. Med.* **2021**, *20*, 126. [CrossRef]
33. Jaspers, A.; De Beéck, T.O.; Brink, M.S.; Frencken, W.G.; Staes, F.; Davis, J.J.; Helsen, W.F. Relationships Between the External and Internal Training Load in Professional Soccer: What Can We Learn from Machine Learning? *Int. J. Sports Physiol. Perform.* **2018**, *13*, 625–630. [CrossRef] [PubMed]
34. Fischer-Sonderegger, K.; Taube, W.; Rumo, M.; Tschopp, M. Physical Load in Soccer: Strengths and Limitations of Three Different Methods. *Int. J. Sports Physiol. Perform.* **2018**, *14*, 627–634. [CrossRef] [PubMed]
35. Akenhead, R.; Nassis, G.P. Training load and player monitoring in high-level football: Current practice and perceptions. *Int. J. Sports Physiol. Perform.* **2016**, *11*, 587–593. [CrossRef]
36. Oliva-Lozano, J.M.; Cuenca-López, J.; Suárez, J.; Granero-Gil, P.; Muyor, J.M. When and How Do Soccer Players from a Semi-Professional Club Sprint in Match Play? *J. Hum. Kinet.* **2023**, *86*, 195–204. [CrossRef]
37. Duthie, G.M.; Thornton, H.R.; Delaney, J.A.; Connolly, D.R.; Serpiello, F.R. Running Intensities in Elite Youth Soccer by Age and Position. *J. Strength Cond. Res.* **2018**, *32*, 2918–2924. [CrossRef] [PubMed]
38. Jaspers, A.; Kuyvenhoven, J.P.; Staes, F.; Frencken, W.G.P.; Helsen, W.F.; Brink, M.S. Examination of the external and internal load indicators' association with overuse injuries in professional soccer players. *J. Sci. Med. Sport* **2018**, *21*, 579–585. [CrossRef] [PubMed]
39. Gabbett, T.J.; Whiteley, R.J. Two Training-Load Paradoxes: Can We Work Harder and Smarter, Can Physical Preparation and Medical be Team-Mates ? *Int. J. Sports Physiol. Perform.* **2017**, *12*, S2-50–S2-54. [CrossRef]
40. Abbott, W.; Brickley, G.; Smeeton, N.J.; Mills, S. Individualizing Acceleration in English Premier League Academy Soccer Players. *J. Strength Cond.* **2018**, *32*, 3503–3510. [CrossRef] [PubMed]
41. Noya Salces, J.; Gómez-Carmona, P.M.; Gracia-Marco, L.; Moliner-Urdiales, D.; Sillero-Quintana, M. Epidemiology of injuries in First Division Spanish football. *J. Sports Sci.* **2014**, *32*, 1263–1270. [CrossRef]
42. Lu, D.; McCall, A.; Jones, M.; Kovalchik, S.; Steinweg, J.; Gelis, L.; Duffield, R. Injury epidemiology in Australian male professional soccer. *J. Sci. Med. Sport* **2020**, *23*, 574–579. [CrossRef]
43. Pulici, L.; Certa, D.; Zago, M.; Volpi, P.; Esposito, F. Injury Burden in Professional European Football (Soccer): Systematic Review, Meta-Analysis, and Economic Considerations. *Clin. J. Sport Med.* **2022**, *33*, 450–457. [CrossRef]
44. Perez, V.; Vázquez, M.; Toscano, J.; Sotos-Martinez, V.J.; López del Campo, R.; Resta, R.; Del Coso, J. Influence of the Weekly and Match-play Load on Muscle Injury in Professional Football Players. *Int. J. Sports Med.* **2022**, *43*, 1533–2110. [CrossRef]

45. Leventer, L.; Eek, F.; Hofstetter, S.; Lames, M. Injury Patterns among Elite Football Players: A Media-based Analysis over 6 Seasons with Emphasis on Playing Position. *Int. J. Sports Med.* **2016**, *37*, 898–908. [CrossRef] [PubMed]
46. Swart, J.; Varekamp, C.; Greyling, J. The pattern of non-contact injuries in a South African professional football team. *S. Afr. J. Sports Med.* **2022**, *34*, 1–5. [CrossRef]
47. Djaoui, L.; Chamari, K.; Owen, A.L.; Dellal, A. Maximal Sprinting Speed of Elite Soccer Players During Training and Matches. *J. Strength Cond. Res.* **2017**, *31*, 1509–1517. [CrossRef]
48. Reardon, C.; Tobin, D.P.; Delahunt, E. Application of individualized speed thresholds to interpret position specific running demands in elite professional rugby union: A GPS Study. *PLoS ONE* **2015**, *10*, e0133410. [CrossRef] [PubMed]
49. Massard, T.; Eggers, T.; Lovell, R. Peak speed determination in football: Is sprint testing necessary? *Sci. Med. Footb.* **2018**, *2*, 123–126. [CrossRef]
50. Mendez-Villanueva, A.; Buchheit, M.; Peltola, E.; Bourdon, P. Does on field sprinting performance in young soccer players depend on how fast they can run or how fast they do run? *J. Strength Cond. Res.* **2011**, *25*, 2634–2638. [CrossRef] [PubMed]
51. Murray, N.B.; Gabbett, T.J.; Townshend, A.D. The use of relative speed zones in Australian Football: Are we really measuring what we think we are? *Int. J. Sports Physiol. Perform.* **2018**, *13*, 442–451. [CrossRef] [PubMed]
52. Núñez-Sánchez, F.J.; Toscano-Bendala, F.J.; Campos-Vázquez, M.A.; Suarez-Arrones, L.J. Individualized speed threshold to analyze the game running demands in soccer players using GPS technology. *Retos Nuevas Tend. Educ. Física Deporte Y Recreación* **2017**, *32*, 130–133.
53. Anderson, L.; Orme, P.; Di Michele, R.; Close, G.L.; Morgans, R.; Drust, B.; Morton, J.P. Quantification of training load during one-, two- and three-game week schedules in professional soccer players from the English Premier League: Implications for carbohydrate periodisation. *J. Sports Sci.* **2016**, *34*, 1250–1259. [CrossRef] [PubMed]
54. Abt, G.; Lovell, R. The use of individualized speed and intensity thresholds for determining the distance run at high-intensity in professional soccer. *J. Sports Sci.* **2009**, *27*, 893–898. [CrossRef]
55. Miguel, M.; Oliveira, R.; Loureiro, N.; García-Rubio, J.; Ibáñez, S.J. Load measures in training/match monitoring in soccer: A systematic review. *Int. J. Environ. Res. Public Health* **2021**, *18*, 2721. [CrossRef] [PubMed]
56. Teixeira, J.E.; Leal, M.; Ferraz, R.; Ribeiro, J.; Cachada, J.M.; Barbosa, T.M.; Monteiro, A.M.; Forte, P. Effects of match location, quality of opposition and match outcome on match running performance in a portuguese professional football team. *Entropy* **2021**, *23*, 973. [CrossRef]
57. Teixeira, J.E.; Forte, P.; Ferraz, R.; Leal, M.; Ribeiro, J.; Silva, A.J.; Barbosa, T.M.; Monteiro, A.M. Monitoring accumulated training and match load in football: A systematic review. *Int. J. Environ. Res. Public Health* **2021**, *18*, 3906. [CrossRef]
58. Guerrero-Calderón, B.; Morcillo, J.A.; Chena, M.; Castillo-Rodríguez, A. Comparison of training and match load between metabolic and running speed metrics of professional Spanish soccer players by playing position. *Biol. Sport* **2022**, *39*, 933–941. [CrossRef] [PubMed]
59. Caro, E.; Campos-Vazquez, M.A.; Lapuente-Sagarra, M.; Caparros, T. Analysis of professional soccer players in competitive match play based on submaximum intensity periods. *PeerJ* **2022**, *10*, e13309. [CrossRef]
60. Al Haddad, H.; Méndez-Villanueva, A.; Torreño, N.; Munguía-Izquierdo, D.; Suárez-Arrones, L. Variability of GPS-derived running performance during official matches in elite professional soccer players. *J. Sports Med. Phys. Fit.* **2018**, *58*, 1439–1445. [CrossRef] [PubMed]
61. Lovell, R.; Fransen, J.; Ryan, R.; Massard, T.; Cross, R.; Eggers, T.; Duffield, R. Biological maturation and match running performance: A national football (soccer) federation perspective. *J. Sci. Med. Sport* **2019**, *22*, 1139–1145. [CrossRef] [PubMed]
62. Díez, A.; Lozano, D.; Arjol-Serrano, J.L.; Mainer-Pardos, E.; Castillo, D.; Torrontegui-Duarte, M.; Nobari, H.; Jaén-Carrillo, D.; Lampre, M. Influence of contextual factors on physical demands and technical-tactical actions regarding playing position in professional soccer players. *BMC Sports Sci. Med. Rehabil.* **2021**, *13*, 157. [CrossRef]
63. Randers, M.B.; Mujika, I.; Hewitt, A.; Santisteban, J.; Bischoff, R.; Solano, R.; Zubillaga, A.; Peltola, E.; Krustrup, P.; Mohr, M. Application of four different football match analysis systems: A comparative study. *J. Sports Sci.* **2010**, *28*, 171–182. [CrossRef] [PubMed]
64. Bradley, P.S.; Di Mascio, M.; Peart, D.; Olsen, P.; Sheldon, B. High-Intensity Activity Profiles of Elite Soccer Players at different Performance Levels. *J. Strength Cond. Res.* **2010**, *24*, 2343–2351. [CrossRef] [PubMed]
65. Harper, D.J.; Carling, C.; Kiely, J. High-Intensity Acceleration and Deceleration Demands in Elite Team Sports Competitive Match Play: A Systematic Review and Meta-Analysis of Observational Studies. *Sports Med.* **2019**, *49*, 1923–1947. [CrossRef] [PubMed]
66. Varley, M.C.; Jaspers, A.; Helsen, W.F.; Malone, J.J. Methodological considerations when quantifying high-intensity efforts in team sport using global positioning system technology. *Int. J. Sports Physiol. Perform.* **2017**, *12*, 1059–1068. [CrossRef]
67. Mallo, J.; Mena, E.; Nevado, F.; Paredes, V. Physical Demands of Top-Class Soccer Friendly Matches in Relation to a Playing Position Using Global Positioning System Technology. *J. Hum. Kinet.* **2015**, *47*, 179–188. [CrossRef] [PubMed]
68. Nakamura, F.Y.; Pereira, L.A.; Loturco, I.; Rosseti, M.; Moura, F.A.; Bradley, P.S. Repeated-Sprint Sequences during Female Soccer Matches Using Fixed and Individual Speed Thresholds. *J. Strength Cond. Res.* **2017**, *31*, 1802–1810. [CrossRef] [PubMed]

69. Bradley, P.S.; Sheldon, W.; Wooster, B.; Olsen, P.; Boanas, P.; Krustrup, P. High-intensity running in English FA Premier League soccer matches. *J. Sports Sci.* **2009**, *27*, 159–168. [CrossRef]
70. Barrera, J.; Sarmento, H.; Clemente, F.M.; Field, A.; Figueiredo, A.J. The effect of contextual variables on match performance across different playing positions in professional Portuguese soccer players. *Int. J. Environ. Res. Public Health* **2021**, *18*, 5175. [CrossRef] [PubMed]
71. Carling, C.; Le Gall, F.; Dupont, G. Analysis of repeated high-intensity running performance in professional soccer. *J. Sports Sci.* **2012**, *30*, 325–336. [CrossRef]
72. Campos-Vazquez, M.A.; Romero-Boza, S.; Toscano-Bendala, F.J.; Leon-Prados, J.A.; Suarez-Arrones, L.J.; Gonzalez-Jurado, J.A. Comparison of the Effect of Repeated-Sprint Training Combined with Two Different Methods of Strength Training on Young Soccer Players. *J. Strength Cond. Res.* **2015**, *29*, 744–751. [CrossRef]
73. Mujika, I.; Spencer, M.; Santisteban, J.; Goiriena, J.J.; Bishop, D. Age-Related Differences in Repeated-Sprint Ability in Highly Trained Youth Football Players. *J. Sports Sci.* **2009**, *27*, 1581–1590. [CrossRef] [PubMed]
74. Girard, O.; Mendez-Villanueva, A.; Bishop, D. Repeated-Sprint Ability—Part I. *Sports Med.* **2011**, *41*, 673–694. [CrossRef]
75. Rampinini, E.; Sassi, A.; Morelli, A.; Mazzoni, S.; Fanchini, M.; Coutts, A.J. Repeated-Sprint Ability in Professional and Amateur Soccer Players. *Appl. Physiol. Nutr. Metab.* **2009**, *34*, 1048–1054. [CrossRef]
76. Buchheit, M.; Mendez-Villanueva, A.; Simpson, B.M.; Bourdon, P.C. Repeated-sprint sequences during youth soccer matches. *Int. J. Sports Med.* **2010**, *31*, 709–716. [CrossRef]
77. Zamparo, P.; Bolomini, F.; Nardello, F.; Beato, M. Energetics (and Kinematics) of Short Shuttle Runs. *Eur. J. Appl. Physiol.* **2015**, *115*, 1985–1994. [CrossRef] [PubMed]
78. Beato, M.; Drust, B. Acceleration intensity is an important contributor to the external and internal training load demands of repeated sprint exercises in soccer players. *Res. Sports Med.* **2021**, *29*, 67–76. [CrossRef]
79. Zamparo, P.; Zadro, I.; Lazzer, S.; Beato, M.; Sepulcri, L. Energetics of shuttle runs: The effects of distance and change of direction. *Int. J. Sports Physiol. Perform.* **2014**, *9*, 1033–1039. [CrossRef] [PubMed]
80. Aziz, A.R.; Mukherjee, S.; Chia, M.Y.H.; Teh, K.C. Validity of the Running Repeated Sprint Ability Test among Playing Positions and Level of Competitiveness in Trained Soccer Players. *Int. J. Sports Med.* **2008**, *29*, 833–838. [CrossRef]
81. Silva, H.; Nakamura, F.Y.; Loturco, I.; Ribeiro, J.; Marcelino, R. Analyzing soccer match sprint distances: A comparison of GPS-based absolute and relative thresholds. *Biol. Sport* **2024**, *41*, 223. [CrossRef]
82. Meylan, C.M.; Trewin, J.; Mckean, K.; Meylan, C. Quantifying Explosive Actions in International Women's Soccer Original Investigation. *Int. J. Sports Physiol. Perform.* **2016**, *12*, 310–315. [CrossRef]
83. Sweeting, A.J.; Cormack, S.J.; Morgan, S.; Aughey, R.J. When is a sprint a sprint? A review of the analysis of team-sport athlete activity profile. *Front. Physiol.* **2017**, *8*, 1–12. [CrossRef]
84. Kavanagh, R.; Di Michele, R.; Oliveira, R.; McDaid, K.; Rhodes, D.; Morgans, R. The relationships between distances covered above generic and relative speed thresholds by male soccer players in English Premier League matches across two competitive seasons. The effects of positional demands and possession. *Biol. Sport* **2024**, *41*, 77–86. [CrossRef] [PubMed]
85. Castellano, J.; Puente, A.; Echeazarra, I.; Usabiaga, O.; Casamichana, D. Number of players and relative pitch area per player: Comparing their influence on heart rate and physical demands in under- 12 and under-13 football players. *PLoS ONE* **2016**, *11*, e0127505. [CrossRef]
86. Sparks, M.; Coetzee, B.; Gabbett, T.J. Internal and External Match Loads of University-Level Soccer Players: A Comparison Between Methods. *J. Strength Cond. Res.* **2017**, *31*, 1072–1077. [CrossRef]
87. Gabbett, T.J. Use of relative Speed Zones Increases the High-speed Running Performed in Team Sport Match Play. *J. Strength Cond. Res.* **2015**, *29*, 3353–3359. [CrossRef]
88. Méndez-Villanueva, A.; Buchheit, M.; Simpson, B.; Bourdon, P. Match play intensity distribution in youth soccer. *Int. J. Sports Med.* **2013**, *34*, 101–110. [CrossRef] [PubMed]
89. Lovell, R.; Barrett, S.; Portas, M.; Weston, M. Re-examination of the post half-time reduction in soccer work-rate. *J. Sci. Med. Sport* **2013**, *16*, 250–254. [CrossRef] [PubMed]
90. Alonso-Callejo, A.; Garcia-Unanue, J.; Perez-Guerra, A.; Gomez, D.; Sanchez-Sanchez, J.; Gallardo, L.; Oliva-Lozano, J.M.; Felipe, J.L. Effect of playing position and microcycle days on the acceleration speed profile of elite football players. *Sci. Rep.* **2022**, *12*, 19266. [CrossRef]
91. Martinez-Cabrera, F.; Núñez-Sánchez, F. The use of metabolic power to assess physical demands in soccer: How does it differ from the traditional approach through speed running? *J. Sports Med. Phys. Fit.* **2017**, *58*, 1403–1411. [CrossRef] [PubMed]
92. Arjol-Serrano, J.L.; Lampre, M.; Díez, A.; Castillo, D.; Sanz-López, F.; Lozano, D. The influence of playing formation on physical demands and technical-tactical actions according to playing positions in an elite soccer team. *Int. J. Environ. Res. Public Health* **2021**, *18*, 4148. [CrossRef]

93. Forcher, L.; Forcher, L.; Jekauc, D.; Woll, A.; Gross, T.; Altmann, S. Center backs work hardest when playing in a back three: The influence of tactical formation on physical and technical match performance in professional soccer. *PLoS ONE* **2022**, *17*, e0265501. [CrossRef]
94. Bradley, P.S.; Carling, C.; Archer, D.; Roberts, J.; Dodds, A.; di Mascio, M.; Paul, D.; Diaz, A.G.; Peart, D.; Krustrup, P. The effect of playing formation on high-intensity running and technical profiles in English FA premier League soccer matches. *J. Sports Sci.* **2011**, *29*, 821–830. [CrossRef]
95. Bradley, P.S.; Noakes, T.D. Match running performance fluctuations in elite soccer: Indicative of fatigue, pacing or situational influences? *J. Sports Sci.* **2013**, *31*, 1627–1638. [CrossRef] [PubMed]
96. Konefał, M.; Chmura, P.; Kowalczuk, E.; Figueiredo, A.J.; Sarmento, H.; Rokita, A.; Chmura, J.; Andrzejewski, M. Modeling of relationships between physical and technical activities and match outcome in elite German soccer players. *J. Sports Med. Phys. Fit.* **2019**, *59*, 752–759. [CrossRef]
97. Bradley, P.S.; Lago-Peñas, C.; Rey, E.; Gomez Diaz, A. The effect of high and low percentage ball possession on physical and technical profiles in English FA Premier League soccer matches. *J. Sports Sci.* **2013**, *31*, 1261–1270. [CrossRef]
98. Andrzejewski, M.; Chmura, P.; Konefal, M.; Kowalczuk, E.; Chmura, J. Match outcome and sprinting activities in match play by elite German soccer players. *J. Sports Med. Phys. Fit.* **2018**, *58*, 785–792. [CrossRef]
99. Chmura, J.; Nazar, K. Parallel changes in the onset of blood lactate accumulation (OBLA) and threshold of psychomotor performance deterioration during incremental exercise after training in athletes. *Int. J. Psychophysiol.* **2010**, *75*, 287–290. [CrossRef] [PubMed]
100. Modric, T.; Versic, S.; Sekulic, D.; Liposek, S. Analysis of the Association between Running Performance and Game Performance Indicators in Professional Soccer Players. *Int. J. Environ. Res. Public Health* **2019**, *16*, 4032. [CrossRef] [PubMed]
101. Akenhead, R.; Hayes, P.R.; Thompson, K.G.; French, D. Diminutions of acceleration and deceleration output during professional football match play. *J. Sci. Med. Sport* **2013**, *16*, 556–561. [CrossRef]
102. Oliveira, R.; Brito, J.P.; Martins, A.; Mendes, B.; Marinho, D.A.; Ferraz, R.; Marques, M.C. In-season internal and external training load quantification of an elite European soccer team. *PLoS ONE* **2019**, *14*, e0209393. [CrossRef]
103. Malone, J.J.; Jaspers, A.; Helsen, W.F.; Frencken, W.G.P.; Brink, M.S. Seasonal training load and wellness monitoring in a profesional soccer goalkeeper. *Int. J. Sports Physiol. Perform.* **2018**, *13*, 672–675. [CrossRef] [PubMed]
104. Di Salvo, V.; Baron, R.; Tschan, H.; Calderon Montero, F.J.; Bachl, N.; Pigozzi, F. Performance characteristics according to playing position in elite soccer. *Int. J. Sports Med.* **2007**, *28*, 222–227. [CrossRef] [PubMed]
105. Vigne, G.; Gaudino, C.; Rogowski, I.; Alloatti, G.; Hautier, C. Activity profile in elite Italian soccer team. *Int. J. Sports Med.* **2010**, *31*, 304–310. [CrossRef] [PubMed]
106. Redwood-Brown, A.J.; O'Donoghue, P.G.; Nevill, A.M.; Saward, C.; Dyer, N.; Sunderland, C. Effects of situational variables on the physical activity profiles of elite soccer players in different score line states. *Scand. J. Med. Sci. Sports* **2018**, *28*, 2515–2526. [CrossRef] [PubMed]
107. Modric, T.; Versic, S.; Sekulic, D. Playing position specifics of associations between running performance during the training and match in male soccer players. *Acta Gymnica* **2020**, *50*, 51–60. [CrossRef]
108. Ingebrigtsen, J.; Dalen, T.; Hjelde, G.H.; Drust, B.; Wisløff, U. Acceleration and sprint profiles of a professional elite football team in match play. *Eur. J. Sport Sci.* **2015**, *15*, 101–110. [CrossRef] [PubMed]
109. Castillo-Rodríguez, A.; Cano-Cáceres, F.J.; Figueiredo, A.; Fernández-García, J.C. Train like you compete? Physical and physiological responses on semi-professional soccer players. *Int. J. Environ. Res. Public Health* **2020**, *17*, 756. [CrossRef] [PubMed]
110. Modrić, T.; Sattler, T.; Morgans, R.; Pavlinovic, V.; Mandic, A. Physical Performance in Highest-Level Soccer: Comparison between FIFA World Cup and UEFA Champions League Matches. *SportMont* **2023**, *21*, 3–7. [CrossRef]
111. Oliva-Lozano, J.M.; Fortes, V.; Krustrup, P.; Muyor, J.M. Acceleration and sprint profiles of professional male football players in relation to playing position. *PLoS ONE* **2020**, *15*, e0236959. [CrossRef] [PubMed]
112. Coutinho, D.; Oliveira, D.; Lisboa, P.; Campos, F.; Nakamura, F.Y.; Baptista, J.; Abade, E. Weekly external load distribution in football teams of different competitive levels. *Biol. Sport* **2024**, *41*, 155–164. [CrossRef]
113. Lago-Peñas, C. The role of situational variables in analysing physical performance in soccer. *J. Hum. Kinet.* **2012**, *35*, 89–95. [CrossRef] [PubMed]
114. Paul, D.J.; Bradley, P.S.; Nassis, G.P. Factors Affecting Match Running Performance of Elite Soccer Players: Shedding Some Light on the Complexity. *Int. J. Sports Physiol. Perform.* **2015**, *10*, 515–519. [CrossRef]
115. Trewin, J.; Meylan, C.; Varley, M.C.; Cronin, J. The influence of situational and environmental factors on match-running in soccer: A systematic review. *Sci. Med. Footb.* **2017**, *1*, 183–194. [CrossRef]
116. Kim, S.; Emmonds, S.; Bower, P.; Weaving, D. External and internal maximal intensity periods of elite youth male soccer matches. *J. Sports Sci.* **2023**, *41*, 547–556. [CrossRef]
117. Morgans, R.; Kweon, D.; Ryan, B.; Ju, W.; Zmijewski, P.; Oliveira, R.; Olthof, S. Playing position and match location affect the number of high-intensity efforts more than the quality of the opposition in elite football players. *Biol. Sport* **2023**, *41*, 29. [CrossRef]

118. Aughey, R.J.; Varley, M.C. Acceleration profiles in elite australian soccer. *Int. J. Sports Med.* **2013**, *34*, 282. [CrossRef]
119. Djaoui, L.; Owen, A.; Newton, M.; Nikolaidis, P.; Dellal, A.; Chamari, K. Effects of congested match periods on acceleration and deceleration profiles in professional soccer. *Biol. Sport* **2022**, *39*, 307–317. [CrossRef] [PubMed]
120. Kovacevic, D.; Elias, G.; Ellens, S.; Cox, A.; Serpiello, F.R. Moving Toward a More Comprehensive Analysis of Acceleration Profiles in Elite Youth Football. *Front. Sports Act. Living* **2022**, *3*, 802014. [CrossRef]
121. Russel, M.; Sparkes, W.; Northeast, J.; Cook, C.J.; Love, T.D.; Bracken, R.M.; Kilduff, L.P. Changes in Acceleration and Deceleration Capacity Throughout Professional Soccer Match-Play. *J. Strength Cond. Res.* **2016**, *30*, 2839–2844. [CrossRef]
122. Stevens, T.G.A.; de Ruiter, C.J.; Twisk, J.W.R.; Savelsbergh, G.J.P.; Beek, P.J. Quantification of in-season training load relative to match load in professional Dutch Eredivisie football players. *Sci. Med. Footb.* **2017**, *1*, 117–125. [CrossRef]
123. Gaudino, P.; Iaia, F.M.; Alberti, G.; Strudwick, A.J.; Gregson, W. Monitoring Training in Elite Soccer Players: Systematic Bias between Running Speed and Metabolic Power Data. *Int. J. Sports Med.* **2013**, *34*, 963–968. [CrossRef] [PubMed]
124. Morin, J.B.; Le Mat, Y.; Osgnach, C.; Barnabò, A.; Pilati, A.; Samozino, P.; di Prampero, P.E. Individual acceleration-speed profile in-situ: A proof of concept in professional football players. *J. Biomech.* **2021**, *123*, 110524. [CrossRef]
125. Osgnach, C.; Poser, S.; Bernardini, R.; Rinaldo, R.; Di Prampero, P.E. Energy cost and metabolic power in elite soccer: A new match analysis approach. *Med. Sci. Sports Exerc.* **2010**, *42*, 170–178. [CrossRef] [PubMed]
126. Dalen, T.; Jørgen, I.; Gertjan, E.; Havard, H.G.; Ulrik, W. Player Load, Acceleration, and Deceleration During Forty-Five Competitive Matches of Elite Soccer. *J. Strength Cond. Res.* **2016**, *30*, 351–359. [CrossRef]
127. Faude, O.; Koch, T.; Meyer, T. Straight Sprinting Is the Most Frequent Action in Goal Situations in Professional Football. *J. Sports Sci.* **2012**, *30*, 625–631. [CrossRef]
128. Hodgson, C.; Akenhead, R.; Thomas, K. Time-motion analysis of acceleration demands of 4v4 small-sided soccer games played on different pitch sizes. *Hum. Mov. Sci.* **2014**, *33*, 25–32. [CrossRef] [PubMed]
129. Kobal, R.; Carvalho, L.; Jacob, R.; Rossetti, M.; de Paula Oliveira, L.; Do Carmo, E.C.; Barroso, R. Comparison among U-17, U-20, and Professional Female Soccer in the GPS Profiles during Brazilian Championships. *Int. J. Environ. Res. Public Health* **2022**, *19*, 16642. [CrossRef] [PubMed]
130. Casamichana, D.; Martín-García, A.; Díaz, A.G.; Bradley, P.S.; Castellano, J. Accumulative weekly load in a professional football team: With special reference to match playing time and game position. *Biol. Sport* **2021**, *39*, 115. [CrossRef]
131. Miguel, M.; Cortez, A.; Romero, F.; Loureiro, N.; García-Rubio, J.; Ibáñez, S.J. Daily and weekly external loads in the microcycle: Characterization and comparison between playing positions on amateur soccer. *Front. Sports Act. Living* **2022**, *4*, 943367. [CrossRef] [PubMed]
132. Sonderegger, K.; Tschopp, M.; Taube, W. The challenge of evaluating the intensity of short actions in soccer: A new methodological approach using percentage acceleration. *PLoS ONE* **2016**, *11*, e0166534. [CrossRef] [PubMed]
133. De Hoyo, M.; Sañudo, B.; Suárez-Arrones, L.; Carrasco, L.; Joel, T.; Domínguez-Cobo, S.; Núñez, F.J. Analysis of the acceleration profile according to initial speed and positional role in elite professional male soccer players. *J. Sports Med. Phys. Fit.* **2018**, *58*, 1774–1780. [CrossRef] [PubMed]
134. Martínez-Cabrera, F.I.; Núñez-Sánchez, F.J.; Losada, J.; Otero-Esquina, C.; Sánchez, H.; De Hoyo, M. Use of individual relative thresholds to assess acceleration in young soccer players according to initial speed. *J. Strength Cond. Res.* **2021**, *35*, 1110–1118. [CrossRef] [PubMed]
135. Kavanagh, R.; McDaid, K.; Rhodes, D.; McDonnell, J.; Oliveira, R.; Morgans, R. An Analysis of Positional Generic and Individualized Speed Thresholds Within the Most Demanding Phases of Match Play in the English Premier League. *Int. J. Sports Physiol. Perform.* **2023**, *19*, 116–126. [CrossRef]
136. Jiménez-Reyes, P.; Garcia Ramos, A.; Párraga Montilla, J.A.; Jos, J.; Morcillo-Losa, J.A.; Cuadrado-Peñ, V.; An Castañ O-Zambudio, A.; Samozino, P.; Morin, J.-B.B. Seasonal Changes in the Sprint Acceleration Force-Velocity Profile of Elite Male Soccer Players. *J. Strength Cond. Res.* **2020**, *3*, 70–74. [CrossRef]
137. Loturco, I.; Pereira, L.A.; Freitas, T.T.; Alcaraz, P.E.; Zanetti, V.; Bishop, C.; Jeffreys, I. Maximum acceleration performance of professional soccer players in linear sprints: Is there a direct connection with change-of-direction ability? *PLoS ONE* **2019**, *14*, e0216806. [CrossRef]
138. Akenhead, R.; Harley, J.A.; Tweddle, S.P. Examining the external training load of an english premier league football team with special reference to acceleration. *J. Strength Cond. Res.* **2016**, *30*, 2424–2432. [CrossRef]
139. Serpiello, F.R.; Duthie, G.M.; Moran, C.; Kovacevic, D.; Selimi, E.; Varley, M. The Occurrence of Repeated High Acceleration Ability (RHAA) in Elite Youth Football. *Int. J. Sports Med.* **2018**, *39*, 502–507. [CrossRef]

140. Barron, D.J.; Atkins, D.S.; Edmundson, A.C.; Fewtrell, A.D. Repeated Acceleration Activity in Competitive Youth Soccer. *J. Sport Sci. Med.* **2016**, *14*, 55–61. [CrossRef]
141. Varley, M.C.; Fairweather, I.H.; Aughey, R.J. Validity and reliability of GPS for measuring instantaneous velocity during acceleration, deceleration, and constant motion. *J. Sports Sci.* **2012**, *30*, 121–127. [CrossRef]

sports

MDPI

Systematic Review

Heading in Female Soccer: A Scoping Systematic Review

Yinhao Shen, Shinting Chen, Qingguang Liu and Antonio Cicchella *

International College of Football, Tongji University, No.1239, Siping Road, Yangpu, Shanghai 200092, China; 11089@tongji.edu.cn (Y.S.); 2132014@tongji.edu.cn (S.C.); qingguang@tongji.edu.cn (Q.L.)
* Correspondence: antonio.cicchella@unibo.it

Abstract: Heading is a key skill in soccer, and it is few investigated in females. Research on heading focused mostly on males and on young players. Data on females' soccer players are sparse and it is difficult to draw firm conclusions. Thus, little is known is known about heading in females. The most investigated aspects of heading are the relationship between heading and play state, training level and anthropometrics. The relationship between the frequency and intensity of headings and long-time outcomes in terms of vigilance, and neuro-cognitive status is also a topic of interest. Aim of this scoping review is to survey the available knowledge about heading in female football to identify possible weaknesses and issues for future research direction in the field. A structured literature search was performed in the main databases. Results show research on heading in female soccer is sparse and to draw firm conclusion on the investigated aspects (effect of play position, occurrence, cognitive impairment, influence of muscle strength, and player's level) is difficult. It emerged mild intensity heading is not dangerous, helmet does not help, play state and player position influences the heading and that high rotational velocities are achieved. The survey identified new directions for research, that should focus on how to ameliorate heading training and skills and develop a more effective and safe heading technique.

Keywords: soccer; female; heading; kinematics; heading exposure; heading skills

1. Introduction

Women's soccer is underrepresented in research, especially in biomechanics research [1]. Most of research investigating biomechanics has been performed in males. Despite the increase in female soccer players, there is a dearth of research in biomechanics in female soccer. Consequently most coaching advice provided to female athletes are solely based on data collected from male players [2], despite Males and females being different for range of motion and flexibility [3] body composition [4], and strength [5]. A large study on over 400 subjects [3], concluded females present greater flexibility (greater hip flexion) and balance than males while males showed higher isokinetic strength of lower limbs. Body fat is also different distributed in females and males' bodies, having the female athletes more fat in the thigh [4]. Higher strength in man is more likely caused by larger muscle fibers than cross-sectional area [5]. The most serious injuries (as consequences) in soccer are those to the head. The general problem of uneven consideration of female injuries to the head was recently highlighted by a paper studying head injuries in crash tests in the automotive industries. This paper described the development of a dummy woman for automotive crash tests [6]. Before this, no such device existed for females, despite more than 50 years of research in crash injuries. For this purpose, was developed a 162 cm and 62 kg dummy, having the inertial characteristics of a mean western, middle aged, female body [6]. Heading in football is a cause of major concussive events, and women are more prone to concussive injuries than men [7]. Despite the high incidence of head injuries and concussive and sub-concussive outcomes, heading in female has been poorly studied from a biomechanical point of view. The microstructural and neurological changes that occur in the brain after continued exposure to heading in soccer players, seems to cause a more pronounced decline in the neurocognitive functions in females [8]. Another review study found biomechanical models of the neck were biased toward males [9]. The same study found female biomechanical research was biased in the height, weight, and BMI distributions [9]. Given the differences in inertial characteristics the head and neck between female and males, these factors influence the heading and its impacts [10].

Heading in soccer can be a frontal, lateral or by vertex impact. Lateral (rotational) heading for goal usually begins with a pre-load stretch [11,12].

The most important muscular motors acting in the heading are the cervical rotator muscles (scalene anterior, longus capitis and longus colli) which gives the highest contribution to the development of the rotational acceleration of the head [13]. In the specific task of lateral heading, before ball contact, there is also a pre-load rotation and a stretch phase of neck muscles [13]. Different indexes can be used to rate the chance of injury after an impact. One of the most accepted is the *HIC*, or head injury criterion.

The head injury criterion is commonly used and is described in the following equation [14]:

$$HIC = \frac{max}{t1, t2}\left\{(t2 - t1)\cdot\left[\frac{1}{t2 - t1}\int_{t1}^{t2} a(t)dt\right]\right\}^{2.5} \quad (1)$$

where $t1$ and $t2$ are the initial and final times (in seconds) chosen to maximize *HIC*, and acceleration a is measured in gs (standard gravity acceleration units). The time duration, $t2 - t1$, can be limited to a maximum value of 36 ms, where the mean impact value is 15 ms [15]. This means that the HIC includes the effects of head acceleration and the duration of the acceleration. Large accelerations can be tolerated for very short times. At a HIC of 1000, there is a 18% probability of a severe head injury, a 55% probability of a serious injury and a 90% probability of a moderate head injury to the average adult [16]. Concussions were found to occur at HIC = 250 in most athletes [17]. The mean HIC found in soccer heading in males was 133.3, thus far away from the critical value [18]. The aim of this scoping review is to analyze the existent literature about female head impact in female's soccer players to provide values for head accelerations and velocities. A second aim is to explore the current directions of research in the field and to identify gaps to be filled in future research.

2. Methods

A comprehensive computerized search was performed: in the following databases: PubMed, Scopus, WoS, Sport Discus (Ebsco).

The following search strings were employed:

"heading in soccer" OR "heading in football" OR "heading in females soccer players" OR "soccer and heading" OR "gender and heading" OR "head impact in soccer" OR "female head impact in soccer" AND "team sport" OR football OR soccer OR futsal" OR "heading biomechanics" AND "female" AND "soccer". The search items were selected for each database consulted. We consulted the MESH terms in PubMed, and searched for the keywords in article type, abstract and keywords in the Scopus database. In Wos we used the Descriptors, Gender, and Mesh headings to retrieve the papers. For Sport Discus we used the thesaurus keywords provided by the database. We found that all databases provided the same relevant keywords. Afterward, the search was performed by substituting soccer with "football" and different combinations of these terms were used.

The reference lists of the studies retrieved were manually searched to identify potentially eligible studies not captured by the electronic searches. Finally, an external expert was contacted to verify the final list of references included in this review and to check if there were any other relevant studies not detected through our search. As suggested by Cochrane's guidelines, the inclusion and exclusion criteria were also provided to the external expert [19]. However, no information was provided about which databases to consult or search strategies to avoid creating a bias in the expert. This process (a double-check by an external expert) is recommended by PRISMA guidelines, to confirm the accuracy of the initial search. The databases searches included papers from the last 15 years up to August

2023. Only papers in scholarly journals indexed in SCIE. were considered. Paper older than 15 years were excluded from the search because the obsolete technologies used in the measurements cannot guarantee reliable data. The search was made in compliance with the PRISMA Checklist (see Supplementary file). Outcomes for which data were sough included head velocities and accelerations in different playing condition in experienced female soccer players. The review was registered in the PROSPERO database with nr. 613726.

2.1. Eligibility Criteria

The inclusion criteria of the present study, were as follows: (i) only head impact in females in soccer; (ii) study that included the mechanics of the heading in females, and outcomes (acute or long term) and (iii) published in the last 15 years. Furthermore, all the studies had to be peer-reviewed, written in English, and provide the full-text. Studies were excluded if they: (i) focused on males; (ii) were narrative reviews, brief reviews, scoping reviews or, methodological proposals; (iii) did not include relevant data in soccer headings; (iv) were not fully written in English; or (v) consisted of abstracts without accompanying full texts. Only studies on female subjects older than 14 years (to exclude pre-pubertal children) and with a sample size greater than 6 were considered. We choose the age range based on a previous study indicating this age is a discriminant in the onset of higher frequency of heading occurrence [20].

The screening of the title, abstract and reference list of each study to locate potentially relevant studies was independently performed by the two authors (AC and YS). Additionally, they reviewed the full version of the included papers in detail to identify articles that met the selection criteria.

2.2. Data Extraction

A data extraction sheet was prepared in Microsoft Excel (Microsoft Corporation, Readmon, WA, USA) in accordance with the Cochrane Consumers and Communication Review Group's data extraction template [21,22]. The Excel sheet was used to assess inclusion requirements and subsequently tested for all selected studies. The process was independently conducted by the two authors. Full text articles excluded, with reasons, were recorded. All the records were stored in the sheet. Data were retrieved and checked by two authors. A specifically designed template for data extraction was developed. For each included heading, the following items were extracted: study citation details, purpose of the study, subject's characteristics and anthropometrics, parameters measured and main outcomes. Means and standard deviations were calculated and reported for the kinematics parameters considered.

2.3. Data Items

The following information was extracted from the included heading studies: number of subjects included (n), age group (>14 years old), sex (women), competitive level (if available), and type of original articles included (experimental, observational analytic or both); identification of the effects if any (acute or adaptations), dimension of analysis (game situation, outcomes, kinematics) and main findings.

The methodological quality of the included studies was evaluated using the AXIS Tool for the Critical Appraisal of Cross-sectional Studies [23]. This tool contains 20 questions, used to assess the study design quality and risk of biases. Each question can be answered as 'Yes', 'No' or 'Unsure/comment'. This assessment was performed independently by two reviewers. Where consensus could not be reached through discussion, a third reviewer was consulted.

3. Results

Study Identification and Selection

The search produced a total of 118 papers. The references were then exported to reference manager software (EndNote^{TM} X9, Clarivate Analytics, Philadelphia, PA, USA).

Duplicates (48 references) were subsequently removed either manually or automatically. The remaining 70 articles were screened for their relevance by reading the titles and the abstracts, and this process resulted in the removal of a further 40 studies. Following the screening procedure, 30 articles were selected for in depth reading and analysis. After reading the full texts, a further 10 studies were excluded due to not being heading studies (n = 3), not being written in English (n = 5), having fewer than six subjects (n1) and being performed with subjects younger than 14 years old (n = 1). Of the 12 papers included in this review, all were biomechanical and considered the outcomes. The AXIS analysis is reported in Figure 1.

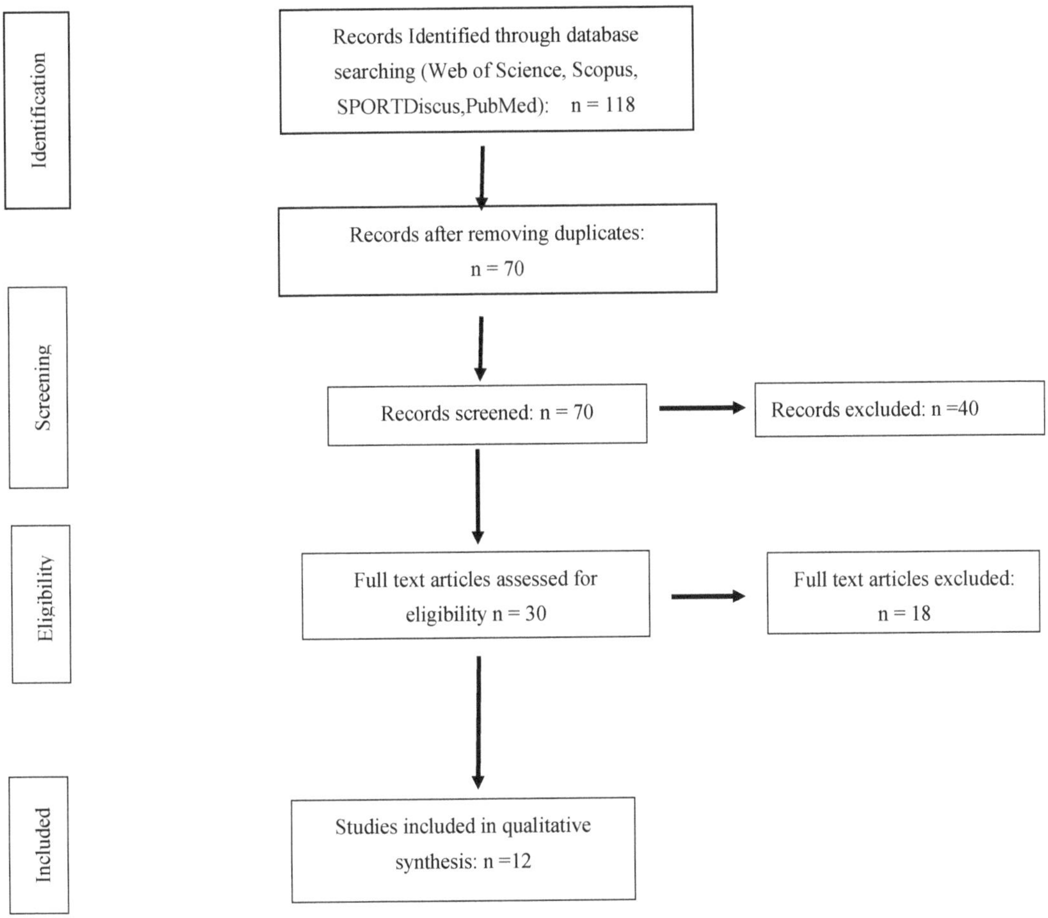

Figure 1. PRISMA flow chart.

In total, 12 studies that met the inclusion criteria were found. We classified the AXIS quality scores according to the number of "Yes" responses for the 20 items for each study. Studies achieving 80% "yes" responses indicated high quality, 60–80% indicated moderate quality, and less than 60% indicated low quality. Thus, studies rated as high quality were 4/12 (36.6%), moderate quality were 5/12 (36.6%), and low quality were 3/12 (27.7%). While the items relating specifically to reporting quality scored quite highly, the detail relating to study design and possible biases are lower and more variable (Figure 2).

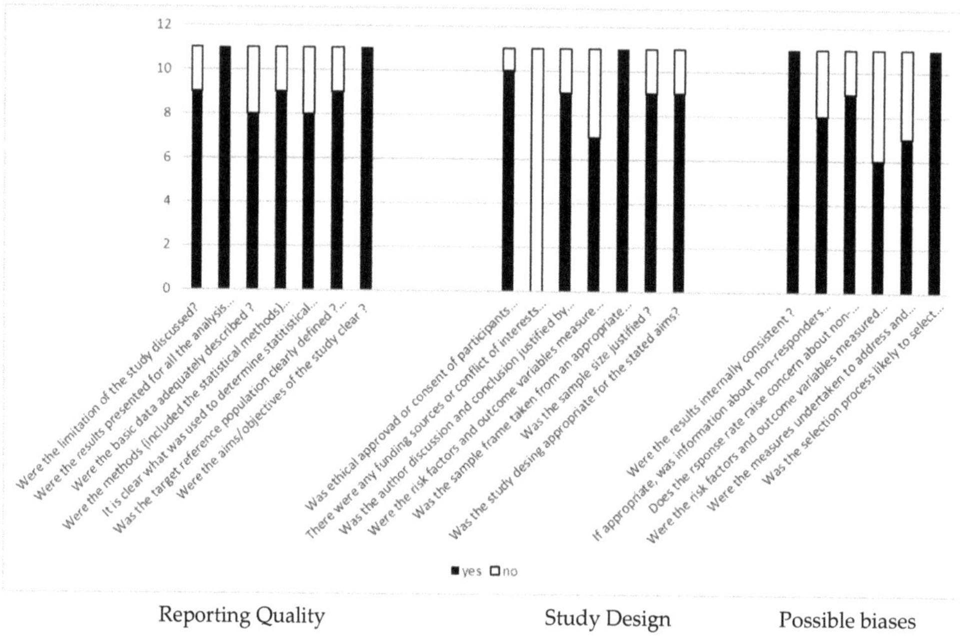

Figure 2. AXIS analysis of the studies. Study characteristics and qualitative synthesis.

The type of study (O = observational, E = experimental) and subjects characteristics are reported in Table 1.

Table 1. Type of Study and subjects characteristics.

Author	Aim of the Study	Study Type	Mean Age (Years)	Weight (kg)	Height (cm)	Gender	Subject Number	Qualification Level
Filben et al. [24]	Categorize head impacts	O	19	62.3	170	F	16	NCAA div 1
Reynolds et al. [25]	Quantify head impactt	O	20.43	n.r.	n.r.	F	7	NCAA div 1
Lynall et al. [26]	Frequency and magnitude of impact	O	19.1	63.7	168	F	22	NCAA
Filben et al. [27]	Difference between younger	E	15.27	61.8	n.r.	F	6	U15
	and experienced	E	20.19	63.08	n.r.	F	13	NCAA div 1
Caccese et al. [28]	Differences in PLA, RV in different heading scenarios		19.6	60.3	167.8	F	16	NCAA div 1
Gutierrez et al. [29]	Effect of heading on neurocognitive function	E	15.9	59	165	F	17	HIGH SCHOOL
Nowak et al. [30]	Assess the reliability of concussion diagnosis	E	19.7	62	168.3	F	23	COLLEGE >5 yrs
Tierney et al. [31]	Headgear effect of PLA	E	19.5	63.2	164	F	29	>5 yrs
Muller et al. [32]	Asses neck and trunk strengthening	E	16.5	56	168	F	7	HIGH SCHOOL
Kenny et al. [33]	Which kick produced more impact	E	19.9	65.5	169.3	F	13	VARSITY
Mihalik et al. [34]	Characterize the impact	E	19.8	64	168.2	F	34	NCAA div 1
Bretzin et al. [35]	Compare PLA and RV with muscle strength	E	20.25	66.9	158.7	F	8	NCAA div 1

Table 2 shows, the instrument used (MMS = Mouth Mounted Sensors; HMS = Head Mounted Sensor) the heading frequency, the main outcomes, and the variables measured. FA: forward acceleration; LA: left acceleration: RA: rotational acceleration; RV: rotational velocity.

Table 2. Instruments used, heading frequencies, outcomes, type of measure and results.

Author	Instrument	Heading	Outcomes	Measures	PLA	RA
		Frequency (if reported)		PLA, PRA, PRV	(G)	(rad/s^2)
Filben et al. [24]	MMS		Goal kicks shows higher PRA	corner	22.9	2189.3
				goal	24.3	2658.9
				free	18	1843.3
				live	18.8	1769.7
Reynolds et al. [25]	MMS	5.7/practice	No difference compared with men in severity	PLA, PRA	19.1	3687
Lynall et al. [26]	MMS	7/90 min game	More impacts during practice	PLA, PRA	12.51	2093
Filben et al. [27]	MMS		Experienced players shows higher PLA, PRA and RV	PLA, PRA, RV	11.7 17.3	9450 1560
Caccese et al. [28]	HMS		Different field scenarios Influence PLA and RA	PLA, RA	28.2	7100
Gutierrez et al. [29]	HMS		descriptive study	FA	5.83	
				LA	6.96	
				RA	6.27	
Nowak et al. [30]	HMS		Head impact predicting concussion outcomes	PLA	16.1	
Tierney et al. [31]	MMS		Head gear increase PLA	PLA	21.52	
Muller et al. [32]	HMS	1.9/90 min	Strength of neck muscle mitigate PLA	PLA	10.9	
Kenny et al. [33]	MMS	1.83/Athlete exposure time	Long kick =higher impact	PLA, RA	22.2	2296
Mihalik et al. [34]	MMS	10/Session	Mild intensity impacts are not dangerous	PLA, RA	19	3457
Bretzin et al. [35]	HMS		Head mass and neck girth negatively correlate with PLA and RV	PLA, RV	24	1416

PLA: peak lateral acceleration; PRA: peak rotational acceleration; PRV: peak rotational velocity.

Among the retrieved studies, 11 were published after 2017, showing an increasing interest in women's safety in football in recent times. The summary of the main evidence found in each review can be found in Table 1. Most studies tested single groups or parallel, non-randomized groups. Seven studies employed a mouthpiece sensor, and five a head mounted sensor. Three studies were observational, and nine were experimental.

Of the included articles, we compared the magnitude of impact between practice and match setting, one studied the differences between male and females, two aimed at characterize the heading in relation to different play scenarios, one studied the differences in impact between young and experienced players, three studied the effect of measured parameters on injury and neurocognitive functions and the relationship between impact characteristics and the likelihood of developing a neurocognitive deficit, two correlated neck muscle and strength with the magnitude of the impact. Two analyzed which kick produced a higher impact in heading and one studied the dumping effect of headgear.

The mean sample size was 16.2 ± 8.7 subjects (range 7–34). Age, weight and height of the studied subjects were respectively: 18.8 ± 1.7 years, 62.3 ± 2.9 kg and 167.1 ± 3.27 cm (BMI 23.3 ± 2.3). 1 study didn't report weight and height. Seven studies used NCAA div 1 players, two used high school players, one used players with >5 years of experience, one used varsity and one used under 15 teams.

The measured impact parameters were: Peak Linear Acceleration (PLA; m/s^2); Mean Rotational Acceleration (RA; m/s^2) and Mean Rotational Velocity (RV; m/s). One study reported frontal acceleration and lateral acceleration (FA; and LA m/s^2). The mean values for PLA, RV and RA were 17.61 ± 6.27 m/s^2; 25.84.6 ± 16.28.41 m/s and 8.27 ± 1.68 m/s^2. Six studies reported the frequency of heading using four different metrics (per training session, per athletes' exposure time, in training and in game). Exposure to heading ranges from 2 to 10 per match/training unit. The measurement devices used were essentially of two types: head and mouth mounted sensors. The main outcomes were that goal heading produced higher rotational acceleration in comparison to other games scenarios [24] and game situations influence heading kinematics [28]. Other results were that no difference was found between males and females in heading kinematics [25], the magnitude of heading was found to be higher during practices than game [26], and experienced players produced higher acceleration and velocities [27]. One study found that medium intensity soccer heading didn't produce significant impairment of neurocognitive function in the short and long term [29,30]. The authors of [31] found that wearing a soft cells helmets increase PLA. Other studies found that head mass and neck girth negatively correlate with PLA and RV [32], and increasing the strength of the neck muscles mitigated PLA [35]. It was also found that the response to long kick produce higher magnitude kinematic response [33,34].

4. Discussion

Although heading is a relatively rare event in a soccer game compared with other skills, the health consequences of heading are of major concern and are the most investigated topic in the literature. Thus, the underlying motivations of several of the examined studies were the short and long-term outcomes of heading exposure. We noticed a comparison of heading frequencies between the studies was difficult, because of the use of different indexes. Rotational acceleration was the most studied parameter of heading. Differently from other sports, soccer is the only situation where maximal rotational acceleration is actively pursued in attempt to score a goal. In other sports, rotational acceleration is passive and caused by an external perturbation which is either expected as in boxing [36] or unexpected, as in a car crash [6]. The heading occurrence we found in females is similar to another study that showed an exposure of 3.6 to 8.6 headings per match [37]. However, within the context of epidemiological studies, it is unclear how to formulate an appropriate exposure metric. It has been proposed that estimates of the cumulative number of heading impacts over a playing career should be used as the main exposure metric in epidemiological studies of professional players [10]. The present state of knowledge does not support the fact that heading in female soccer players is deleterious and this result align with other review studies that focused on long term outcomes [38]. However, due to the relevance of the topic for health and safety, further studies focusing on female players are necessary: the existing studies on females are too few to draw a firm conclusion. Also, it concerns the question of how much risk is personally and socially acceptable, given that heading can also cause fatalities or permanent disabilities and cognitive problems at older ages. It emerged from the literature that mastering the heading skill was found in more experienced players. Although little is known about neck muscle in females, it was shown that when normalized for body mass, the neck muscle mass of females does not differ from males [39]. Protocols for strengthening the neck muscle has been evaluated in different sports [40], but we only found two studies on this topic, that showed the need to increase the muscle strength of the neck in females. On-field tactics during a match influence heading occurrence, thus suggesting adopting different tactical arrangement in the presence of a strong heading player. A player's skills are also reflected in heading kinematics.

The available data about kinematics of the soccer heading in females are very scarce and dealt with the heterogenous aspects of heading. A limitation of our review was that we could not access non-English literature, and we did not review the coaching literature, which may contain some suggestion for further studies. For each direction of research, we found a maximum of two papers. The investigated aspects are sparse and there is no sound body of knowledge on the different aspects of heading in female football players. However, some evidence suggests that mild impact heading is not dangerous, head gears would not help in preventing injuries, and the match situation influences heading. It remains a problem that heading can cause serious outcomes in females. Further research is necessary to constitute a clear body of knowledge on female soccer players heading. We identified the following research directions for female soccer headings: (1) research connected to safety, and especially long-term observational studies of heading outcomes and the effect of the use of protective devices; (2) research connected to performance, e.g., intervention studies aimed at modifying of the heading biomechanics by increasing the strength of the neck muscles or ameliorating the pose before heading in response to different games situation (heading techniques interventions).

5. Conclusions

Further research is needed on female soccer players, to improve the existing knowledge about heading safety and improve performance. Furthermore, the gap between males and females' players in this research field must be filled. Future research on biomechanics of headings on females should consider a more in-depth analysis of the effects on soft tissue, using simulation methods to build reliable models of a female's head and implement the measured accelerations. This approach could reduce the need for direct measurement on the field and allow for broader and more complex experimental conditions in vivo.

Supplementary Materials: The following supporting information can be downloaded at: https://www.mdpi.com/article/10.3390/sports12120327/s1, Supplementary File: Reporting checklist for systematic review.

Author Contributions: Y.S.: funding acquisition, analysis, and interpretation of data; A.C.: acquisition, analysis, interpretation of data and writing, S.C. performed the literature search, Q.L. summarized the results. All authors agree to be personally accountable for the author's own contributions and for ensuring that questions related to the accuracy or integrity of any part of the work, even ones in which the author was not personally involved, are appropriately investigated, resolved, and documented in the literature. All authors have read and agreed to the published version of the manuscript.

Funding: This study was supported by the Education Research and Reform Cultivation Project of Tongji University and PA2023000337.

Conflicts of Interest: The authors declare no conflict of interest.

References

1. Okholm, K.; Wang, A.; Mehta, R.; Impellizzeri, F.M.; Massey, A.; McCall, A. Research on women's football: A scoping review. *Sci. Med. Footb.* **2022**, *6*, 549–558. [CrossRef]
2. Sakamoto, K.; Asai, T. Comparison of kicking motion characteristic at ball impact between female and male soccer players. *Int. J. Sports Sci. Coach.* **2013**, *8*, 63–76. [CrossRef]
3. Allison, K.F.; A Keenan, K.; Sell, T.C.; Abt, J.P.; Nagai, T.; Deluzio, J.; McGrail, M.; Lephart, S.M. Musculoskeletal, biomechanical, and physiological gender differences in the US military. *U.S. Army Med. Dep. J.* **2015**, 22–32.
4. Mascherini, G.; Castizo-Olier, J.; Irurtia, A.; Petri, C.; Galanti, G. Differences between the sexes in athletes' body composition and lower limb bioimpedence values. *Muscles Ligaments Tendons J.* **2018**, *7*, 573–581. [CrossRef]
5. Miller, A.E.J.; MacDougall, J.D.; Tarnopolsky, M.A.; Sale, D.G. Gender differences in strength and muscle fiber characteristics. *Eur. J. Appl. Physiol. Occup. Physiol.* **1993**, *66*, 254–262. [CrossRef]
6. Carlsson, A.; Davidsson, J.; Linder, A.; Svensson, M.Y. Design and Evaluation of the Initial 50th Percentile Female Prototype Rear Impact Dummy, BioRID P50F-Indications for the Need of an Additional Dummy Size. *Front. Bioeng. Biotechnol.* **2021**, *9*, 687058. [CrossRef]
7. Lipton, M.L.; Kim, N.; Zimmerman, M.E.; Kim, M.; Stewart, W.F.; Branch, C.A.; Lipton, R.B. Soccer heading is associated with white matter microstructural and cognitive abnormalities. *Radiology* **2013**, *268*, 850–857. [CrossRef]
8. Maerlender, A.; Smith, E.; Brolinson, P.G.; Crisco, J.; Urban, J.; Ajamil, A.; Rowson, S.; Campolettano, E.T.; Gellner, R.A.; Bellamkonda, S.; et al. Neuropsychological Change After a Single Season of Head Impact Exposure in Youth Football. *J. Int. Neuropsychol. Soc.* **2020**, *27*, 113–123. [CrossRef]
9. Booth, G.R.; Cripton, P.A.; Siegmund, G.P. The Lack of Sex, Age, and Anthropometric Diversity in Neck Biomechanical Data. *Front. Bioeng. Biotechnol.* **2021**, *9*, 684217. [CrossRef]
10. Basinas, I.; McElvenny, D.M.; Pearce, N.; Gallo, V.; Cherrie, J.W. A Systematic Review of Head Impacts and Acceleration Associated with Soccer. *Int. J. Environ. Res. Public Health.* **2022**, *19*, 5488. [CrossRef]
11. Luxbacher, J.A. Combining fitness training with technique training—Heading and shooting skills. *Perform. Cond. Soccer* **1999**, *6*, 7–8.
12. Ost, R.; Schum, T.; Stanley, K.; Vennell, J. Heading: Proper technique, as taught at the NSCAA Academy, begins with the fundamentals. *Soccer J.* **1996**, *41*, 37–40.

13. Wismans, J.; Philippens, M.; van Oorschot, E.; Kallieris, D.; Mattern, R. Comparison of Human Volunteer and Cadaver Head-Neck Response in Frontal Flexion. In Proceedings of the 31st Stapp Car Crash Conference, New Orleans, LA, USA, 9–11 November 1987; p. 872194. [CrossRef]
14. Marjoux, D.; Baumgartner, D.; Deck, C.; Willinger, R. Head injury prediction capability of the HIC, HIP, SIMon and ULP criteria. *Accid. Anal. Prev.* **2008**, *40*, 1135–1148. [CrossRef]
15. Chichester, C.; Bass, C.; Sanderson, E.; Di Marco, G. A Test Methodology for Assessing Demining Personal Protective Equipment. US Army Cecom Report. May 2001, pp. 1–73. Available online: https://web.archive.org/web/20130409222827/http://www.dtic.mil/cgiin/GetTRDoc?AD=ADA458677 (accessed on 1 September 2024).
16. Henn, H.W. Crash Tests and the Head Injury Criterion. *Teach. Math. Its Appl.* **1998**, *17*, 162–170. [CrossRef]
17. Ewing, C.L.; Thomas, D.J. *Human Head and Neck Response to Impact Acceleration*; NAMRL Monograph, 21; Naval Aerospace Medical Research Laboratory, Naval Aerospace Medical Institute: Pensacola, FL, USA, 1972.
18. Viano, D.C. Head Impact Biomechanics in Sport. IUTAM Symposium on Impact Biomechanics: From Fundamental Insights to Applications. *Solid Mech. Its Appl.* **2005**, *124*, 121–130. Available online: https://link.springer.com/content/pdf/bfm:978-1-4020-3796-2/1 (accessed on 1 September 2024).
19. Moritz, E.F.; Haake, S.; Self, B.P.; Beck, J.; Schill, D.; Eames, C.; Knox, T.; Plaga, J. Head Accelerations During Soccer Heading. In *The Engineering of Sport 6*; Springer: New York, NY, USA, 2006; pp. 81–86. [CrossRef]
20. Harriss, A.; Johnson, A.M.; Walton, D.M.; Dickey, J.P. The number of purposeful headers female youth soccer players experience during games depends on player age but not player position. *Sci. Med. Footb.* **2019**, *3*, 109–114. [CrossRef]
21. Cochrane Handbook for Systematic Reviews of Interventions. Available online: https://training.cochrane.org/handbook/current (accessed on 1 September 2024).
22. Cochrane Consumers and Communication Review Group Data Extraction Template. Available online: https://studylib.net/doc/7648732/data-extraction-template---cochrane-consumers-and-communi... (accessed on 1 September 2024).
23. Downes, M.J.; Brennan, M.L.; Williams, H.C.; Dean, R.S. Development of a critical appraisal tool to assess the quality of crosssectional studies (AXIS). *BMJ Open* **2016**, *6*, e011458. [CrossRef]
24. Filben, T.M.; Pritchard, N.S.; Hanes-Romano, K.E.; Miller, L.E.; Miles, C.M.; Urban, J.E.; Stitzel, J.D. Comparison of women's collegiate soccer header kinematics by play state, intent, and outcome. *J. Biomech.* **2021**, *126*, 110619. [CrossRef]
25. Reynolds, B.B.; Patrie, J.; Henry, E.J.; Goodkin, H.P.; Broshek, D.K.; Wintermark, M.; Druzgal, T.J. Effects of Sex and Event Type on Head Impact in Collegiate Soccer. *Orthop. J. Sports Med.* **2017**, *5*, 2325967117701708. [CrossRef]
26. Lynall, R.C.; Clark, M.D.; Grand, E.E.; Stucker, J.C.; Littleton, A.C.; Aguilar, A.J.; Petschauer, M.A.; Teel, E.F.; Mihalik, J.P. Head Impact Biomechanics in Women's College Soccer. *Med Sci Sports Exerc.* **2016**, *48*, 1772–1778. [CrossRef]
27. Filben, T.M.; Pritchard, N.S.; Miller, L.E.; Miles, C.M.; Urban, J.E.; Stitzel, J.D. Header biomechanics in youth and collegiate female soccer. *J. Biomech.* **2021**, *128*, 110782. [CrossRef]
28. Caccese, J.B.; Buckley, T.A.; Tierney, R.T.; Arbogast, K.B.; Rose, W.C.; Glutting, J.J.; Kaminski, T.W. Head and neck size and neck strength predict linear and rotational acceleration during purposeful soccer heading. *Sports Biomech.* **2017**, *17*, 462–476. [CrossRef]
29. Gutierrez, G.M.; Conte, C.; Lightbourne, K. The Relationship between Impact Force, Neck Strength, and Neurocognitive Performance in Soccer Heading in Adolescent Females. *Pediatr. Exerc. Sci.* **2014**, *26*, 33–40. [CrossRef]
30. Nowak, M.K.; Bevilacqua, Z.W.; Ejima, K.; Huibregtse, M.E.; Chen, Z.; Mickleborough, T.D.; Newman, S.D.; Kawata, K. NeuroOphthalmologic Response to Repetitive Subconcussive Head Impacts: A Randomized Clinical Trial. *JAMA Ophthalmol.* **2020**, *138*, 350–357. [CrossRef]
31. Tierney, R.T.; Higgins, M.; Caswell, S.V.; Brady, J.; McHardy, K.; Driban, J.B.; Darvish, K. Sex Differences in Head Acceleration During Heading While Wearing Soccer Headgear. *J. Athl. Train.* **2008**, *43*, 578–584. [CrossRef]
32. Müller, C.; Zentgraf, K. Neck and Trunk Strength Training to Mitigate Head Acceleration in Youth Soccer Players. *J. Strength Cond. Res.* **2020**, *35*, S81–S89. [CrossRef]
33. Kenny, R.; Elez, M.; Clansey, A.; Virji-Babul, N.; Wu, L.C. Head Impact Exposure and Biomechanics in University Varsity Women's Soccer. *Ann. Biomed. Eng.* **2022**, *50*, 1461–1472. [CrossRef]
34. Mihalik, J.P.; Amalfe, S.A.; Roby, P.R.; Ford, C.B.; Lynall, R.C.; Riegler, K.E.; Teel, E.F.; Wasserman, E.B.; Putukian, M. Sex and Sport Differences in College Lacrosse and Soccer Head Impact Biomechanics. *Med. Sci. Sports Exerc.* **2020**, *52*, 2349–2356. [CrossRef]
35. Bretzin, A.C.; Mansell, J.L.; Tierney, R.T.; McDevitt, J.K. Sex Differences in Anthropometrics and Heading Kinematics Among Division I Soccer Athletes. *Sports Health* **2017**, *9*, 168–173. [CrossRef]
36. Lota, K.S.; Malliaropoulos, N.; Blach, W.; Kamitani, T.; Ikumi, A.; Korakakis, V.; Maffulli, N. Rotational head acceleration and traumatic brain injury in combat sports: A systematic review. *Br. Med. Bull.* **2022**, *141*, 33–46. [CrossRef]
37. Langdon, S.; Goedhart, E.; Oosterlaan, J.; Königs, M. Heading Exposure in Elite Football (Soccer): A Study in Adolescent, Young Adult, and Adult Male and Female Players. *Med. Sci Sports. Exerc.* **2022**, *54*, 1459–1465. [CrossRef]
38. McCunn, R.; Beaudouin, F.; Stewart, K.; Meyer, T.; MacLean, J. Heading in Football: Incidence, Biomechanical Characteristics and the Association with Acute Cognitive Function—A Three-Part Systematic Review. *Sports Med.* **2021**, *51*, 2147–2163. [CrossRef]

39. Rankin, G.; Stokes, M.; Newham, D. Size and shape of the posterior neck muscles measured by ultrasound imaging: Normal values in males and females of different ages. *Man. Ther.* **2005**, *10*, 108–115. [CrossRef]
40. Hrysomallis, C. Neck Muscular Strength, Training, Performance and Sport Injury Risk: A Review. *Sports Med.* **2016**, *46*, 1111–1124. [CrossRef]

MDPI AG
Grosspeteranlage 5
4052 Basel
Switzerland
Tel.: +41 61 683 77 34

Sports Editorial Office
E-mail: sports@mdpi.com
www.mdpi.com/journal/sports

www.ingramcontent.com/pod-product-compliance
Lightning Source LLC
Chambersburg PA
CBHW061440210926
51850CB00008B/1563
9783725859030